Neuroradiology
A Core Review

Take a look at all of the titles in the
Core Review Series
Available wherever quality medical references are sold

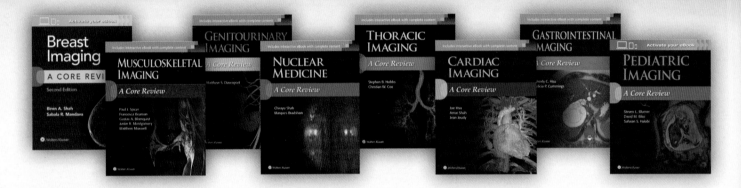

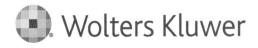

Neuroradiology
A Core Review

EDITORS

Prachi Dubey, MBBS, MPH
Senior Editor

Department of Radiology
Columbia University Medical Center
New York-Presbyterian/Columbia Hospital
New York, New York

Sathish Kumar Dundamadappa, MBBS

Department of Radiology
University of Massachusetts Medical School
Worcester, Massachusetts

Daniel Thomas Ginat, MD, MS

Department of Radiology
University of Chicago
Pritzker School of Medicine
Chicago, Illinois

Rafeeque Bhadelia, MD

Department of Radiology
Beth Israel Deaconess Medical Center
Harvard Medical School
Boston, Massachusetts

Gul Moonis, MD
Senior Editor

Department of Radiology
Columbia University Medical Center
New York-Presbyterian/Columbia Hospital
New York, New York

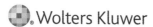 Wolters Kluwer

Philadelphia • Baltimore • New York • London
Buenos Aires • Hong Kong • Sydney • Tokyo

Senior Acquisitions Editor: Sharon Zinner
Editorial Coordinator: Lauren Pecarich
Marketing Manager: Dan Dressler
Production Project Manager: David Saltzberg
Design Coordinator: Steve Druding
Manufacturing Coordinator: Beth Welsh
Prepress Vendor: SPi Global

Library of Congress Cataloging-in-Publication Data
Names: Dubey, Prachi, editor. | Dundamadappa, Sathish Kumar, editor. | Ginat, Daniel Thomas, editor. | Bhadelia, Rafeeque, editor. | Moonis, Gul, editor.
Title: Neuroradiology : a core review / editors, Prachi Dubey, Sathish Kumar Dundamadappa, Daniel Ginat, Rafeeque Bhadelia, Gul Moonis.
Other titles: Core review series.
Description: Philadelphia : Wolters Kluwer, [2018] | Series: Core review series | Includes bibliographic references and index.
Identifiers: LCCN 2017036846 | ISBN 9781496372505
Subjects: | MESH: Central Nervous System Diseases—diagnostic imaging | Neuroradiography—methods
Classification: LCC RC348 | NLM WL 141.5.N47 | DDC 616.8/0475—dc23 LC record available at https://lccn.loc.gov/2017036846

To my loving family, for being my rock, and to all the wonderful radiology residents, you are my inspiration

—PRACHI

To family, teachers, and patients who taught me radiology

—SATHISH

To my parents, Roselyne and Jonathan

—DANIEL

To my wife and children for their unwavering support throughout my life

—RAFEEQUE

To my parents, Shehla and Moonis Raza, for inspiring me not only to be a lifelong educator but also a student, and to Jafar and Zohran for their support, encouragement, and patience during the long gestation period of this book

—GUL

Aly H. Abayazeed, MD

Department of Radiology
University of Massachusetts Medical School
Worcester, Massachusetts

Syed Adil Aftab, MD

Department of Radiology
University of Chicago
Chicago, Illinois

Rafeeque Bhadelia, MD

Department of Radiology
Beth Israel Deaconess Medical Center
Harvard Medical School
Boston, Massachusetts

Yu-Ming Chang, MD, PhD

Department of Radiology
Beth Israel Deaconess Medical Center
Harvard Medical School
Boston, Massachusetts

David Choi, MD

Department of Radiology
University of Massachusetts Medical School
Worcester, Massachusetts

Daniel Chow, MD

Department of Radiology
University of California Irvine
Irvine, California

Hisham M. Dahmoush, MBBCh, FRCR

Department of Radiology
Stanford University
Stanford, California

Robert Darflinger, MD

Department of Radiology
UCSF School of Medicine
San Francisco, California

Prachi Dubey, MBBS, MPH

Department of Radiology
Columbia University Medical Center
New York-Presbyterian/Columbia Hospital
New York, New York

Sathish Kumar Dundamadappa, MBBS

Department of Radiology
University of Massachusetts Medical School
Worcester, Massachusetts

Lee Finkelstone, MD

Department of Radiology
Columbia University Medical Center
New York-Presbyterian/Columbia Hospital
New York, New York

Ernst Garcon, MD

Department of Radiology
Columbia University Medical Center
New York-Presbyterian/Columbia Hospital
New York, New York

Daniel Thomas Ginat, MD, MS

Department of Radiology
University of Chicago
Pritzker School of Medicine
Chicago, Illinois

Gaurav Jindal, MD

Department of Radiology
Brown University
Providence, Rhode Island

David B. Khatami, MD, PhD

Department of Radiology
Beth Israel Deaconess Medical Center
Harvard Medical School
Boston, Massachusetts

Jonathan Youngsuk Kim, MD

Department of Radiology
Beth Israel Deaconess Medical Center
Harvard Medical School
Boston, Massachusetts

Pritesh Mehta, MD

Department of Radiology
Beth Israel Deaconess Medical Center
Harvard Medical School
Boston, Massachusetts

Gul Moonis, MD
Department of Radiology
Columbia University Medical Center
New York-Presbyterian/Columbia Hospital
New York, New York

Lidia Mayumi Nagae, MD, PhD
Department of Radiology
University of Colorado, School of Medicine
Denver, Colorado

Pamela H. Nguyen, DO
Department of Radiology
Columbia University Medical Center
New York-Presbyterian/Columbia Hospital
New York, New York

Andrea Poretti, MD
Department of Radiology
Johns Hopkins School of Medicine
Baltimore, Maryland

Rafael Rojas, MD
Department of Radiology
Beth Israel Deaconess Medical Center
Harvard Medical School
Boston, Massachusetts

Shyam Sabat, MD
Department of Radiology
Penn State Health
Hershey, Pennsylvania

Archana Siddalingappa, MD
Department of Radiology
Beth Israel Deaconess Medical Center
Harvard Medical School
Boston, Massachusetts

Scott Sorenson, MD
Department of Radiology
University of Chicago
Chicago, Illinois

Neuroradiology: A Core Review covers the vast field of neuroradiology in a way that I am confident will serve as a useful guide for residents to assess their knowledge and review the material in a question style format that is similar to the core examination.

Dr. Prachi Dubey, Dr. Gul Moonis, Dr. Sathish Dundamadappa, Dr. Daniel Ginat, and Dr. Rafeeque Bhadelia have succeeded in presenting a very challenging topic in a manner that exemplifies the philosophy and goals of the *Core Review Series*. They have done a magnificent job in distilling the essential facts and concepts of neuroradiology in a manner that is straightforward with many multipart questions that cover the subject matter very well. The multiple-choice questions have been divided into chapters that correspond to how board exams are organized so as to make it easy for learners to work on particular topics as needed. There are also references provided for each question for those who want to delve more deeply into a specific subject.

The intent of the *Core Review Series* is to provide the resident, fellow, or practicing physician a review of the important conceptual, factual, and practical aspects of a subject by providing approximately 300 multiple-choice questions, in a format similar to the core examination. For *Neuroradiology: A Core Review*, there are additional questions that can be found in the eBook version. The *Core Review Series* is not intended to be exhaustive but to provide material likely to be tested on the core exam and that would be required in clinical practice.

As series editor of the *Core Review Series*, it has been rewarding to not only be an author of one of the books but also be able to work with many outstanding individuals in the profession of radiology across the country who contributed to the series. This series represents countless hours of work and involvement by so many that it could not have come together without their participation. It has been very gratifying to see the growing popularity and positive feedback the authors of the *Core Review Series* have received from many reviews.

Dr. Prachi Dubey, Dr. Gul Moonis, Dr. Sathish Dundamadappa, Dr. Daniel Ginat, Dr. Rafeeque Bhadelia, and their contributors are to be commended on doing an outstanding job. I believe *Neuroradiology: A Core Review* will serve as an excellent resource for residents during their board preparation and a valuable reference for fellows and practicing radiologists.

Biren A. Shah, MD, FACR
Director, Breast Imaging
Director, Breast Imaging Fellowship
Associate Professor of Radiology
School of Medicine
Virginia Commonwealth University
Richmond, Virginia

PREFACE

The certification examination by American Board of Radiology (ABR) requires targeted preparation for a timed, computerized, image-based, multiple-choice testing platform. The main purpose of this book is to serve as a consolidated resource by providing practice questions and relevant study material to bridge any gaps in knowledge. In addition, this book covers topics in sufficient detail to serve as a reference guide for practice and aid in preparation for Neuroradiology Certificate of Added Qualifications examinations.

The book is divided in three sections, one for each part of neuroradiology, Brain, Spine, and Head and Neck, in a single volume. The chapters within these sections cover all relevant topics following the ABR blue print as a guide. The questions have subparts designed with the aim of addressing key concepts, misconceptions, and areas of ambiguity through questions that highlight these nuances. The discussion provides images with explanations to serve as an independent reference source and aid in quickly revising concepts prior to the examination. The study material, while focused on the certification requirement, also provides conceptual understanding of important topics with references for additional reading based on the reader's interest.

We would like to express our sincere gratitude to Wolters Kluwer, Dr. Biren Shah (series editor), and our numerous contributors from academic institutions across the country for their dedication to this project and enthusiasm toward the shared goal of training the best radiologists, who further the field of radiology and serve as role model physicians for the coming generation.

We are also grateful to our families for lasting support and encouragement through this long and tedious process requiring countless hours of work. We sincerely hope this book will serve as a useful comprehensive resource for future radiologists and neuroradiologists.

Prachi Dubey
Sathish Kumar Dundamadappa
Daniel Thomas Ginat
Rafeeque Bhadelia
Gul Moonis

ACKNOWLEDGMENTS

We would like to thank Dr. Angela Lignelli for providing support and encouragement during this project and Ms. Zainab Noor Rizvi for working with us on formatting the images. Last but not the least, we would like to thank our patients for inspiring us to do our best and the numerous radiology technologists and nurses across the nation whose dedication and hard work make this work possible.

CONTENTS

1 Neoplastic Abnormalities

SATHISH KUMAR DUNDAMADAPPA • LIDIA MAYUMI NAGAE • PRACHI DUBEY

QUESTIONS

1 A 55-year-old male presents for further workup of a right frontal lobe calcified mass incidentally discovered on CT for altered mental status.

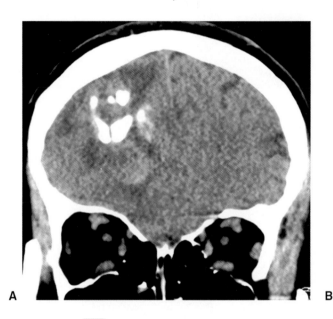
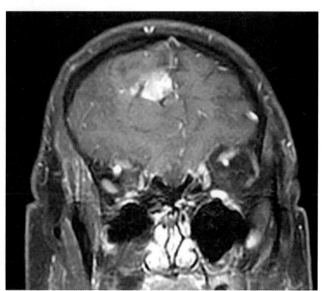

A   B

1a What is the most likely diagnosis?

    A. Meningioma

    B. Oligodendroglioma

    C. Metastasis

    D. Primitive neuroectodermal tumor

1b Which of the following is a rare manifestation of oligodendroglioma?

    A. Involvement of cortical/subcortical white matter

    B. Presence of coarse intratumoral calcification

    C. None or subtle enhancement on postcontrast MRI

    D. Intraventricular location

2   A 67-year-old hypertensive otherwise healthy man presents with new-onset seizure to the emergency department. A noncontrast head CT was performed to evaluate for intracranial hemorrhage.

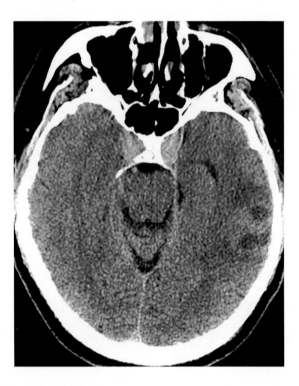

2a   What should be the next step?

    A. Normal; no further imaging is needed
    B. CT angiogram of head and neck
    C. MRI of brain without and with contrast
    D. FDG PET/CT

2b   What should be the most likely diagnosis?

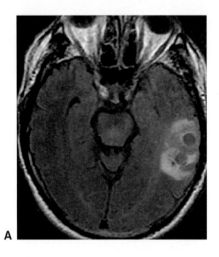 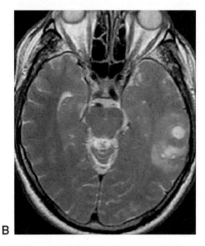 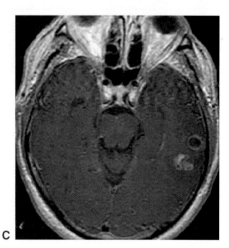

A   B   C

    A. Glial neoplasm, such as glioblastoma
    B. Primary CNS lymphoma
    C. Metastasis
    D. Herpes encephalitis

3 A surveillance MRI performed for a known condition. Key images are shown below:

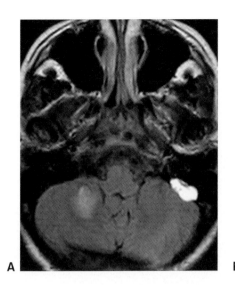
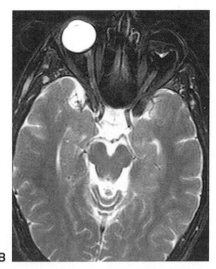
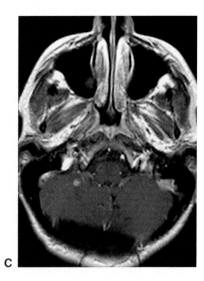

A   B   C

3a Which of the following is likely to occur in these patients?

A. Pancreatic neuroendocrine tumors
B. Plexiform neurofibroma
C. Port-wine stain
D. Renal angiomyolipoma

4 A 40-year-old woman presents with a history of dizziness.

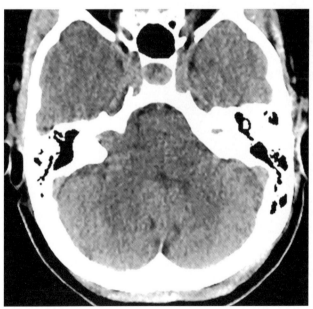
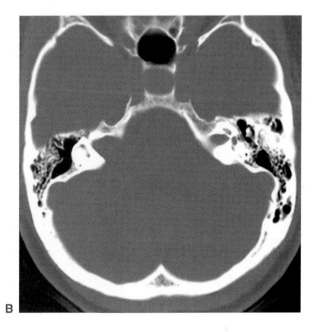

A   B

4a What is the next best step?

    A. A contrast-enhanced CT scan

    B. A contrast-enhanced MRI

    C. CT angiogram of the head

    D. No further follow-up evaluation is needed.

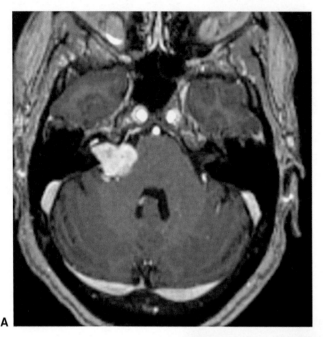

A

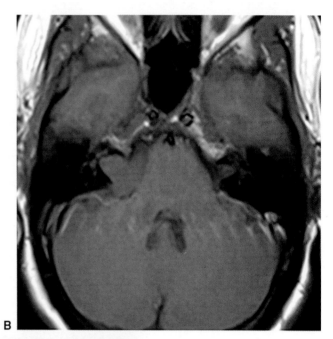

B

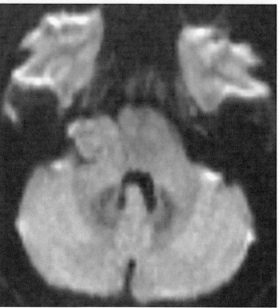

C

4b What is the most likely diagnosis based on the contrast enhanced MRI performed on this patient?

    A. Vestibular schwannoma

    B. CP angle meningioma

    C. Neurofibroma

    D. Epidermoid lesion

5 A 20-year-old male presents with gait disturbances and abnormal NECT. An MRI with contrast was performed for further assessment. Key images are shown below:

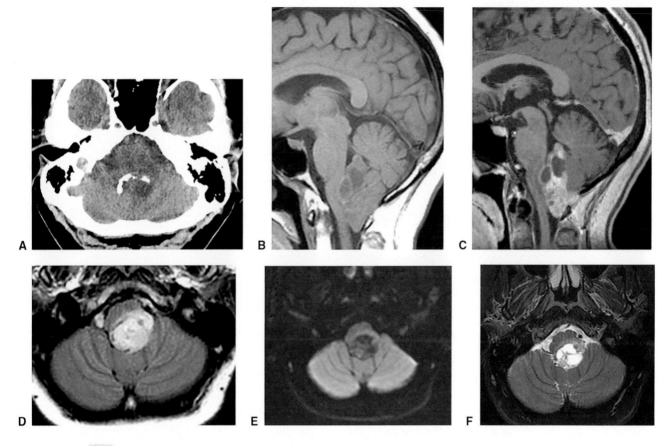

5a What is the most likely diagnosis?

    A. Ependymoma

    B. Subependymoma

    C. Oligodendroglioma

    D. Metastasis

5b These tumors originate from which of the following cell types?

    A. Ependymal cells

    B. Astrocytes

    C. Oligodendrocytes

    D. Cell type outside the CNS.

6   Provided below are key images from an MRI performed for a known intraventricular mass seen on CT.

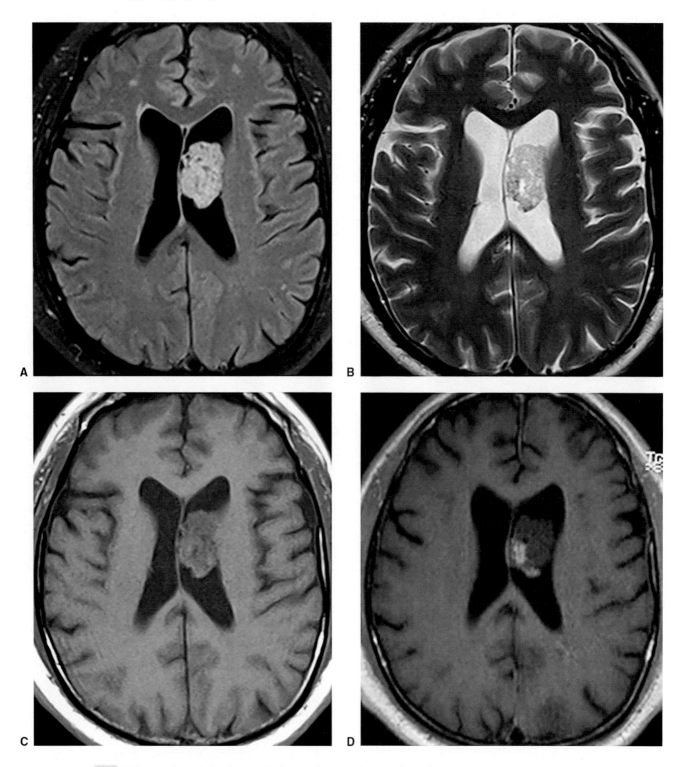

6a   What is the likely diagnosis for the lesion shown above?

     A.   Central neurocytoma

     B.   Ependymoma

     C.   Subependymal giant cell astrocytoma

     D.   Intraventricular metastasis

6b Which is the common anatomic site for these lesions?

   A. Lateral ventricle attached to the septum pellucidum or ventricular wall
   B. Choroid plexus in the fourth ventricle
   C. Third ventricle
   D. Commonly extraventricular in location.

7 A 10-year-old male with abnormal head CT performed for progressive difficulty in swallowing, facial weakness, and visual abnormalities. An MRI was performed for further assessment; key images are shown below:

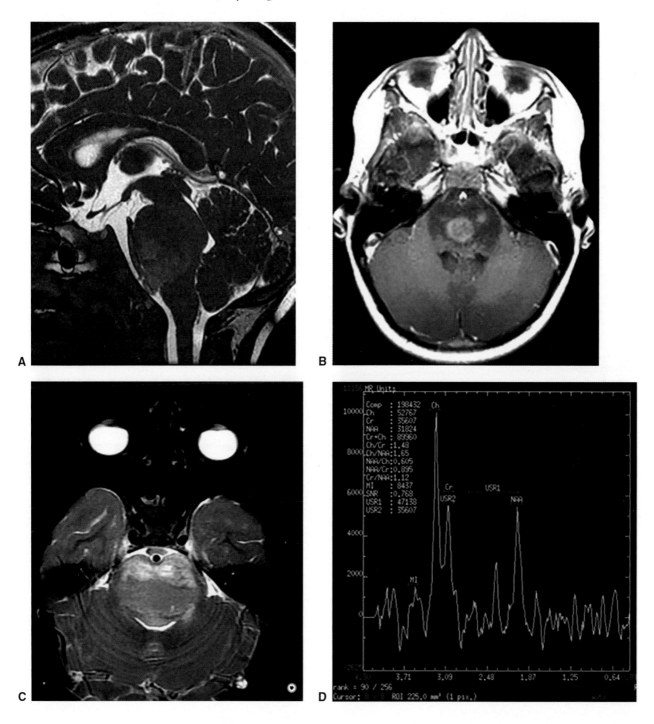

7a Based on the above images, what is the most likely etiology for the above changes?

    A. Primary CNS glial neoplasm
    B. Metastatic disease
    C. Osmotic demyelination
    D. Neuro-Behcet disease

7b What specific metabolite abnormality is depicted on the proton MRS?

    A. Elevated choline and reduction in NAA
    B. Elevated lactate
    C. Reduced choline and elevated NAA
    D. No abnormality is depicted with physiologic metabolite pattern.

8 CT and MRI were performed for further workup of left-sided trigeminal neuralgia. Key images are shown below:

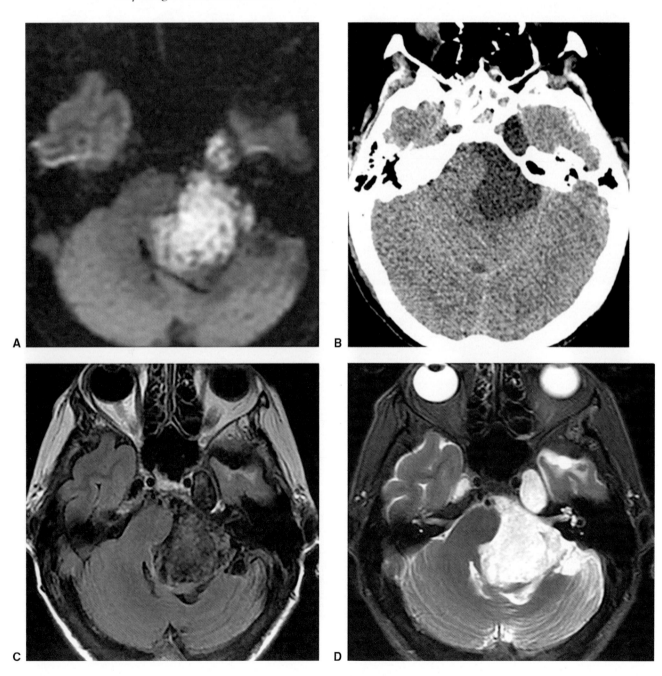

8a Which of the provided signal features are characteristics for this abnormality?

A. Extra-axial, T2 shine through on DWI, low attenuation on CT.

B. Extra-axial, restricted diffusion, low attenuation on CT, incomplete suppression on FLAIR

C. Intra-axial, T2 shine through on DWI, low attenuation on CT.

D. Extra-axial, T2 shine through on DWI, complete suppression on FLAIR

8b Which of the above characteristics help differentiate this lesion from an arachnoid cyst?

A. T2 shine through on DWI

B. Restricted diffusion on DWI

C. Low attenuation on CT

D. High attenuation on CT

9 A 55-year-old male, previously healthy, presents with altered mental status. Key images from CT and MRI are shown below:

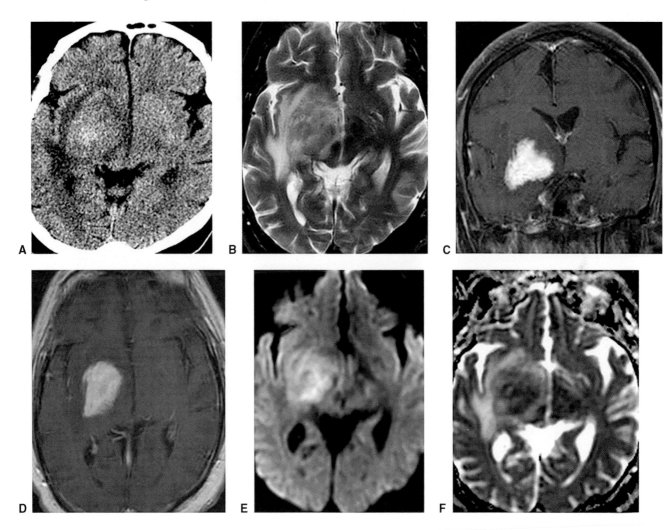

9a Based on the above images what is the most likely diagnosis in an immunocompetent adult?

A. Primary CNS lymphoma

B. Subacute infarction

C. Cerebral abscess

D. Tumefactive demyelination

10 A 35-year-old male with long-standing medically intractable seizures presents for initial evaluation with an abnormal MRI. No other comorbidities.

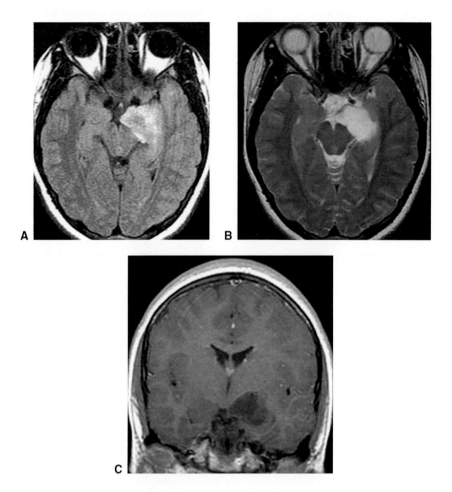

10a What is the best next step?

    A. Neurosurgical consultation

    B. Antiviral therapy

    C. No further intervention is needed.

    D. Routine annual follow-up can be performed.

10b Which of the following is true about the above entity?

    A. Temporal lobe intracortical location is common for this lesion (DNET).

    B. This is an aggressive malignant process.

    C. White matter location is common.

    D. This is a lesion typically seen in older <70 age group.

11   A 13-year-old male who presents with constant suboccipital headache, blurring of vision, and truncal ataxia on examination. An MRI with contrast was performed; the images are provided below:

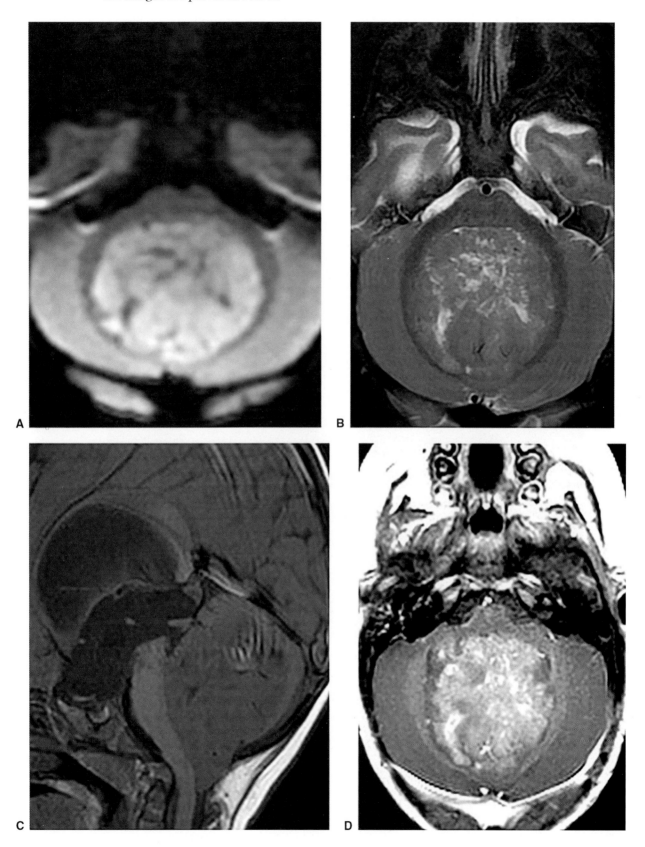

A

B

C

D

11a Based on these views, the abnormality showed above is centered in which of the following structures in the posterior fossa?

    A. Midline cerebellar vermis

    B. Brainstem

    C. Lateral cerebellar hemispheres

    D. Tentorium

11b In this age group and location, which is the most common malignant neoplasm?

    A. Medulloblastoma

    B. Juvenile pilocytic astrocytoma

    C. Metastasis

    D. Hemangioblastoma

12 A 10-year-old male presents with headache and blurring of vision with an abnormal MRI shown below.

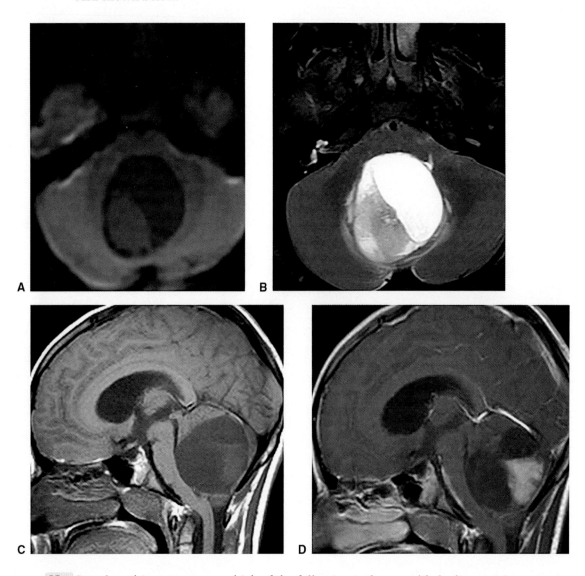

12a Based on this appearance, which of the following is the most likely diagnosis?

    A. Pilocytic astrocytoma

    B. Hemangioblastoma

    C. Ganglioglioma

    D. Ependymoma

12b Which of the following statements is true regarding the above lesion?

    A. It may have different morphologic features based on location.

    B. Radiation is the mainstay of therapy for cerebellar lesions in children < 5 years age.

    C. Overall prognosis is poor with low 10-year survival rate.

    D. This entity has been associated in patients with neurofibromatosis type 2.

13 A patient with known tuberous sclerosis presents for surveillance MRI, shown below.

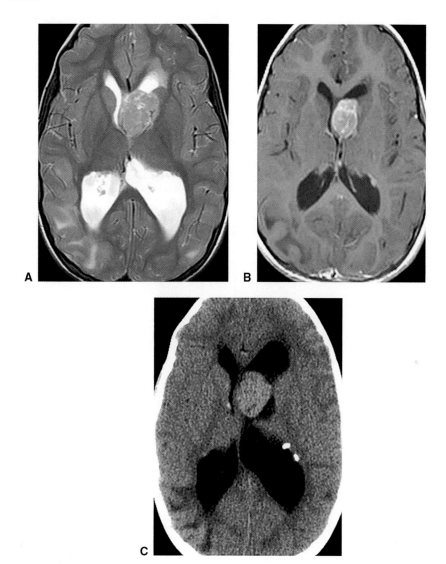

13a Which of the following best describes the anatomic location for this lesion?

    A. Foramen of Monro

    B. Atria of the lateral ventricle

    C. Roof of the third ventricle

    D. Forniceal pillars

13b Which of the following findings helps differentiate the above from subependymal nodules also seen with TS?

    A. Growth on follow-up MRI

    B. Calcification within the nodule

    C. Size <1 cm

    D. Presence of enhancement within the nodule.

14 A patient presents for preoperative evaluation of a mass noted on CT. Key images are shown below:

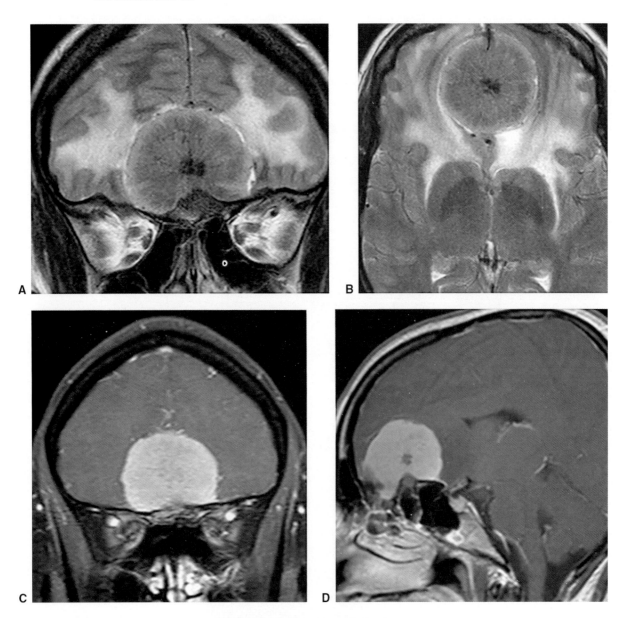

14a Based on the coronal plane and axial plane T2-weighted sequence, which is the most likely location of this lesion and why?

A. Intra-axial because of lack of CSF cleft
B. Extra-axial because of presence of a CSF cleft
C. Intra-axial with exophytic growth
D. Extra-axial lesion with cortical invasion

14b Of the following, which is the most accurate terminology for describing the above lesion?

A. Anterior cranial fossa, planum sphenoidale meningioma
B. Middle cranial fossa, sphenoid wing meningioma
C. Intraosseous meningioma
D. Tuberculum sellae meningioma

15 A 42-year-old male with sudden onset of left face and hand numbness. An MRI of the brain is performed.

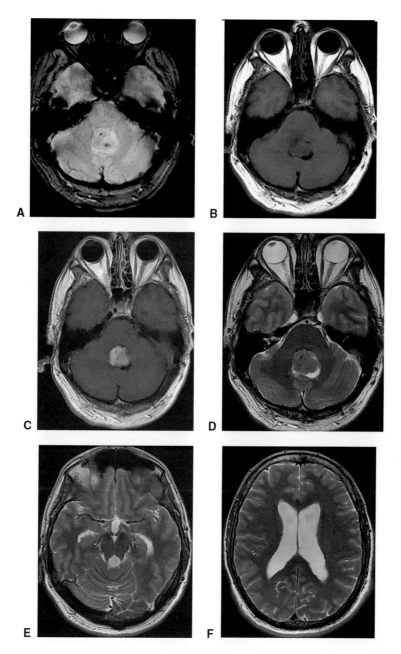

15a What imaging finding shown above is most critical regarding patient management acutely?

A. Upward transtentorial herniation
B. Presence of secondary lesions
C. Obstructive hydrocephalus
D. CSF dissemination of neoplasm

15b Which of the following entities is more likely to be supratentorial in location in this age group?

A. Choroid plexus papilloma
B. Medulloblastoma
C. Subependymal giant cell astrocytoma
D. Hemangioblastoma

16   A previously healthy 15-year-old male presents with diplopia evolving to isolated left-sided cranial nerve palsy in the course of 2 weeks. An MRI of the brain is performed.

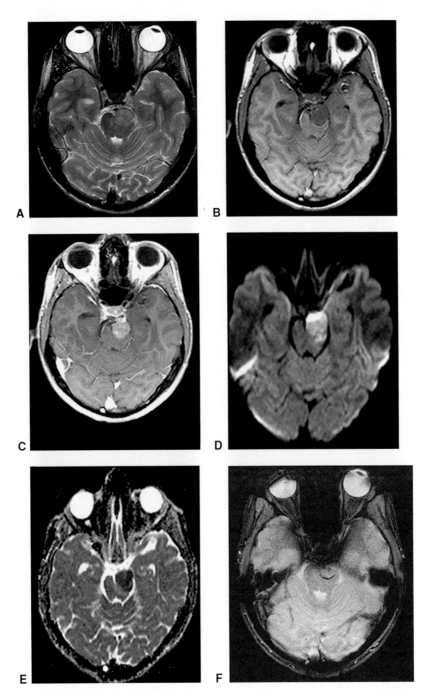

16a   Which of the following lesions are likely to demonstrate hyperattenuation on CT and restricted diffusion on DWI?

   A. Oligodendroglioma
   B. Anaplastic astrocytoma
   C. Pilocytic astrocytoma
   D. Atypical teratoid rhabdoid tumor

16b Which of the following is likely to be the isolated cranial nerve palsy in this patient?

    A. CN V
    B. CN II
    C. CN IV
    D. CN III

17 A 60-year-old male with 3-week history of progressive headaches, nausea, vomiting, dizziness, and ataxia. An MRI of the brain was performed. Key images are shown below.

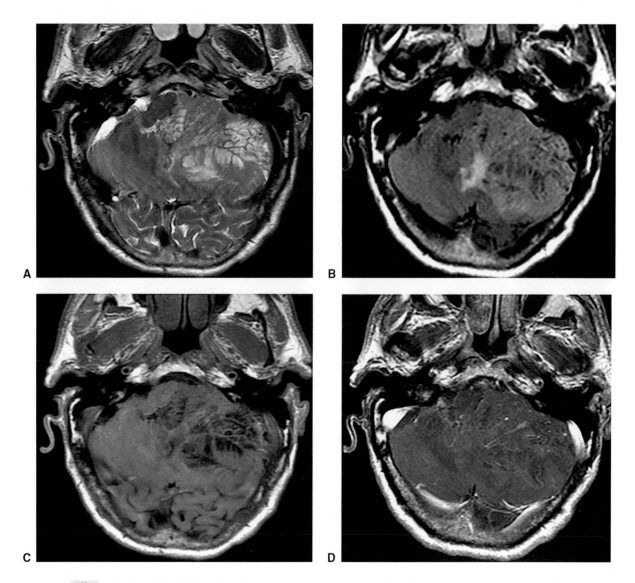

17a Which of the following characteristics is associated with this lesion?

    A. Tigroid appearance
    B. Nodular heterogeneous enhancement
    C. Necrosis and cystic change
    D. Meningeal infiltration

17b What is the most likely diagnosis?

    A. Acute left PCA infarct

    B. Organizing left cerebellar hemorrhage with mass effect

    C. Lhermitte-Duclos disease

    D. Cerebellar glioblastoma

18 A 51-year-old male presented with headaches and ataxia. An MRI was performed. Key images are shown below:

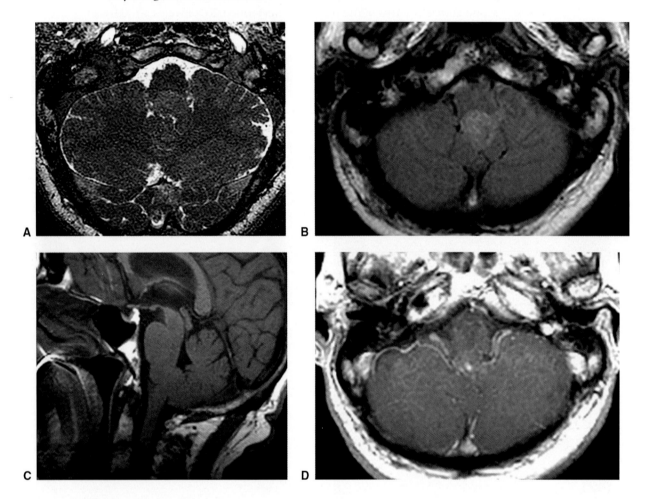

18a What is the most likely diagnosis for the lesion shown above?

    A. Ependymoma

    B. Subependymoma

    C. Choroid plexus papilloma

    D. Metastasis

18b In view of this lesion's location, what poses the greatest risk for neurologic compromise?

    A. CSF obstruction

    B. Cervicomedullary invasion

    C. Tonsillar herniation

    D. No foreseeable risk, therefore managed conservatively.

19 A 26-year-old female with medically refractory complex partial seizures presents
for MRI. Key images from a contrast enhanced MRI are provided below.

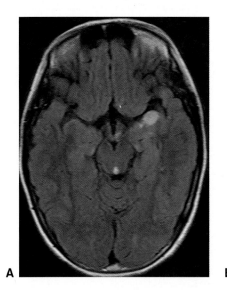

A

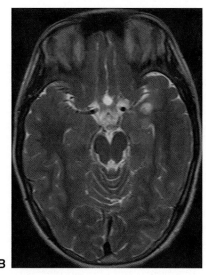

B

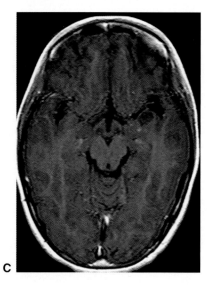

C

19a Which of the following is the most common neoplasm associated with chronic
intractable epilepsy?

A. Pleomorphic xanthoastrocytoma

B. Dysembryoplastic neuroepithelial tumor

C. Ganglioglioma

D. Angiocentric glioma

19b This lesion is likely slow growing and nonaggressive in nature. Which of the
following imaging features favor those characteristics?

A. Lack of vasogenic edema

B. Peripheral superficial cortical location

C. Necrotic foci

D. Osseous erosion

ANSWERS AND EXPLANATIONS

1a **Answer B.**   Oligodendroglioma. The most appropriate choice would be oligodendroglioma. A meningioma is typically an extra-axial dural-based lesion. A metastasis will be an appropriate differential possibility; however, a metastatic lesion of this size and in such a location is likely to incite more vasogenic edema (note that it is possible for a metastatic lesion to not incite large amount of vasogenic edema, typically when a lesion is present peripherally in the cortical or juxtacortical location).

1b **Answer D.**   Intraventricular location. The presence of an intraventricular oligodendroglioma is possible but rare, approximately 3% to 8%. These tumors when present have different imaging features compared to parenchymal oligodendrogliomas; for example, presence of enhancement, tumor blush on angiography, and high attenuation on CT relative to brain parenchyma are seen with these lesions but not with parenchymal oligodendroglioma. The other more typical intraventricular neoplasms are meningioma, central neurocytoma, ependymoma/subependymoma, and choroid plexus papilloma.

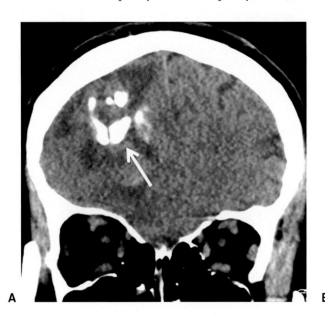
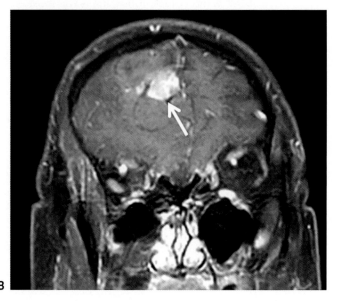

A   B

Imaging Findings: Noncontrast head CT showing calcifications within a right frontal lobe cortical based mass (A) and contrast enhanced T1w MRI in coronal plane showing heterogenous enhancement (B). This location and calcification are typical for oligodendroglioma.

Discussion: Oligodendroglioma is a tumor of neuroglial origin with variable prognostic features, ranging from relatively low aggressive potential relative to a similar-grade astrocytoma to very aggressive behavior similar to higher grade glial neoplasms. It is the third most common glioma, accounting for 5% to 18% of all glial neoplasms.

Calcification within oligodendroglioma may range from 20% to 90%; occasionally cystic degeneration and hemorrhage may also be seen. On MR, most commonly heterogenous signal intensity is noted; vasogenic edema although present is typically not as striking or common as the higher grade astrocytoma, and the ADC values on diffusion-weighted imaging might be low, such as seen with other higher grade glial neoplasm, purported to have resulted from lowered extracellular hyaluronic acid.

Differential Diagnosis: Other primary CNS glial neoplasm, metastasis, or less likely meningioma. Although other primary CNS glial neoplasms and metastasis cannot be excluded, the presence of calcification, peripheral cortical location, and lack of significant vasogenic edema are most typical for oligodendroglioma. Meningioma is not likely because this is a peripheral but intra-axial lesion instead of an extra-axial lesion.

References: Koeller KK, et al. From the archives of the AFIP: oligodendroglioma and its variants: radiologic-pathologic correlation. *Radiographics* 2005;25(6):1669–1688.

Smith AB, et al. From the radiologic pathology archives: intraventricular neoplasms: radiologic-pathologic correlation. *Radiographics* 2013;33(1):21–43.

2a **Answer C.**   MRI of brain without and with contrast. There is a heterogenous mass-like lesion in the left temporal lobe; the best way to assess this will be MRI with contrast because of higher soft tissue detail. FDG PET and CTA will not be appropriate modalities in this case.

2b **Answer A.**   Glial neoplasm, such as glioblastoma. The location, heterogeneous enhancement, and necrotic foci favor glioblastoma.

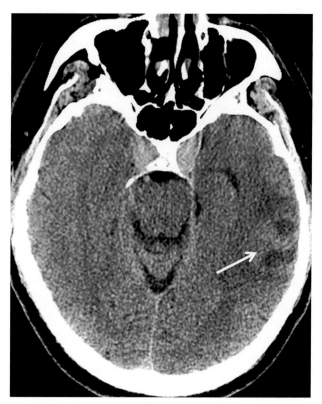

Figure 1

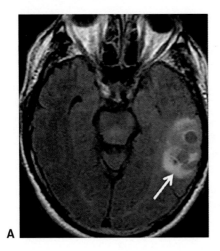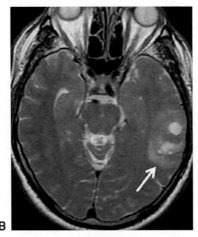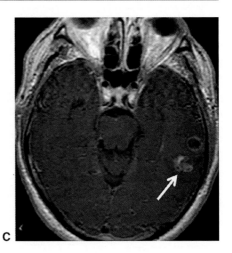

Figure 2

Imaging Findings: Figure 1. A mass-like cortical-based lesion in the left temporal lobe with necrotic/cystic foci on noncontrast head CT.

Figure 2. The same lesion on FLAIR (A), T2w (B), and contrast-enhanced T1w (C) sequences, with a heterogenously enhancing morphology, cystic/necrotic foci, and nonenhancing T2/FLAIR hyperintensity. These features are most consistent with a glial neoplasm with heterogenous enhancement pattern and potential necrosis favoring a relatively aggressive behavior.

Discussion: The above case shows an example of an aggressive primary CNS glial neoplasm, glioblastoma. It is the most common primary CNS neoplasm (~15% of all intracranial neoplasms).

In distribution, it is frequently supratentorial, predominantly involving ages 40 to 70 years. When it is rarely found in children, it may be more commonly infratentorial compared to adults.

The majority of these lesions have a rapid clinical course, have an abrupt presentation, and arise de novo within the brain, that is, without a preexisting lower grade precursor lesion. However, a few lesions may result from de-differentiation of a preexisting lower grade glial neoplasm; typically, the latter is seen in younger population (mean age, 40 years) and has a longer clinical course.

Proton MR spectroscopy typically demonstrates elevation of choline (3.2 ppm) and lactate peak (1.3 ppm). MR perfusion (either DSC or DCE) shows elevated CBV within the lesion, as would have been the case with any other aggressive neoplasm and occasionally with aggressive demyelination/inflammation. However, it is noteworthy that both MR perfusion and proton MR spectroscopy, are nonspecific in isolation and should be interpreted in conjunction with lesion morphology on other sequences and clinical presentation.

Differential Diagnosis: Metastasis, primary CNS lymphoma, herpes encephalitis, are differential consideration; however as explained above, the most likely diagnosis will be primary CNS glial neoplasm.

There has been a recent update in the glial neoplasm classification as of June 2016 with incorporation of the specific molecular profile. This was necessary because the histopathologic classification alone did not accurately predict clinical course or treatment response. For example, presence of IDH mutation, and ATRX loss are associated with a favorable prognosis.

References: Altman DA, Atkinson DS Jr, Brat DJ. Best cases from the AFIP: glioblastoma multiforme. *Radiographics* 2007;27(3):883–888.

Brat DJ, et al. Comprehensive, integrative genomic analysis of diffuse lower-grade gliomas. *N Engl J Med* 2015;372(26):2481–2498.

Louis DN, et al. The 2016 World Health Organization Classification of Tumors of the Central Nervous System: a summary. *Acta Neuropathol* 2016;131(6):803–820.

3a **Answer A.** Pancreatic neuroendocrine tumors. This is a case of von Hippel-Lindau syndrome with evidence of globe enucleation secondary to retinal hemangioblastoma, a left-sided endolymphatic sac tumor, and a right cerebellar hemangioblastoma. This entity has multisystem involvement with one of the manifestations being pancreatic neuroendocrine tumor (or islet cell tumor), seen in 5% to 17% of these patients.

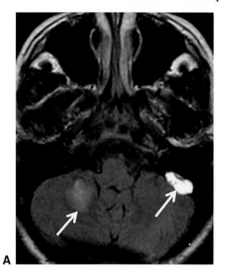
A

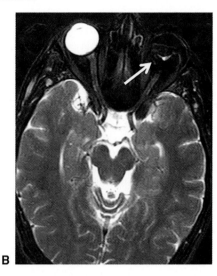
B

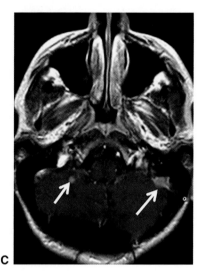
C

Imaging Findings: Axial FLAIR sequence demonstrating a focus of hyperintensity in the right anterior cerebellum (A) with corresponding punctate enhancement seen on postcontrast T1w sequence (C) and a left petromastoid FLAIR hyperintense ovoid lesion, (A); there is enucleation of the left eye seen on axial T2w sequence (B). Constellation of findings suggest a right cerebellar hemangioblastoma, left endolymphatic sac tumor and left globe enucleation due to prior retinal hemangioblastoma, this is compatible with the diagnosis of von Hippel-Lindau syndrome.

Discussion: Hemangioblastoma is a benign slow-growing tumor of vascular origin. Its pathogenesis and cell of origin are not known. About two-thirds of these are sporadic, and the rest are seen in association with von Hippel-Lindau syndrome (VHL). Multiple tumors are almost always associated with VHL. A rare non-VHL form of multiple hemangioblastomas has been reported, known as leptomeningeal hemangioblastomatosis. Metastasis is extremely rare, but has been reported.

They are primarily seen in third to fifth decade of life; the presentation is earlier by a decade in VHL-associated tumors. They account for about 2% of intracranial tumors and 10% of posterior fossa tumors. They are the most common primary brain tumor of the posterior fossa in an adult. Most are located in the posterior fossa (cerebellum, vermis, and medulla in that order), followed by the spinal cord. Supratentorial location is rare, seen in about 5% to 10%. The growth pattern can be "stuttered" with periods of quiescence and growth.

The most common tumor morphology is peritumoral cyst with an intensely enhancing tumor nodule, seen in about 60%. About 30% of tumors are purely solid. Solid tumors, intratumoral cysts, and tumors with intra- and peritumoral cyst are rare patterns.

On CT, the cyst is hypodense and the nodule is almost isodense to the parenchyma. On MRI, the cyst shows fluid signal on T2 images. The solid nodule shows moderate hyperintensity on T2 and hypointensity on T1. Intense contrast enhancement of the nodule is typical. Tortuous vessels can be demonstrated in the vicinity of the tumor in precontrast, postcontrast, and CTA/MRA images. The surrounding edema is variable and can be disproportionately large compared to the nodule size. In larger nodules and solid masses, the enhancement can be heterogeneous. The cyst wall either shows no enhancement or minimal thin enhancement.

Differential diagnosis for cerebellar hemangioblastoma:

In children, pilocytic astrocytoma.

In adults, metastatic disease. In patients with VHL, metastasis from renal cell cancer can be hypervascular and may pose diagnostic difficulty.

References: Naidich TP, ed. *Imaging of the brain. Expert radiology series.* Philadelphia, PA: Saunders/Elsevier, 2013.

Osborn AG. *Osborn's brain: imaging, pathology, and anatomy,* 1st ed. Salt Lake City, UT: Amirsys Pub., 2013.

4a **Answer B.**   A contrast-enhanced MRI. Given there is an abnormality within the right IAC, best seen with obvious expansion of the IAC on bone window (Figure 1B), the best way to evaluate this will be an MRI with contrast.

4b **Answer A.**   Vestibular schwannoma. The most likely explanation for this enhancing mass without restricted diffusion will be a vestibular schwannoma. Neurofibroma, also a nerve sheath tumor, has greater risk of malignant transformation but is exceedingly rare as a primary intracranial lesion, even in patients with type 1 neurofibromatosis, making this a very unlikely diagnosis for CP angle masses. CP angle meningioma is a differential possibility and cannot be reliably excluded on imaging alone. However, meningioma typically presents with a dural tail and adjacent reactive osseous hyperostosis and may also have restricted diffusion due to high cellularity, not seen in this case. Epidermoid lesion typically follows CSF appearance on both CT and MRI; however, it also demonstrates restricted diffusion. Enhancement if any is typically peripheral in nature.

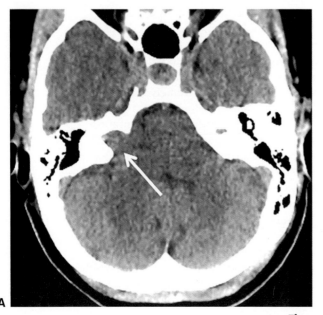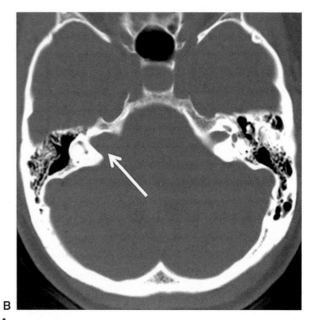

Figure 1

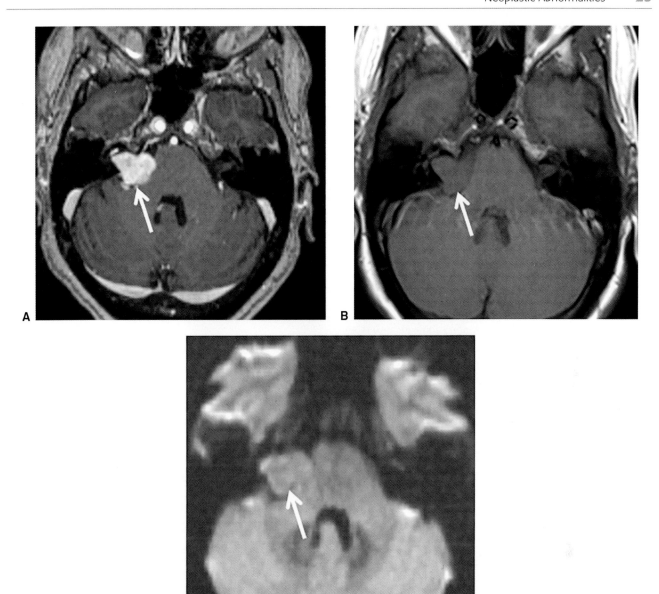

Figure 2

Imaging Findings: Figure 1. Axial noncontrast CT demonstrates a mass in the right cerebellopontine angle (CP angle) with extension into the right internal auditory canal (IAC). Note, on the bone windows (B), there is expansion of the right-sided IAC (it is key to carefully scrutinize the IAC on bone windows to detect any masses or space-occupying lesions that may remain occult on standard brain window).

Figure 2. A subsequent contrast-enhanced MRI confirms presence of an enhancing mass involving the right IAC and right CP angle, (A). No evidence of restricted diffusion to suggest high cellularity (C).

Discussion: Vestibular schwannoma is the most common mass in the CP angle, accounting for 85% of CP angle masses. Schwannoma is a benign, slowly growing neoplasm. CP angle schwannomas most commonly involve the inferior division of the vestibular nerve (vestibular branch of CN VIII). A majority of the intracranial schwannomas are sporadic. Less than 20% of these may be associated with neurofibromatosis type 2. Intracranial schwannomas most commonly occur along sensory nerve fibers, of which CN VIII is most common, followed by trigeminal nerve.

Patients commonly present with hearing loss, rarely with vertigo and imbalance. Management of such lesions can include observation, Gamma Knife surgery, or microsurgical resection. Various factors influence the treatment choices, and therefore further subspecialty consultation will be warranted to better understand treatment options.

Differential Diagnosis: Mengingioma (a dural tail, reactive hyperostosis in the underlying bone, and potentially restricted diffusion due to higher cellularity may be seen as differentiating features; however oftentimes this is difficult to definitively differentiate, particularly because meningiomas may have canalicular AND labyrinthine extension); epidermoid (follows CSF signal and shows restricted diffusion); metastasis (rare in isolation; typically seen with leptomeningeal disease, prior history of a primary).

References: Fisher JL, et al. Loud noise exposure and acoustic neuroma. *Am J Epidemiol* 2014;180(1):58–67.

Silk PS, et al. Surgical approaches to vestibular schwannomas: what the radiologist needs to know. *Radiographics* 2009;29(7):1955–1970.

Smirniotopoulos JG, et al. Cerebellopontine angle masses: radiologic-pathologic correlation. *Radiographics* 1993;13:1131–1147.

5a **Answer A.** Ependymoma.

5b **Answer A.** Ependymal cells. These tumors originate from the ependymal lining of ventricles and spinal cord central canal, hence the name "ependymoma"; however, it should be noted that extraventricular variants of this tumor have also been reported.

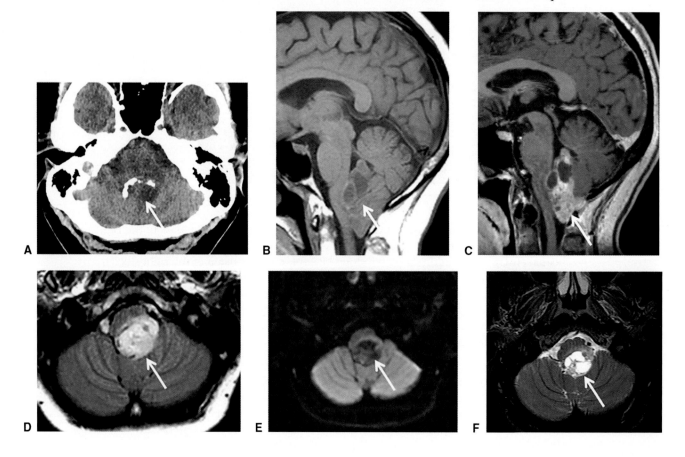

Imaging Finding: A calcified lesion on NECT (A) centered in the fourth ventricle with cystic foci on T2w sequences (F). There is no significant vasogenic edema on FLAIR (D) or evidence of restricted diffusion (E). Pre- and postcontrast images (B and C, respectively) show heterogeneous enhancement and elongated appearance that appears to squeeze through the foramen magnum on the sagittal plane, compressing the dorsal aspect of the cervicomedullary junction.

Discussion: Ependymoma is a type of primary CNS neoplasm that arises from the ependymal lining. They are within the subtype of neuroepithelial neoplasms unlike astrocytomas, which are primary neuroglial subtype of tumors.

These tumors can be seen at any age. Typically, younger patients tend to have posterior fossa and older patients tend to have supratentorial ependymoma. These can be found in the fourth, lateral, and third ventricles. These can also be extraventricular in location particularly when seen in a supratentorial location in children. These are classified as WHO grade II lesions. Variant of higher grade or anaplastic ependymomas have also been reported (WHO grade III).

Imaging features on MR are typically hyperintensity on T2-weighted images and isointensity on T1-weighted images with intense contrast enhancement within the soft tissue components. Calcification, hemorrhage, and cystic components are commonly seen that lead to morphologic heterogeneity within this lesion. These lesions are classically defined as soft or plastic lesions; when seen in the fourth ventricle, these can squeeze through the foramen of Luschka, foramen of Magendie, and foramen magnum.

Postoperative imaging is key in determining survival rate with residual disease associated with a lower overall survival.

References: Cage TA, Clark AJ, Aranda D, et al. A systematic review of treatment outcomes in pediatric patients with intracranial ependymomas. *J Neurosurg Pediatr* 2013;11(6): 673–681.

Smith AB, Smirniotopoulos JG, Horkanyne-Szakaly I. From the radiologic pathology archives: intraventricular neoplasms: radiologic-pathologic correlation. *Radiographics* 2013;33(1):21–43.

6a   **Answer A.**   Central neurocytoma.

6b **Answer A.** Lateral ventricle attached to the septum pellucidum or ventricular wall.

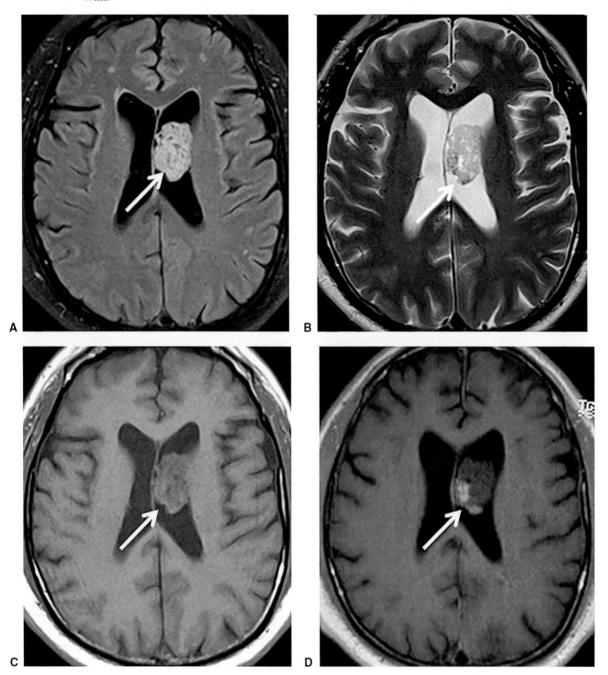

Imaging Findings: Axial images from a contrast-enhanced MRI demonstrate a FLAIR/T2-hyperintense septal-based intraventricular mass attached to the septum pellucidum with cystic foci (A and B), no intrinsic T1 hyperintensity on precontrast T1w sequence (C), and few foci of nodular enhancement on the medial edge (D). The lesion has a bubbly appearance because of the numerous small cysts and overall features most consistent with a central neurocytoma.

Discussion: Central neurocytomas are WHO grade II lesions that are commonly seen in young adults and adolescents within the intraventricular location, predominantly in the lateral ventricle attached to the wall or septum pellucidum. Rarely, extraventricular occurrences of neurocytoma have been reported; however, the term "central" neurocytoma is reserved for the former. Complete surgical excision is standard management with role of postsurgical radiation therapy in selected cases such as incomplete resection. Given the propensity of this lesion to attach to the septum pellucidum adjacent to the Monro foramen, these lesions are associated with obstructive hydrocephalus and typically need ventriculostomy catheter for extraventricular CSF drainage for decompression along with gross total resection. Although extremely rare, central neurocytomas can occur in the spinal cord as a primary intramedullary lesion.

On Imaging, these are lobulated masses with frequent cystic foci giving it a bubbly appearance. About half of these lesions may also have calcifications. These are isointense to gray matter on T1w and hyperintense on T2w sequences. On postcontrast T1w, these lesions can show moderate to intense heterogenous enhancement. Periventicular T2 hyperintensity and prominent flow voids may also be present.

Reference: Chen CL, Shen CC, Wang J, et al. Central neurocytoma: a clinical, radiological and pathological study of nine cases. *Clin Neurol Neurosurg* 2008;110(2):129–136.

7a **Answer A.**   Primary CNS glial neoplasm. Sagittal FIESTA and axial T2w images show infiltrative ill-defined T2-hyperintense pontine mass with an expansile morphology and heterogeneous enhancement. This appearance is very typical for a brainstem glioma.

7b **Answer A.**   Elevated choline and reduction in NAA. The findings on MR spectroscopy show elevated choline and reduced NAA. Typically, on physiologic spectra the choline peak is less than NAA peak; here, as we note, the pattern is reversed.

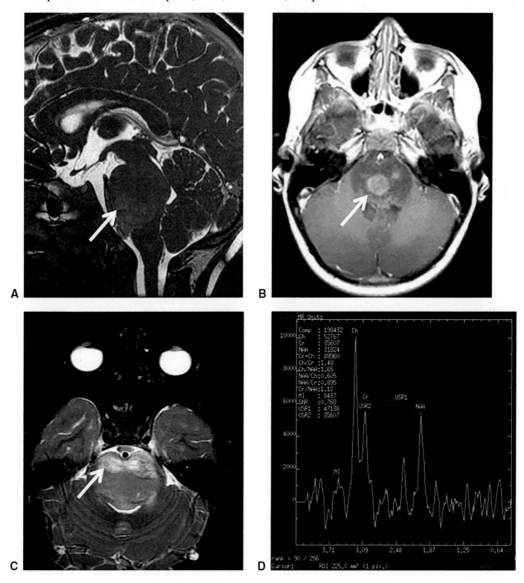

Imaging Findings: Sagittal high-resolution FIESTA image (A) shows a partially exophytic expansile lesion centered in the pons; the lesion is hyperintense on T2w sequence (C) and enhances on postcontrast T1w sequence (B). Single-voxel MR spectroscopy with spectra obtained from the lesion itself shows abnormal elevation of choline and reduced *N*-acetylaspartate. A definite lactate peak is not visualized.

Discussion: Brainstem gliomas (BSG) are a heterogeneous group of tumors with distinct subtypes with variable prognosis. They account for 10% to 20% of all intracranial tumors in children. They can uncommonly be seen in adults (median age of 30 to 35 years). In adults, the behavior and prognosis are similar to those of supratentorial gliomas. The rest of the discussion here is focused on pediatric BSG.

They are broadly classified into diffuse infiltrating type (about 80% of BSG) and focal gliomas. The prognosis largely depends on the site of origin. Also, BSG that are associated with NF1 have better prognosis.

Midbrain gliomas (tectal or tegmental) are generally low grade (pilocytic/grade II astrocytoma or ganglioglioma) and tend to be indolent. The treatment is often just shunting and imaging surveillance. Tumor-specific treatment is pursued in the unlikely event of tumor growth.

Most pontine gliomas are infiltrating fibrillary astrocytomas with poor prognosis. Irrespective of histologic grading, these have an aggressive course with a mean survival of 4 to 15 months. They tend to show extension into the midbrain superiorly and medulla inferiorly and through the middle cerebellar peduncle into the cerebellar hemisphere.

Less commonly, focal tumors can arise in the pons, and they show a good prognosis. Medullary tumors commonly show lower grade and better prognosis and have a higher incidence of exophytic growth compared to pontine tumors.

On CT, one-third of pontine tumors are hypodense, one-third are isodense, and most of the remainder show mixed density. In case of hemorrhage, tumors can have high density. Smaller midbrain tumors may not be well seen on CT. On MRI, BSGs are hypointense on T1 and hyperintense on T2/FLAIR. Patchy, focal, or ring enhancements within pontine tumors are common (either at presentation or developing during the course of the disease) as is hemorrhage; these features suggest an aggressive tumor. But enhancement in focal tumors and medullary tumors do not necessarily mean bad prognosis. Expanded brainstem that obliterates the prepontine cistern, compresses the fourth ventricle, and envelops the basilar artery is a strong indicator for BSG. Obstructive hydrocephalus occurs commonly with midbrain and medullary tumors and less commonly with pontine tumors. In case of aqueductal pattern of hydrocephalus, MRI is the investigation of choice to evaluate for midbrain tumors as smaller tumors may not be evident on CT and the patient may carry a diagnosis of just "aqueductal stenosis" instead. Midbrain tumor is better demonstrated with thin slices through this region, preferably a 3D T2 or steady-state sequence in sagittal plane.

Differential Diagnosis:

Demyelinating disease: Clinical picture is usually distinct with often multiphasic episodes; often multifocal in involvement with supra- and infratentorial lesions.
Infection (abscess and cerebritis): Tuberculosis
Neuro-Behcet syndrome: Generally in young adult population

References: Atlas SW, ed. *Magnetic resonance imaging of the brain and spine*, 4th ed. Philadelphia, PA: Lippincott Williams & Wilkins, 2008.

Gupta N, Banerjee A, Haas-Kogan D, eds. *Pediatric CNS tumors*, 2nd ed. Berlin, Germany: Springer, 2010.

8a   **Answer B.**   Extra-axial, restricted diffusion, low attenuation on CT, incomplete suppression on FLAIR.

8b   **Answer B.**   Restricted diffusion on DWI. The low attenuation on CT will be seen with both epidermoid and arachnoid cysts.

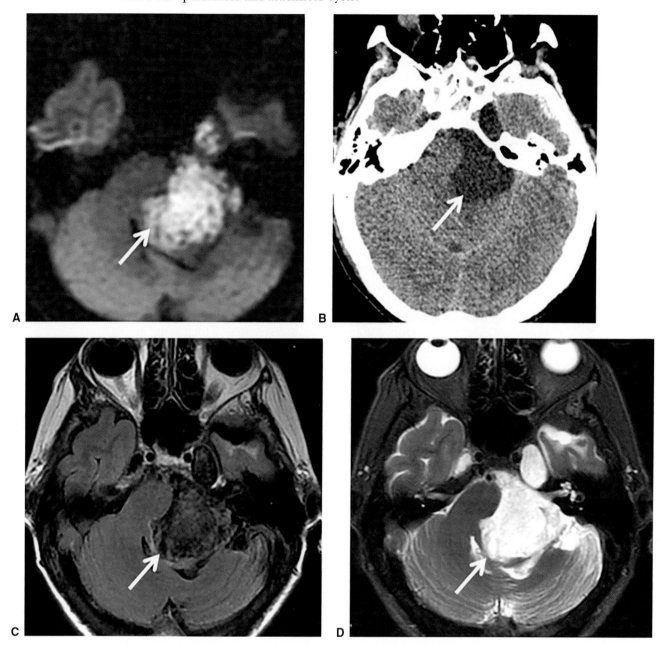

Imaging Findings: Axial DWI image showing restricted diffusion within an extra-axial mass in the left CP angle (A). This lesion has fluid intensity on CT and axial T2w sequence (B and D) with dilated appearance of the left Meckel cave and shows incomplete suppression on FLAIR (C), contrast the right Meckel cave CSF signal and signal within the globes on FLAIR to appreciate the incomplete fluid suppression within this lesion.

Discussion: Intracranial epidermoids are congenital tumor-like inclusion cysts and constitute about 1% of intracranial tumors. They are believed to be the result of sequestration of ectodermal element within the neural tube during the 3rd to 5th week of embryonic development. Acquired epidermoid is rare in the brain.

They are well-marginated lesions with irregular nodular surface and composed of a wall made up of stratified keratinized squamous epithelium surrounded by connective tissue. The cyst content is mainly derived from desquamated epithelial cells and includes debris, keratin, water, and cholesterol. These lesions do not contain dermal appendages.

The clinical presentation depends on the location and the degree of mass effect on adjacent neural structures. There may also be chemical meningitis secondary to leakage of cyst contents into subarachnoid space. The common locations are CP angle cistern (40% to 50% of lesions), fourth ventricle, sellar region, and less commonly intraparenchymal. Ten percent of tumors are extradural.

On imaging, they are thinly marginated, but irregular lesions, insinuating within the CSF space encasing and surrounding adjacent vessels and nerves. Calcification can be seen in 10% to 25% of cases. Rarely, intralesional hemorrhage can be present. On CT, the lesions are well circumscribed and hypodense and often show near CSF density, similar in appearance to arachnoid cyst. MRI is the investigation of choice. On T1 and T2 images, they look somewhat similar to an arachnoid cyst showing near CSF intensity or slight hyperintensity relative to CSF. On FLAIR images, these show incomplete signal suppression and can show some degree of heterogeneity. Diffusion images show restriction, which is the most useful MR imaging feature for diagnosis. Most of the lesions show no contrast enhancement; about a quarter show minimal rim enhancement.

Epidermoid can be hyperdense on CT because of hemorrhage or proteinaceous content (white epidermoid). These lesions can be hyperintense on T1 images and show variable signal on T2 images. Diffusion restriction is typically present. Malignant degeneration of epidermoid is extremely rare, but reported.

Differential Diagnosis:

Arachnoid cyst: especially on CT. On MRI, the differentiation is easy as epidermoids show incomplete FLAIR suppression and diffusion restriction unlike arachnoid cysts.

References: Chen CY, Wong JS, Hsieh SC, et al. Intracranial epidermoid cyst with hemorrhage: MR imaging findings. *AJNR Am J Neuroradiol* 2006;27(2):427–429.

Forghani R, Farb RI, Kiehl TR, et al. Fourth ventricle epidermoid tumor: radiologic, intraoperative, and pathologic findings. *Radiographics* 2007;27(5):1489–94. doi: 10.1148/rg.275075011.

9a **Answer A.** Primary CNS lymphoma. This lesion has classic characteristics of primary CNS lymphoma.

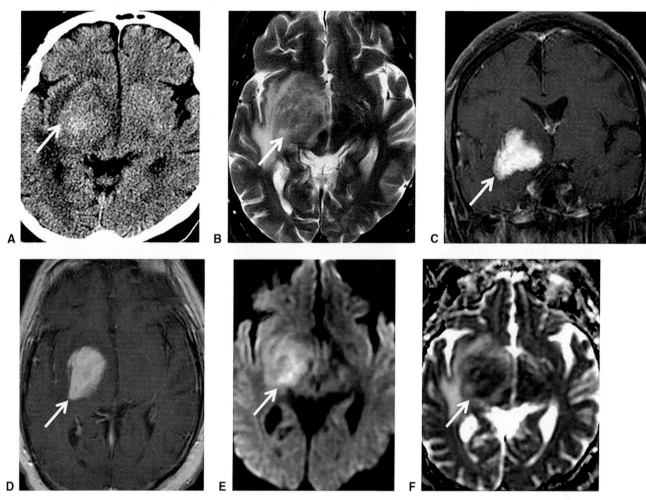

Image Findings: There is a right basal ganglia/thalamic mass, which is hyperattenuating on CT (A), is heterogeneously hypointense on T2w (B), and shows homogenous intense enhancement on postcontrast T1w sequence (C and D) and restricted diffusion (E and F). These features are typical for primary CNS lymphoma.

Discussion: Primary CNS lymphoma (PCNSL) is an extranodal non-Hodgkin lymphoma that affects the brain and is rarely isolated to the spinal cord, meninges, and orbit. It is usually of the large B-cell variety, which represents 5% to 7% of all primary brain tumors. By definition, extra-CNS disease is absent at the time of diagnosis.

Cerebral hemispheres are the commonest site with predilection of periventricular region and corpus callosum, followed by basal ganglia, thalami, and rarely posterior fossa. Lymphoma is a differential consideration for "butterfly" tumor. Leptomeningeal involvement occurs in about 12% tumors; dural involvement is rare. They tend to show angiocentric growth pattern. Most of the tumors tend to abut the CSF surface (either ventricular margin or the pia) with a tendency for subependymal spread. The mass effect is less pronounced for their size.

Over half of the tumors are solitary. The internal imaging characteristics depend on the immune status.

In immunocompetent patients, the tumors occur in older age group with a mean age of about 60 years. The most common presentation is solid uniformly enhancing lesion showing high cellularity and prominent perilesional edema. The high cellularity results in hyperdensity of CT, iso- to only mild hypointensity on T1-weighted images, intermediate to low signal on T2-weighted images, and restricted diffusion. Untreated lesions do not show calcification. Less commonly, they can be infiltrative and rarely can show necrosis, hemorrhage, and even no enhancement.

In immunocompromised patients, the lesions tend to occur at an earlier age (mean age of about 40 years). They show a higher incidence of necrosis, hemorrhage, and inhomogeneous enhancement.

Secondary lymphomas tend to involve dura and leptomeninges and only rarely present as isolated parenchymal mass.

PCNSL show increase in CBV on perfusion studies, but less than what is seen with glioblastomas. Reduction in ADC is more dramatic than what can be seen with tumefactive demyelination. Spectroscopy shows "tumor signature." They are FDG avid.

Differential Diagnosis:

Glioblastoma: hemorrhage and necrosis are the hallmark, which are rare in PCNSL of immunocompetent patients. Abutment of CSF surface is more common with lymphoma. Uniform restricted diffusion is rare with glioblastoma.

Metastases: History and multiplicity are helpful. Diffusion restriction is less common with metastatic disease. They tend to be located at gray-white junction as opposed to near the CSF surface with lymphoma. Mass effect is disproportionately less for lesion site with lymphomas, as opposed to metastasis.

Tumefactive demyelination: Enhancement is more commonly peripheral, incomplete ring shaped, or comma shaped. Concentric rings of differing signal on T2-weighted images favor demyelination. Diffusion restriction can occasionally be seen with acute demyelination, but tends to be more pronounced with lymphoma. In difficult cases, follow-up is the key.

Toxoplasmosis: This is a differential consideration in the immunocompromised. Eccentric target sign favors toxoplasmosis. As opposed to lymphoma, toxoplasmosis is non-avid on PET and on thallium scan.

References: Lu SS, Kim SJ, Kim N, et al. Histogram analysis of apparent diffusion coefficient maps for differentiating primary CNS lymphomas from tumefactive demyelinating lesions. *AJR Am J Roentgenol* 2015;204(4):827–834. doi: 10.2214/AJR.14.12677.

Naidich TP, ed. *Imaging of the brain*. Expert Radiology Series. Philadelphia, PA: Saunders/Elsevier, 2013.

Tsiouris AJ, Sanelli PC, Comunale J. *Case-based brain imaging*, 2nd ed. New York, NY: Thieme, 2013.

10a **Answer A.** Neurosurgical consultation. Given this is a chronic refractory epilepsy that has an identifiable structural substrate on imaging, a neurosurgical consultation with further relevant workup may be considered. In this case, this lesion is likely to represent dysembryoplastic neuroepithelial tumor.

10b **Answer A.** Temporal lobe intracortical location is common for this lesion (DNET). The other choices are untrue for this lesion, because it is commonly cortical, commonly in younger age group, and typically has a relatively benign clinical course.

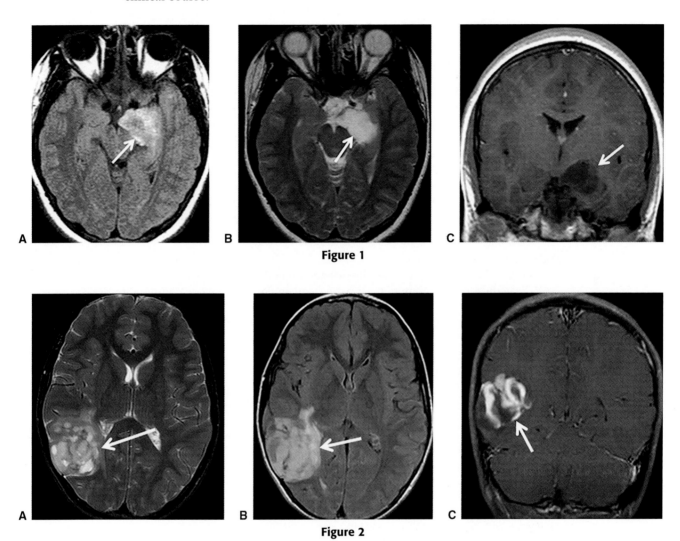

Figure 1

Figure 2

Image Findings: Figure 1. There is left medial temporal lobe mass that expands the cortex with heterogeneous FLAIR hyperintensity (A), T2 hyperintensity (B), and lack of enhancement on postcontrast sequences (C). This appearance is most consistent with DNET. Ganglioglioma is a differential possibility; however, contrast enhancement is more commonly seen with the latter.

Figure 2. Companion case. There is a T2-hyperintense partly cystic lesion with a "bubbly" morphology in the right temporoparietal region (A); note that the bubbly foci do not suppress on FLAIR (B). There is heterogeneous enhancement (C).

Discussion: Dysembryoplastic neuroepithelial tumor (DNET) is a benign grade I glial–neuronal neoplasm, commonly seen in the second and third decades of life with male preponderance and presenting with intractable seizures.

It is peripherally located in the cortex with gyral expansion. Underlying white matter is often involved. Temporal lobe is the most common location followed by frontal lobe. Deeper location is uncommon and includes the basal ganglia, thalamus, pons, and cerebellum. Clinicoradiologic criteria for diagnosis include seizure onset before 20 years of age, absence of neurologic deficit, cortical location of the lesion and absence of mass effect/peritumoral edema. Typical radiologic features include a cortical-based wedge-shaped well-demarcated mass pointing toward the ventricle, presence of internal septations, absence of contrast enhancement, and scalloping of the overlying bone. On CT, these lesions are hypo- to isodense. On MRI, these lesions are T2 hyperintense, are generally T1 hypointense, and show "bubbly" appearance. Up to a third of lesions can show enhancement, generally nodular in morphology. Thin hyperintense rim on FLAIR images (seen in nearly three-fourths of cases) and high ADC values are other useful imaging features. Cystic changes are occasionally seen. Calcification can be seen but is rare. Associated cortical dysplasia is common.

These tumors generally do not show growth. Surgical resection is for seizure control and is curative. The histologic picture can occasionally be confusing; it is important to suggest the diagnosis based on preoperative imaging.

Differential Diagnosis:

Ganglioglioma: Cystic lesion with enhancing nodule is typical. Unlike DNET, calcification is common. Contrast enhancement is also more common in ganglioglioma.

Cortical dysplasia: Relatively non–mass-like appearance, cystic foci are unusual.

Low-grade astrocytoma: Tend to be centered in the white matter. Overlying bony change is unusual. May appear ill defined.

References: Fernandez C, Girard N, Paz Paredes A, et al. The usefulness of MR imaging in the diagnosis of dysembryoplastic neuroepithelial tumor in children: a study of 14 cases. *AJNR Am J Neuroradiol* 2003;24(5):829–834.

Gupta N, Banerjee A, Haas-Kogan D, eds. *Pediatric CNS tumors*, 2nd ed. Berlin, Germany: Springer, 2010.

Koeller KK, Henry JM. From the archives of the AFIP: superficial gliomas: radiologic-pathologic correlation. Armed Forces Institute of Pathology. *Radiographics* 2001;21(6):1533–1556. doi: 10.1148/radiographics.21.6.g01nv051533.

Raz E, Kapilamoorthy TR, Gupta AK, et al. Case 186: dysembrioplastic neuroepithelial tumor. *Radiology* 2012;265(1):317–320. doi: 10.1148/radiol.12100118.

11a Answer A. Midline cerebellar vermis.

11b Answer A. Medulloblastoma. The most common malignant neoplasm in children is medulloblastoma, and it most commonly occurs in the posterior fossa.

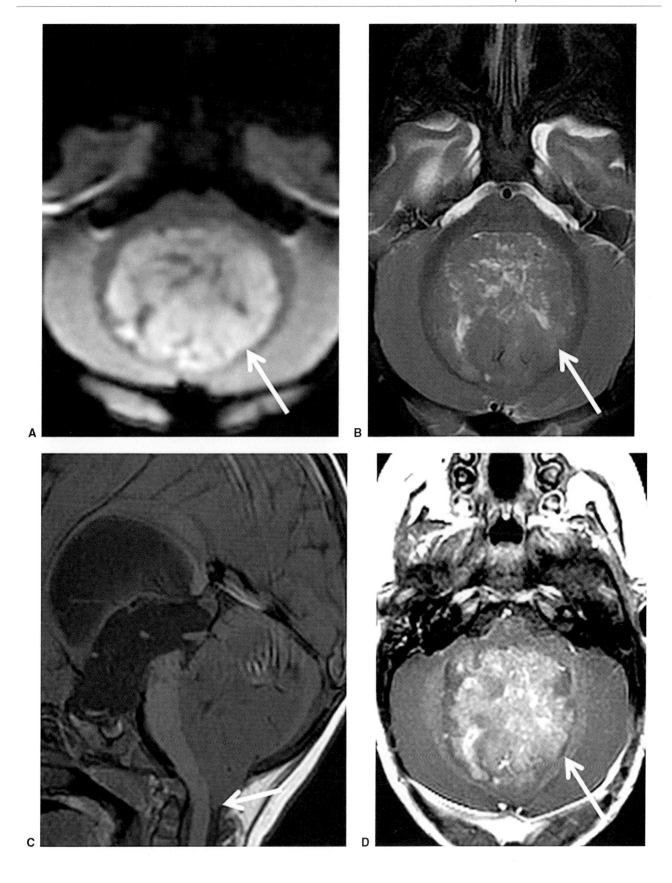

Imaging Findings: There is a large mass centered in the fourth ventricle with restricted diffusion (A) and small cystic foci on T2w (B) and obstructive hydrocephalus (C). It is relatively hypointense on sagittal precontrast T1 (C) and shows intense heterogeneous enhancement on axial postcontrast T1w image (D). This appearance in the current age group is most consistent with a medulloblastoma.

Discussion: Medulloblastoma is the most common malignant pediatric brain tumor, but may also occur in adults. It is considered a primitive neuroectodermal tumor of the posterior fossa. Together with pilocytic astrocytoma, it forms the bulk of posterior fossa tumors in children. A majority of the tumors are seen in the first decade, the peak being 5 to 7 years of age. A small percentage of these tumors is seen with genetic tumor syndromes (Gorlin syndrome, Turcot syndrome, Li-Fraumeni syndrome, ataxia telangiectasia, Coffin-Siris syndrome).

Several histologic subtypes of medulloblastoma have been identified, the most common type being classic medulloblastoma. The other subtypes include desmoplastic/nodular medulloblastoma, medulloblastoma with extensive nodularity, large cell medulloblastoma, anaplastic medulloblastoma, and much rarer variants of medullomyoblastoma and melanotic medulloblastoma.

The majority of the tumors are in the midline involving the vermis. The inferior medullary velum thought to be the primary site of origin. Hemispheric location is more commonly seen in the older age group and shows a higher incidence of desmoplastic variety. Less commonly, the tumor can be purely intraventricular. Most of the tumors appear fairly circumscribed with surrounding edema. Hydrocephalus is a common feature.

On CT, these tumors are hyperdense related to high cellularity. On MRI, the lesions are T1 isointense and generally show intermediate to low signal on T2. Diffusion restriction is a key feature and is seen in 95% of tumors. Cysts if present are smaller in size, as opposed to pilocytic astrocytoma. About two-thirds show moderate to intense contrast enhancement. In rest, the enhancement can be streaky, marginal, or minimal.

Over a third of patients have CSF dissemination at the time of initial diagnosis. Contrast-enhanced MRI with diffusion-weighted imaging is the investigation of choice. Screening of the spine is routinely done at initial presentation.

If prominent dural calcifications are present, the patient should be investigated for Gorlin syndrome, which has treatment implications, and radiation may be avoided. Spectroscopy shows elevated choline to NAA ratio, occasionally elevated lipid/lactate and characteristic taurine peak at 3.35 ppm in short TE spectrum.

The combination of surgery and radiotherapy is the common treatment. Survivors have an increased risk for secondary malignancies (meningioma, basal cell carcinoma, glioblastoma, thyroid cancer, cervical cancer, uterine cancer, and acute leukemia) attributable to radiotherapy/chemotherapy.

References: Koeller KK, Rushing EJ. From the archives of the AFIP: medulloblastoma: a comprehensive review with radiologic-pathologic correlation. *Radiographics* 2003;23(6):1613–1637.

Perreault S, Ramaswamy V, Achrol AS, et al. MRI surrogates for molecular subgroups of medulloblastoma. *AJNR Am J Neuroradiol* 2014;35(7):1263–1269.

Osborn, Anne G. *Osborn's brain: imaging, pathology, and anatomy*, 1st ed. Salt Lake City, Utah: Amirsys Publishing, Inc., 2013.

12a   Answer A.   Pilocytic astrocytoma. In the current age group, this is the most common neoplasm in cerebellum (as opposed to medulloblastoma that is the most common malignant neoplasm in the same age group). In addition, the cystic mass with mural nodule appearance is classic for this lesion in this location.

12b **Answer A.**   It may have different morphologic features based on location. It is accurate that this lesion may have different morphologic appearance based on location (as described below in discussion). Whereas a cyst with mural nodule is seen in tumors within the cerebellum and cerebral hemispheres, solid and infiltrative appearance may be seen with hypothalamic and optic apparatus.

The remaining statements are false, because radiation is avoided in children younger than 5 because of high morbidity with surgical resection being the mainstay for cerebellar lesions. Ten-year survival for this lesion is highly favorable reaching up to 94%. There is an association with NF1 (instead of NFII).

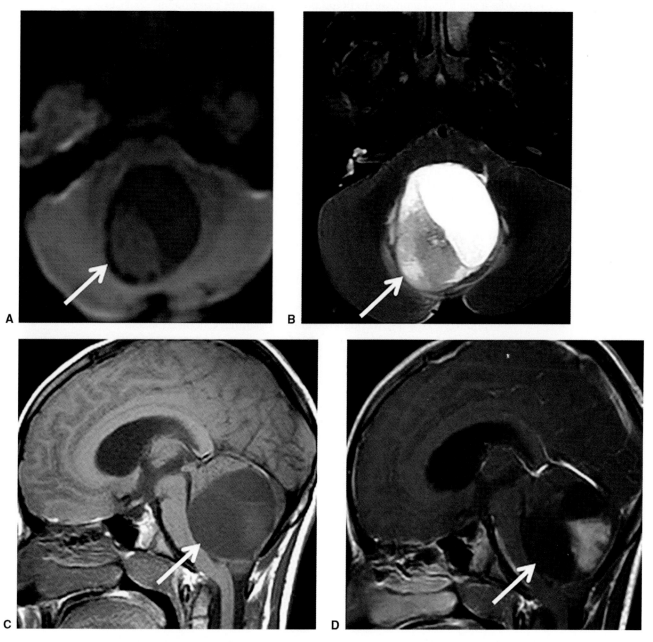

Imaging Findings: There is a mixed cystic and solid mass involving the fourth ventricle (B) without restricted diffusion (A) completely obstructing the fourth ventricle and leading to obstructive hydrocephalus (C and D). This mass shows enhancement within the peripherally located solid component (D). In the current age group, this lesion is most consistent with a pilocytic astrocytoma.

Discussion: Pilocytic astrocytoma (PA) is the most common pediatric primary brain tumor. They are grade I tumors with excellent prognosis and mostly manifest in the first two decades of life. In children, the cerebellum, optic nerve chiasm, and hypothalamic regions are the most common locations, in that order. In adults, the tumor is more common in cerebral hemispheres.

Optic–hypothalamic pilocytic astrocytomas have known association with NF1. Imaging features vary with tumor location.

Posterior fossa PA commonly arises from the vermis or the hemisphere, and typical morphology is cystic lesion with solid enhancing portion (size can vary from a small mural nodule to being the predominant component). They are generally well circumscribed, and the enhancing nodule tends to be away from the pial surface (unlike hemangioblastoma). Surrounding edema is generally absent or small. The nodule is T1 hypointense, T2 hyperintense, and mildly hypodense on CT and shows intense enhancement. The enhancement in cyst wall varies from none to moderate.

Optic–hypothalamic and tectal PAs are generally solid, infiltrating, and less well marginated; the contrast enhancement is variable. The tumors anterior to the chiasm tend to be iso- to less T2 hyperintense and show no/minimal enhancement, and chiasmal and posterior optic pathway tumors tend to be T2 hyperintense and show more intense enhancement and these occur in adolescent and young adults. The tectal PAs are nonenhancing.

Though these are grade I tumors and curable whenever the surgery is feasible, they sometimes show alarming imaging features, but still with a benign course.

Differential Diagnosis:

Posterior fossa PA:

Medulloblastoma—generally more solid tumor. Diffusion restriction is a key feature.

Ependymoma—located in the region of the fourth ventricle and has "toothpaste" morphology extruding through the outlet foramina. Calcification and hemorrhage are common.

Hemangioblastoma—the enhancing nodule is generally based on the pia. This is an adult tumor. Also, known association with von Hippel-Lindau disease.

Hypothalamic PA:

Pilomyxoid astrocytoma; tends to occur in younger children; hemorrhage is common and shows a more aggressive appearance.

Hemispheric PA:

Other lesions with cystic-solid morphology (ganglioglioma, pleomorphic xanthoastrocytoma)

References: Koeller KK, Rushing EJ. From the archives of the AFIP: pilocytic astrocytoma: radiologic-pathologic correlation. *Radiographics* 2004;24(6):1693–1708.

Osborn AG. *Osborn's brain: imaging, pathology, and anatomy*, 1st ed. Salt Lake City, UT: Amirsys Pub., 2013.

13a **Answer A.**   Foramen of Monro. Foramen of Monro will be the best location to describe the location of this lesion.

13b **Answer A.**   Growth on follow-up MRI. Of all these features, growth is the most reliable indicator of SEGA. Size >1 cm favors SEGA. Enhancement and calcification are seen in both the entities.

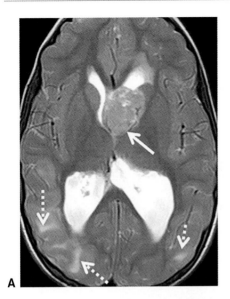
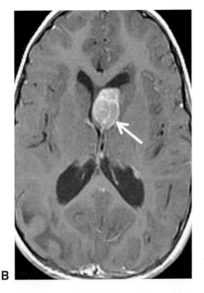
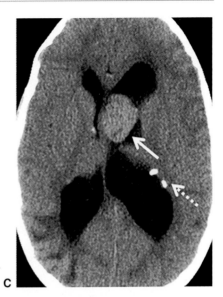

A   B   C

Imaging Findings: Within the frontal horn of the left lateral ventricle adjacent to the Monro foramen, there is a mass that is iso- to hyperintense to gray matter on T2w with small cystic foci (A) and shows intense enhancement on T1w post contrast (B) and hyperdense appearance on CT (C). Notice calcified subependymal nodules along the atria of the left lateral ventricle, which is also dilated because of obstruction at the left Monro foramen (dotted arrow C). In addition, T2 hyperintensity is noted along the subcortical region of the right parieto-occipital location suggesting cortical tubers (dotted arrow A).

The constellation of these findings is most consistent with tuberous sclerosis with the Monro foramen lesion likely representing a subependymal giant cell astrocytoma.

Discussion: Subependymal giant cell astrocytoma (SEGA) is a grade I localized tumor that happens in about 15% of tuberous sclerosis (TSC) patients. It can rarely be seen on non-TSC patients as well. Subependymal giant cell tumor is probably a better term as these are of mixed glioneuronal lineage.

The classic location is caudothalamic groove at the foramen of Monro, thought to arise from the subependymal nodule of TSC. These tumors can be asymptomatic or present with obstructive hydrocephalus. There is a wide range for age of presentation, the mean being 11 years. They tend to show slow growth. There is an intact ependymal lining, which makes CSF seeding unlikely.

The major differential is hamartomatous subependymal nodule of TSC. Size of over a centimeter favors SEGA. Enhancement and calcification are seen in both the entities. Growth is an indicator of tumor. The enhancing nodules at the foramen of Monro need to be followed up to assess growth, the presence of which would indicate SEGA.

The mass is iso- to hypodense on CT, hypointense on T1 images, and hyperintense on T2 images. Calcification is common. The tumor shows avid contrast enhancement. Circumscribed tumor is the rule; rarely, there can be invasion of adjacent structures. Gradient sequence helps in visualization of calcified subependymal nodules, and FLAIR sequence is extremely useful in demonstrating the rest of TSC stigmata.

References: Osborn AG. *Osborn's brain: imaging, pathology, and anatomy,* 1st ed. Salt Lake City, UT: Amirsys Pub., 2013.

Smith AB, Smirniotopoulos JG, Horkanyne-Szakaly I. From the radiologic pathology archives: intraventricular neoplasms: radiologic-pathologic correlation. *Radiographics* 2013;33(1):21–43. doi: 10.1148/rg.331125192.

14a **Answer B.** Extra-axial because of presence of a CSF cleft. Extra-axial because of presence of a CSF cleft separating the lesion from the overlying cortex.

14b **Answer A.** Anterior cranial fossa, planum sphenoidale meningioma. This is an anterior cranial fossa, dural-based extra-axial mass, and likely to represent a planum sphenoidale meningioma (associated with body of sphenoid bone). On the other hand, the middle cranial fossa meningiomas are commonly associated with the greater sphenoid wing.

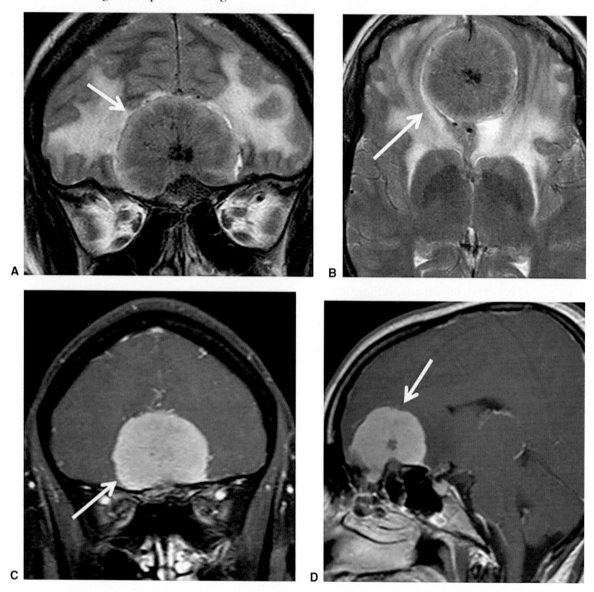

Imaging Findings: There is a large anterior cranial fossa mass with dural-based morphology and T2-hyperintense cleft seen surrounding this lesion (A and B) indicating extra-axial location and intense enhancement (C and D). This is most consistent with a planum sphenoidale meningioma.

Discussion: The first and the most important factor in tumor imaging is deciding whether the lesion is intra-axial or extra-axial in location.

MRI is the investigation of choice for localization.

The definitive signs of extra-axial location are

- CSF cleft between the mass and the brain
- Superficial vessels between the mass and the brain

- Dura between the mass and the brain
- Multiplanar or 3D T2-weighted sequences are extremely helpful in demonstrating these definitive signs.

    Suggestive signs are as follows:

- Broad base toward the calvarium/dura
- Changes in the overlying bone
- "Dural tail" sign
- Apparent brain displacement from the calvarium/dura
- Caution should be exercised while making the distinction solely based on these suggestive signs. Many of the superficial intraaxial masses can exhibit these signs.

15a **Answer C.**   Obstructive hydrocephalus. Presence of hydrocephalus should be evaluated in any lesion of the fourth ventricle. There is mild enlargement of the supratentorial ventricular system, with bulging of the temporal horns of the lateral ventricles, of concern for hydrocephalus. No definite transependymal edema is seen. Findings should be communicated to the ordering physician, as obstructive hydrocephalus is potentially fatal.

15b **Answer C.**   Subependymal giant cell astrocytoma. This lesion is a WHO grade I neoplasm arising from subependymal nodules located in the foramen of Monro, therefore supratentorial in location, and is typically associated with tuberous sclerosis. All the other entities are reasonable differential diagnosis for this lesion. Note that in the adult population, choroid plexus papilloma is more likely to be in the fourth ventricle as opposed to the pediatric age group where they are seen in the lateral ventricles.

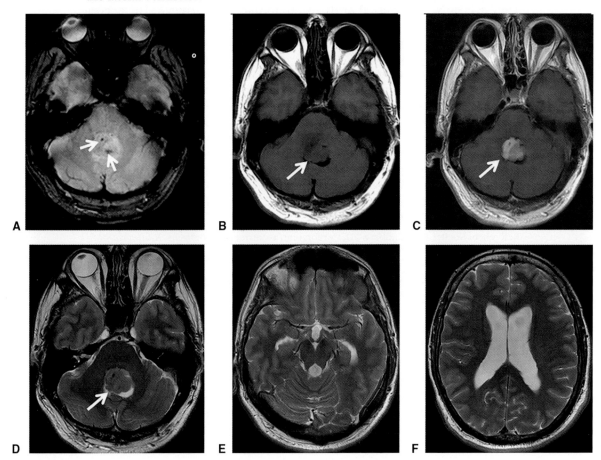

Imaging Findings: Axial GRE, pre- and postcontrast T1- and axial T2-weighted images are shown. There is a solid, avidly enhancing mass with lobulated contours within the fourth ventricle (B, C, and D) with punctate foci of hypointensity on GRE (arrows A), likely representing calcifications or blood products. The mass causes partial obstruction of the fourth ventricle, with mild supratentorial hydrocephalus (E and F). In this case, this lesion represent a choroid plexus papilloma of the fourth ventricle.

Discussion: Choroid plexus papillomas (CPP) and carcinomas (CPC) constitute 0.4%–0.6% of all intracranial neoplasms, most commonly seen in the pediatric population. The most common sites for CPP and CPC are in the lateral ventricles (50%), fourth ventricle (40%), and third ventricle (5%), with 5% in more than one location. Rarely, CPP and CPC may be found in an extraventricular site. The age range for fourth ventricle location is wide, 0 to 50 years of age, most commonly in males. Similar to the ones in other locations, they usually present as avidly enhancing lobulated masses with a cauliflower-like appearance, with associated cysts, and hemorrhage. Parenchyma invasion and necrosis may suggest CPC over CPP; however, this diagnosis is many times difficult even on histology. Some reports support that MR spectroscopy demonstrating increased choline, decreased *N*-acetylaspartate (NAA), and increased lactate should support carcinoma. CPP and CPC may produce CSF, which contributes to hydrocephalus.

Differential Diagnosis: Ependymoma is typically seen in children with a mean age of 6 years. It arises from the floor or roof of the fourth ventricle and frequently extends through the foramina of Luschka and Magendie with a "toothpaste" appearance. Blood products and calcifications are often associated. They may be WHO grades II or III and are prone to recurrence. The majority of subependymoma are WHO grade I, occur in the fourth ventricle, occur in males older than 15 years, and are commonly asymptomatic. They are usually slow-growing, avascular neoplasms, in which gross surgical resection is usually curative. Subependymoma may be associated with cysts, calcifications, or hemorrhage, and may present variable behavior postcontrast, from absent to minimal to intense enhancement. Metastasis to the choroid plexus is rare, with incidence between 0.9% and 4.6%, most commonly secondary to renal cell carcinoma and lung cancer, followed by melanoma, gastric and colon carcinoma, and lymphoma. Intraventricular meningiomas are rare, even more so when arising in the fourth ventricle. On MR spectroscopy, decreased *N*-acetylaspartate (NAA) and creatinine, increased choline, and variable lactate and lipids may be seen, with the presence of alanine thought to be more characteristic.

Reference: Koeller KK, Sandberg GD. Cerebral intraventricular neoplasms. *Radiographics* 2002;22:1473–1505.

16a **Answers D.** Atypical teratoid rhabdoid tumor. Atypical teratoid rhabdoid tumor being a small blue cell neoplasm is likely to have restricted diffusion.

16b **Answers D.** CN III. This lesion is exophytic from the left pontomesencephalic junction and partly occupies the interpeduncular cistern. This location is the expected site for left-sided third CN nerve or oculomotor nerve. This lesion is an atypical teratoid/rhabdoid tumor and has been reported to occur in this location as a distinct clinicoradiologic entity in infants/young children. For this reason, it often has been mistaken for a schwannoma or peripheral nerve sheath tumor. More commonly, however, this lesion is seen in the posterior fossa.

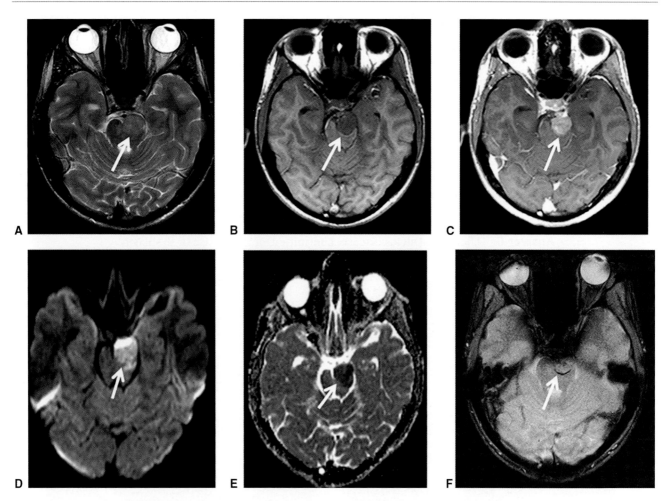

Imaging Findings: There is a T2-hyperintense (A) and T1-hypointense (B) enhancing mass as seen on postcontrast T1w (C) with restricted diffusion (D and E) centered in the left pontomesencephalic junction. GRE demonstrates peripheral susceptibility, suggestive of associated hemorrhage. These features, in a young patient, suggests a small blue cell tumor.

Discussion: Small blue cell tumor: atypical teratoid/rhabdoid tumor (ATRT).

A hyperdense mass on CT with associated restricted diffusion should lead to the differential diagnosis of small blue cell tumor. This is a result of hypercellularity, with big nuclei and scant cytoplasm leading resulting in high nuclear-to-cytoplasmic ratio. For the same reasons, there is commonly associated T2 hypointensity. This category of tumors include lymphomas, germinomas, medulloblastomas, Ewing sarcoma, rhabdomyosarcoma, neuroblastoma, and ATRT. Small cell lung cancer and meningioma can also present with restricted diffusion. Glioblastomas may present with restricted diffusion in areas of hypercellularity.

ATRT are typically pediatric tumors, of embryonal origin, usually diagnosed before age 5. This is a highly aggressive malignant neoplasm, rarely seen in adults. Ninety-five percent of the tumors occur in the posterior fossa of children; however, they may be found in any location throughout the brain and spine. When large tumors are seen in the supratentorial compartment, a thick, wavy heterogeneously enhancing wall surrounding cystic portions of the mass has been described. When small, they may be circumscribed. MR spectroscopy reports describe increased choline and decreased N-acetylaspartate (NAA). Described cases in the literature are usually case reports or small series, and there has been suggestion for a distinct clinicoradiologic entity involving cranial nerve III in young infants.

Prognosis is dismal despite radiation, when feasible, and chemotherapy.

Differential Diagnosis: Lymphomas rarely present with hemorrhage prior to treatment. Schwannoma of the third cranial nerve is usually well circumscribed and slow growing.

References: Oh CC, et al. Atypical teratoid/rhabdoid tumor (ATRT) arising from the 3rd cranial nerve in infants: a clinical-radiologic entity? *J Neurooncol* 2015;124:175–183.

Wu WW, et al. Adult atypical teratoid/rhabdoid tumors. *World Neurosurg* 2014;85:197–204.

Yong AK, et al. How specific is the MRI appearance of supratentorial atypical teratoid/rhabdoid tumor? *Pediatr Radiol* 2013;43:347–354.

17a **Answer A.**   Tigroid appearance. Tigroid appearance is classically seen with this entity.

17b **Answer C.**   Lhermitte-Duclos disease. Lhermitte-Duclos disease or dysplastic gangliocytoma is the most likely diagnosis for this appearance.

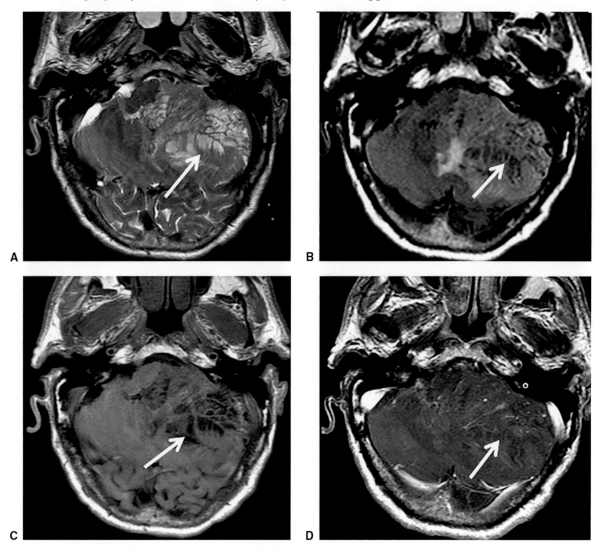

Imaging Findings: Axial T2, FLAIR, and pre- and postcontrast T1-weighted images are shown. There is a heterogeneous expansile non-enhancing lesion in the left cerebellar hemisphere with mass effect upon the medulla. There is a peculiar appearance of the lesion, with a "tiger-striped" or striated foliar pattern, which should suggest the diagnosis of Lhermitte-Duclos disease.

Discussion: Lhermitte-Duclos disease (LDD) or dysplastic gangliocytoma is considered a WHO grade I dysplastic gangliocytoma of the cerebellum. It may be part of Cowden syndrome, which is an autosomal dominant neoplastic syndrome associated with mucocutaneous lesions, systemic hamartoma, and malignant neoplasms of the breast, thyroid, and genitourinary and gastrointestinal tracts. It is associated with phakomatoses, multiple congenital malformations including hamartoma in the brain or body, malformations of cortical development, and meningiomas. LDD was described in 1920; however, it has been called by different names since then, such as ganglioneuroma of the cerebellar cortex, purkinjoma, and cerebellar hamartoma. It presents in young adults, but may be seen at any age.

Symptomatic cases may present with ataxia, nausea, vomiting, and hydrocephalus. A T1-hypointense, T2-hyperintense nonenhancing expansile mass is seen, which may infiltrate the brainstem and cause mass effect on the fourth ventricle with hydrocephalus. A tigroid pattern is very typical and should lead to the diagnosis.

Differential Diagnosis: Low-grade glioma, although the striated pattern is very unusual for this entity. Additional consideration is, pseudotumoral hemicerebellitis (PTHC) is a transitory inflammatory process of with T1-hypointense and T2-hyperintense signal abnormality of the involved unilateral cerebellar hemisphere with associated mass effect. The characteristic foliar pattern, infiltration of the brainstem, and presence of other malformations of cortical development or hamartoma in the brain or body favor LDD. Pial enhancement outlining the cerebellar folia favors PTHC. Enhancement of vessels in between the cerebellar folia may be seen in LDD. Increased choline levels are described in PTHC; however, choline levels are normal or decreased in LDD. Lactate may be present in LDD. Follow-up with resolution of T2 hyperintensity and atrophy in PTHC is seen over weeks or months.

References: Bosemani T, et al. Pseudotumoral hemicerebellitis as a mimicker of Lhermitte-Duclos disease in children: does neuroimaging help to differentiate them? *Childs Nerv Syst* 2016;32:865–871.

Thomas B, et al. Advanced MR imaging in Lhermitte-Duclos disease: moving closer to pathology and pathophysiology. *Neuroradiology* 2007;49:733–738.

18a **Answer B.** Subependymoma. This lesion is likely to represent a subependymoma. All the other options are reasonable differential etiologies. But relatively older age group and low level enhancement (typically more intense enhancement seen with other entities) is most characteristic for subependymoma.

18b **Answer A.** CSF obstruction. This lesion poses the greatest risk from CSF obstruction, with obstructive hydrocephalus and raised intracranial pressure. Neurosurgical consultation is therefore warranted with this lesion. It is a slow-growing benign entity; therefore, cervicomedullary invasion is not seen with this lesion. The small size and lack of mass effect argue against a foreseeable risk of tonsillar herniation.

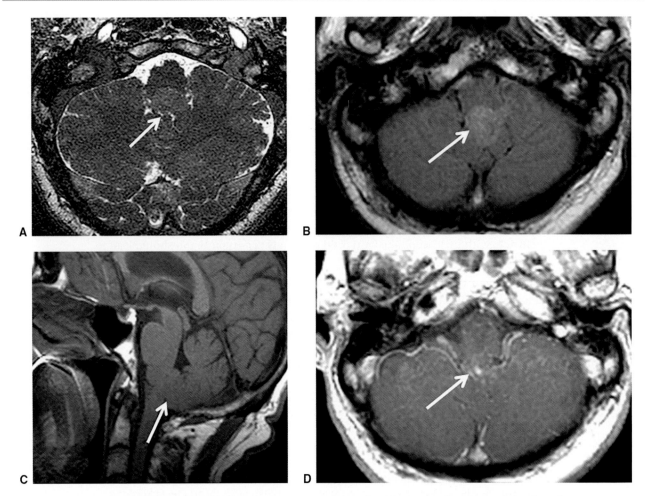

Imaging Findings: There is a well-circumscribed lesion at the obex of the fourth ventricle with (A) with no surrounding vasogenic edema in the brainstem or cerebellum (B). It is isointense on T1w sequence (C) with minimal enhancement on the postcontrast sequence (D).

Discussion: Subependymoma is a benign slow-growing WHO grade I neoplasm of ependymal origin; the majority are intraventricular in location, commonly seen in patients who are older than 15 years of age. These lesions may be incidentally discovered in asymptomatic patients or be symptomatic usually because of obstruction to CSF flow.

On CT, these lesions are iso- to hypoattenuating, well circumscribed, with most of them having a cystic component. Occasionally, they may have calcification or hemorrhage although not as common as the microcysts. These lesions show variable, but typically mild to no enhancement on postcontrast T1w MRI. Occasionally, moderate heterogeneous enhancement may be seen.

Rarely, these are extraventricular parenchymal in location. Those lesions are very difficult to differentiate from low-grade glioma and often misdiagnosed as such.

These can be managed with surgical total or partial resection with microsurgical techniques with excellent prognosis. Typically, the surgical goal is restoration of CSF flow because these lesions do not have an aggressive or invasive nature.

Differential Diagnosis: Ependymoma; although both may have cystic foci, ependymoma tends to have more intense heterogeneous enhancement with frequent coarse calcifications. Unlike subependymoma, these lesions can invade adjacent parenchyma, are prone to CSF seeding, and may be associated with vasogenic edema within adjacent brain.

Central neurocytoma; these can also be seen around the Monro foramen but tend to have a speculated peripheral margin, bubbly lobulated appearance, and moderate to intense enhancement.

Low-grade glioma; these lesions show none to minimal enhancement similar to subependymoma; however, microcystic pattern is less common in these lesions.

Medulloblastoma; this is a differential for lesions in the fourth ventricle; however, typically more intense enhancement and restricted diffusion are seen in medulloblastoma.

References: Amit J, Amin AG, Jain P, et al. Subependymoma: clinical features and surgical outcomes. *Neurol Res* 2012;34(7):677–684.

Smith AB, Smirniotopoulos JG, Horkanyne-Szakaly I. From the radiologic pathology archives: intraventricular neoplasms: radiologic-pathologic correlation. *Radiographics* 2013;33(1):21–43.

19a **Answer C.** Ganglioglioma. Ganglioglioma is the most common neoplasm associated with chronic intractable epilepsy. It can also be seen in superficial cortical location with solid/cystic or mixed morphology, most frequently in the temporal lobe. On diffusion weighted imaging, the ADC values have been found to be lower for pleomorphic xanthoastrocytoma compared to ganglioglioma, both of which are possible considerations for the lesion shown here.

19b **Answer A.** Lack of vasogenic edema. Lack of vasogenic edema suggests slow growth and relatively nonaggressive low-grade nature.

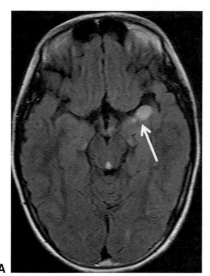

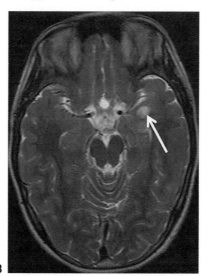

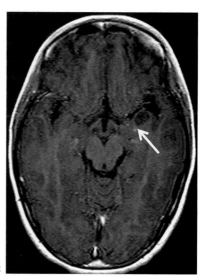

A   B   C

Imaging Findings: A superficial predominantly cystic cortical based lesion in the left anterior temporal lobe without associated vasogenic edema seen on FLAIR and T2w sequences (A and B). No intralesional or pial enhancement is noted on the postcontrast T1w sequence (C).

Discussion: Pleomorphic xanthoastrocytoma (PXA); the lesion shown here is PXA, a rare WHO grade II neoplasm with primarily astrocytic differentiation and limited neuronal differentiation. It has a relatively good prognosis and is seen commonly in children and young adults. It is commonly cortical superficial (subpial, with commonly pial contact seen) supratentorial lesion, most commonly seen in the temporal lobe. On MRI, this can be cystic, solid, or mixed in morphology with intense enhancement of the solid component on postcontrast T1-weighted sequences. The degree of peritumoral edema is variable, with most slow-growing lesions showing none to little peritumoral edema. It is notable here that presence of peritumoral edema alone does not necessarily confer an aggressive nature to the tumor.

Differential Diagnosis includes ganglioglioma, gangliocytoma, and DNET and pilocytic astrocytoma.

Both ganglioglioma/gangliocytoma are more likely to have little to no peritumoral edema and more likely to have macroscopic calcification compared to PXA.

Other than the optic chiasm location of pilocytic astrocytoma, it is frequently infratentorial as opposed to PXA, which is most commonly supratentorial and hemispheric in nature.

DNET may also have a similar appearance; presence of associated cortical dysplasia may help in differentiating it from PXA.

Complete surgical resection is the mainstay for treatment with favorable prognosis and low rate of recurrence. Adjuvant postoperative chemotherapy may be considered for patients with subtotal or partial resection.

References: Moore W, Mathis D, Gargan L, et al. Pleomorphic xanthoastrocytoma of childhood: MR imaging and diffusion MR imaging features. *AJNR Am J Neuroradiol* 2014;35(11):2192–2196.

Yu S, He L, Zhuang X, et al. Pleomorphic xanthoastrocytoma: MR imaging findings in 19 patients. *Acta Radiol* 2011;52(2):223–228.

Inflammatory and Demyelinating Conditions

SATHISH KUMAR DUNDAMADAPPA • ALY H. ABAYAZEED • SHYAM SABAT • PRACHI DUBEY

QUESTIONS

1. A 40-year-old previously healthy female presents with acute-onset right lower extremity weakness. NECT head shows a mass in the left perirolandic region, for which an MRI was recommended. Key images from the MRI are provided below.

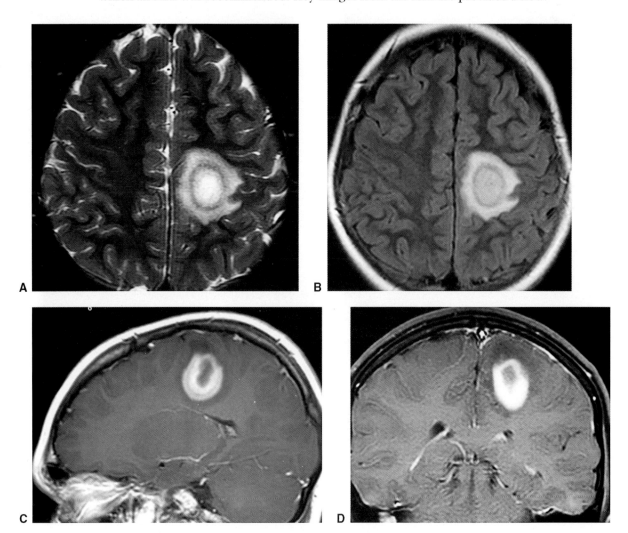

1a What is the most likely diagnosis?

    A. Glioblastoma

    B. Primary CNS lymphoma

    C. Balo concentric sclerosis

    D. Metastatic disease

1b Which of the following imaging features is typical for the above entity as shown in this case?

    A. Lamellar demyelination with concentric morphology

    B. Incomplete horseshoe shape of enhancement

    C. Central necrosis and hemorrhage

    D. Gray and white matter junction location.

2 An 18-year-old female with encephalopathy, dysmetria, paresthesia, and clonus presents for initial evaluation to the ER. Following are some key images from her MRI.

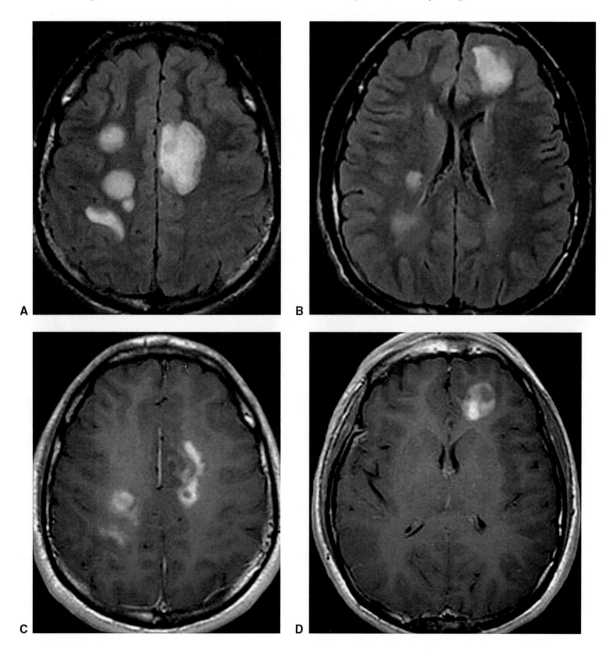

2a Which of the following is a relevant past medical history that may be associated with this entity?

    A. Recent viral infection, fever, or immunization

    B. IV drug use

    C. Recent high-speed motor vehicle accident

    D. Immunocompromised state

2b In the clinical setting of recent upper respiratory tract infection, what is the most likely diagnosis?

    A. Multiple sclerosis

    B. Meningoencephalitis

    C. Acute disseminated encephalomyelitis

    D. Multifocal GBM

3 A 22-year-old female presents with long-standing history of drug-resistant partial complex seizures and progressive cognitive decline. Key images are shown below:

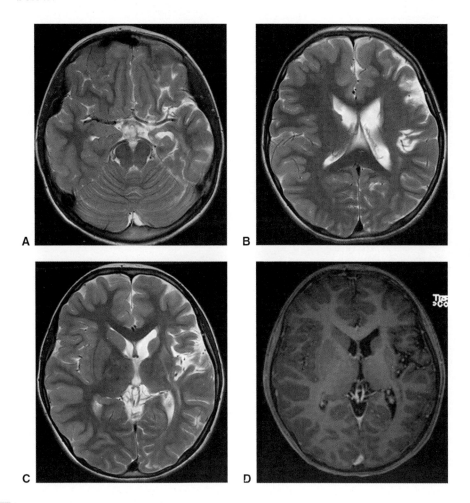

3a What is the most likely diagnosis?

    A. Sturge-Weber syndrome

    B. Rasmussen encephalitis

    C. Dyke-Davidoff-Masson syndrome

    D. Focal cortical dysplasia

3b What are the most common changes expected on MRI during the prodromal phase of this illness?

    A. Normal brain MRI

    B. Cortical edema and enhancement.

    C. Cortical restricted diffusion

    D. Parenchymal petechial microhemorrhages

4 A 19-year-old male with lymphoma presents with acute mental status change.

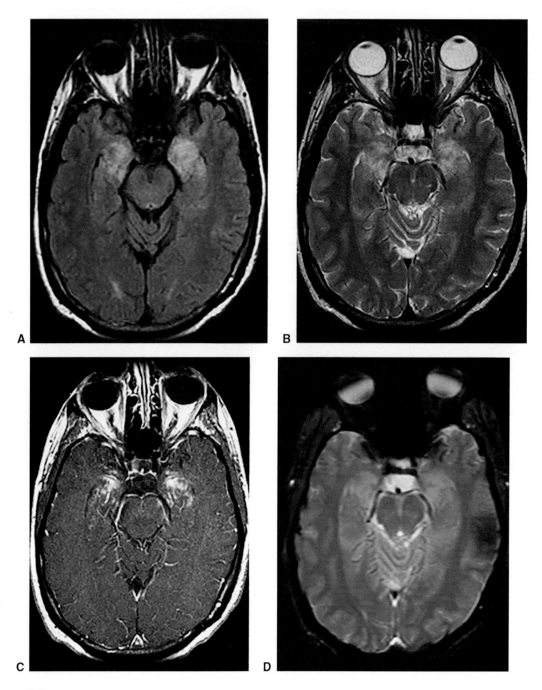

4a What is the most likely diagnosis?

    A. Status epilepticus

    B. Low-grade glioma

    C. Herpes encephalitis

    D. Autoimmune paraneoplastic limbic encephalitis

4b Which of the following have been implicated as a cause for nonneoplastic autoimmune limbic encephalitis?

    A. Anti–glutamic acid decarboxylase (GAD) antibodies
    B. Anti-Hu antibodies
    C. Anti-Yo antibodies
    D. Anti-Ri antibodies

5 A 55-year-old male with HIV positive status, noncompliant with antiretroviral treatment, presented with disorientation. Key images from an MRI are shown below:

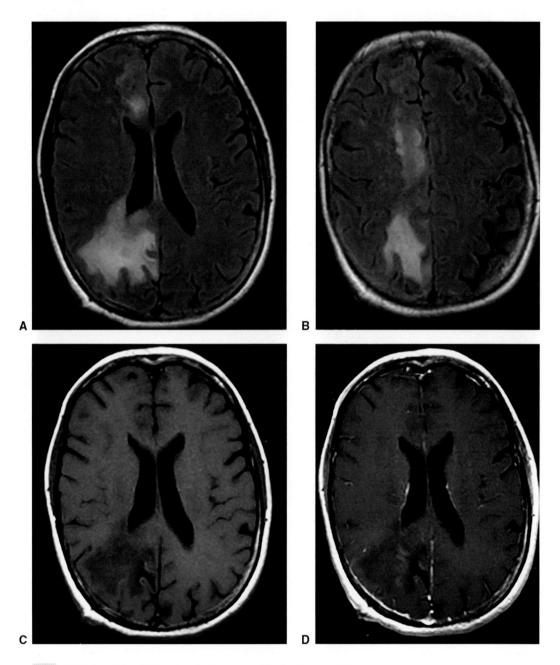

5a Which of the following is the most likely diagnosis?

    A. Lymphoma
    B. Progressive multifocal leukoencephalopathy (PML)
    C. HIV encephalitis
    D. Toxoplasmosis

A lumbar puncture was performed and the patient was started on antiretroviral therapy, and appropriate treatment was started. After treatment, CD4 counts improved; however, there was further deterioration of clinical status. A repeat MRI was performed, and key images are provided below:

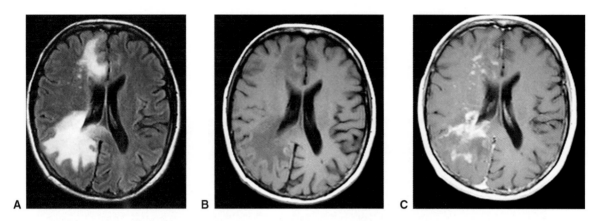

5b   Based on the above scenario, what is the most likely diagnosis?

A. Lymphoma
B. Progressive multifocal leukoencephalopathy (PML)
C. Kaposi sarcoma
D. Immune reconstitution inflammatory syndrome (IRIS)

6   A 37-year-old previously healthy female presents with recent-onset memory loss and headaches. Key images from her MRI are provided below.

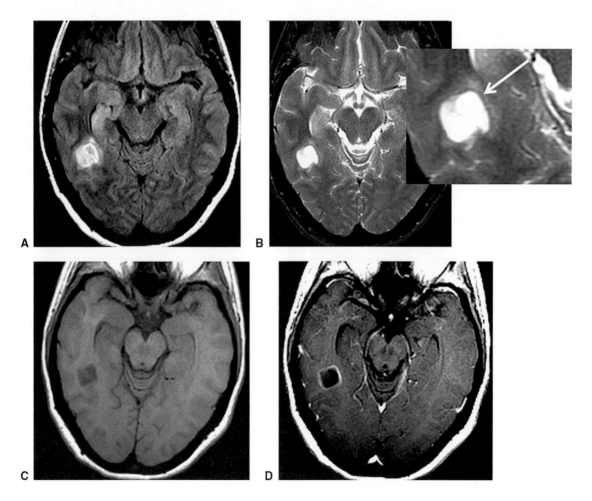

6a A ring-enhancing lesion was seen in the right periventricular posterior temporal lobe without restricted diffusion, (diffusion images not shown). What is the most likely diagnosis?

A. Abscess
B. Tumefactive demyelinating lesion
C. Low-grade astrocytoma
D. Primary CNS lymphoma

6b A lumbar puncture was performed, and CSF studies were normal. The patient was started on IV steroids with excellent clinical response. Which of following is the best next step in management?

A. No further follow-up is needed.
B. FDG-PET
C. Routine clinical follow-up and an MRI within 6 to 8 weeks
D. Surgical biopsy

7 Following are the key images from a contrast-enhanced MRI of a 40-year-old female with diabetes.

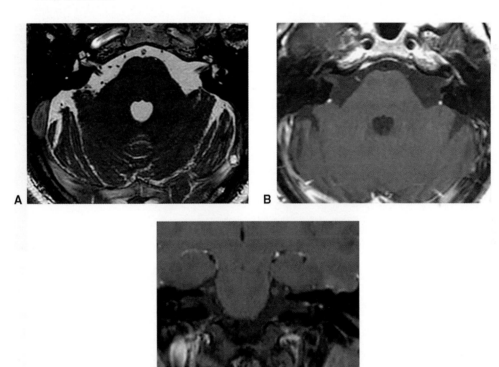

7a Based on the above images, which of the following is the most likely symptom expected in this patient?

A. Left-sided facial paralysis
B. Right-sided facial pain and paresthesia
C. Left-sided sensorineural hearing loss
D. Fever, neck stiffness, and left-sided ear discharge

7b Which segment of the facial nerve most commonly exhibits physiologic enhancement?

    A. Cisternal segment
    B. Meatal or canalicular segment
    C. Tympanic segment
    D. Parotid segment

8 A 36-year-old female with headaches and left upper extremity paresthesias presented for initial evaluation. An MRI was performed, and key images are provided below.

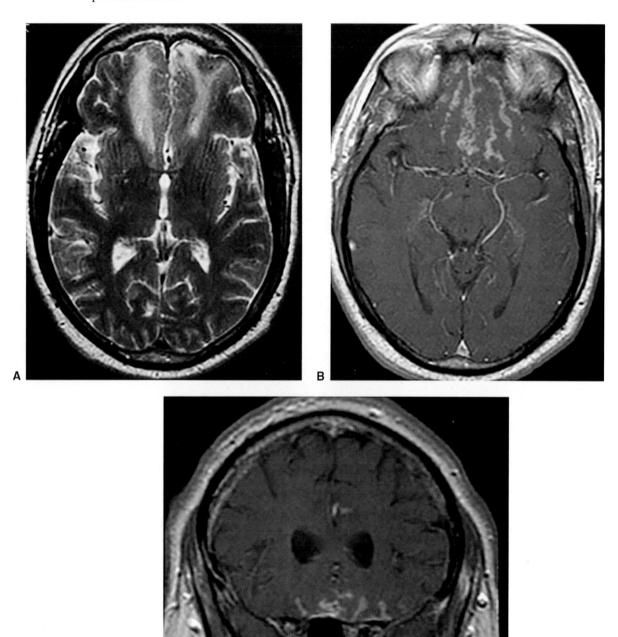

8a Initial workup revealed an abnormal chest x-ray and elevated serum angiotensin-converting enzyme (ACE) levels. Lumbar puncture was normal. Which of the following is the most likely diagnosis?

A. Multiple sclerosis
B. Subacute embolic infarction
C. Metastasis
D. Neurosarcoidosis

8b How common is isolated neurosarcoidosis without systemic manifestations of sarcoidosis?

A. <1% of cases
B. 25% to 50% of cases
C. 50% to 75% of cases
D. >75% of cases

9 A 45-year-female with multiple sclerosis presents for routine follow-up MRI.

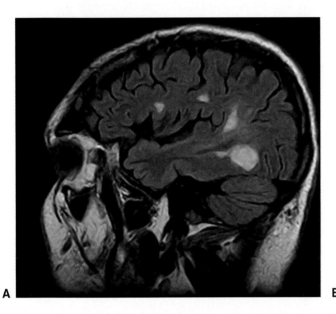 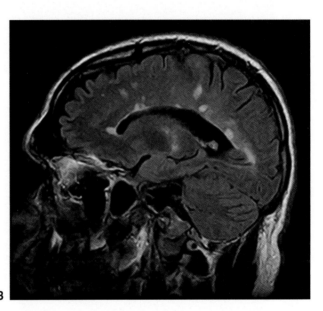

A   B

9a According to the 2010 revised McDonald diagnostic criteria for multiple sclerosis, which of the following is defined as "dissemination in space"?

A. Clustered perpendicular periventricular lesions, (Dawson fingers)
B. Presence of an enhancing T2 hyperintense lesion
C. One or more lesion in at least two of four designated areas of CNS
D. Presence of T1 hypointense lesions at the callososeptal interface

9b What can be a potentially lethal complication of treatment with natalizumab, (Tysabri) in MS patients?

A. Drug-induced thrombocytopenia
B. Progressive multifocal leukoencephalopathy
C. Fulminant renal failure
D. Profound ototoxicity

10   The below images are typical for which of following potentially fatal type of demyelination?

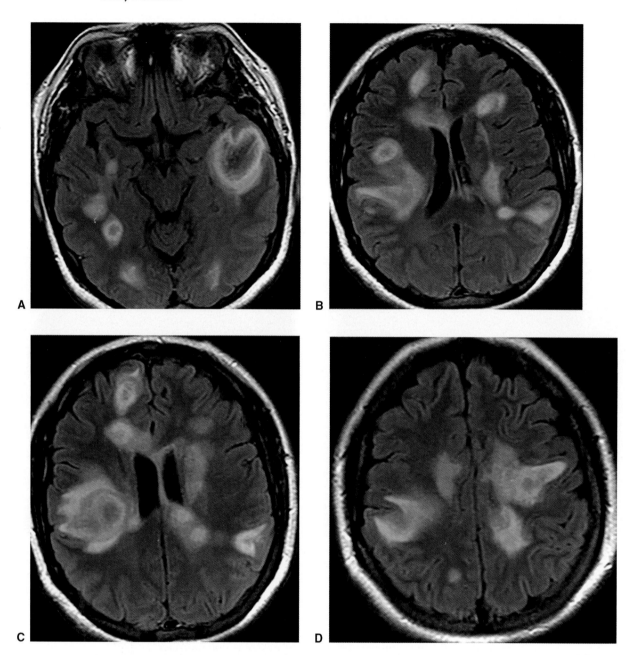

A. Balo concentric sclerosis (BCS)
B. Neuromyelitis optica (NMO)
C. Marburg variant of multiple sclerosis
D. Susac syndrome

11 A 35 year old male with acute onset encephalopathy, key images from an MRI are shown below:

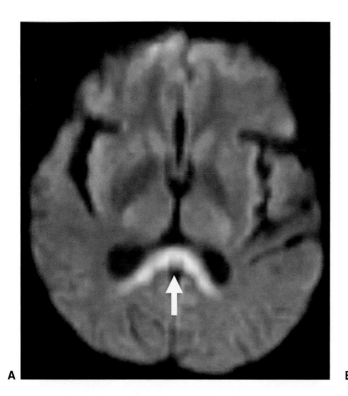

A

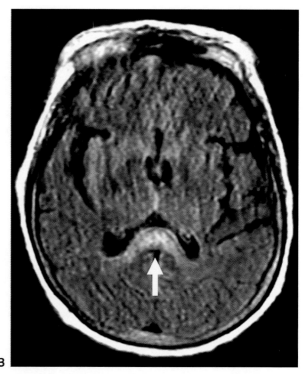

B

11a Which of the following phrases best describes the abnormality, pointed by the arrow, on the above images?

   A. Restricted diffusion within the splenium of corpus callosum
   B. Vasogenic edema within the splenium of corpus callosum
   C. Necrosis within the splenium of corpus callosum
   D. Hypercellularity within the splenium of corpus callosum

11b What is the most likely diagnosis in the setting of acute alteration of mental status, chronic alcoholism, malnutrition, and hepatic cirrhosis?

   A. Wernicke encephalopathy
   B. Hyperammonemic hepatic encephalopathy
   C. Korsakoff psychosis
   D. Marchiafava-Bignami disease (MBD)

12 A 37-year-old female who presented with seizures undergoes an MRI for initial evaluation. Key images are shown below:

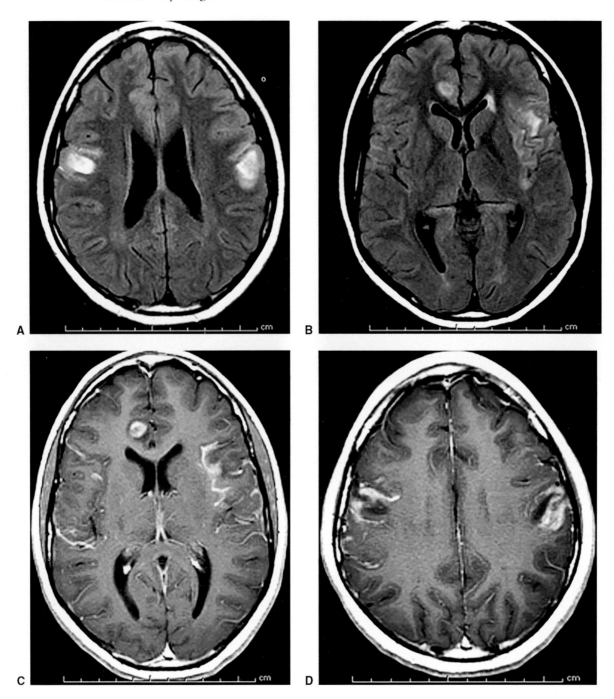

12a Further workup revealed positive ANA and dsDNA titers. Which of the following is the most likely diagnosis?

A. CNS lupus
B. Neurosarcoidosis
C. Meningoencephalitis
D. Primary CNS angiitis

12b The patient was started on steroids and immunosuppressive therapy with excellent response. Which other complication is this patient at increased risk for?

A. Cerebral abscess
B. Stroke
C. Obstructive hydrocephalus
D. Malignancy

13

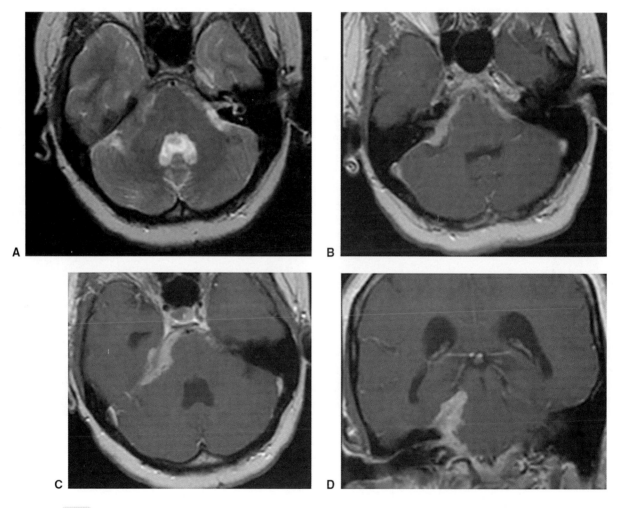

A

B

C

D

13a Based on the above images, which is a possible clinical feature expected in this patient?

A. Hemiparesis
B. Multiple cranial neuropathies
C. Isolated oculomotor palsy
D. Horner syndrome

13b Basal meningeal enhancement is most commonly seen with which of the following
entities?

A. Tuberculous meningitis
B. Carcinomatous meningitis
C. Intracranial hypotension
D. CNS lymphoma

13c Which of the following entities is a noninfectious cause with predilection for basal
meningeal involvement?

A. Carcinomatous meningitis
B. Intracranial hypotension
C. CNS lymphoma
D. Neurosarcoidosis

14 A 60-year-old male presents with weight loss, abdominal pain and fever.
Pancreatitis was noted on the CT abdomen. Patient subsequently developed
seizures. Key images from MRI brain are shown below.

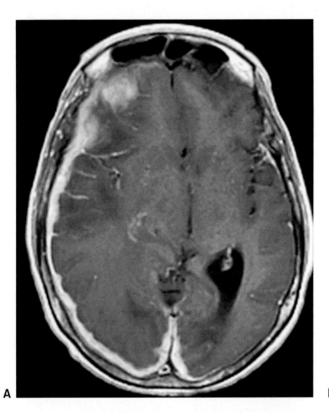
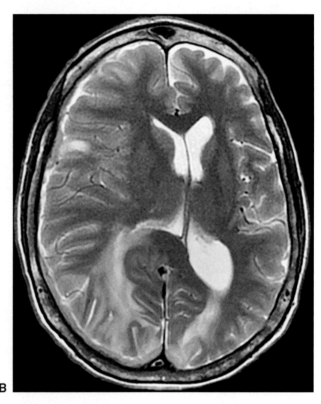

A   B

What is the most likely diagnosis in this case?

A. Septic meningoencephalitis
B. IgG4-related disease
C. Metastatic adenocarcinoma
D. CNS lymphoma

15 A 52-year-old male presents with headache, weakness, and progressive gait abnormality. A contrast-enhanced MRI was performed, and key images are shown below:

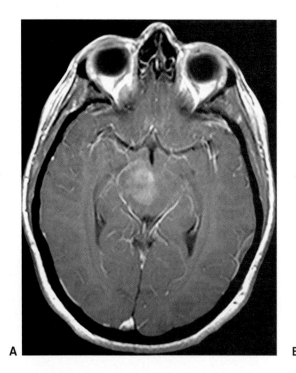

A

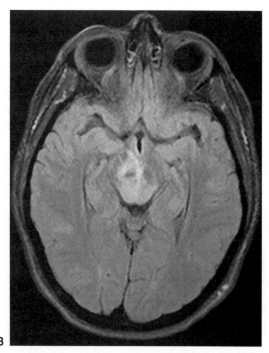

B

15a What can be done noninvasively to better characterize this lesion?

A. Proton MR spectroscopy

B. Short interval follow-up MRI

C. MR angiogram

D. CT perfusion

Single proton MR spectroscopy was performed from the voxel centered in the midbrain signal abnormality; spectra are shown below.

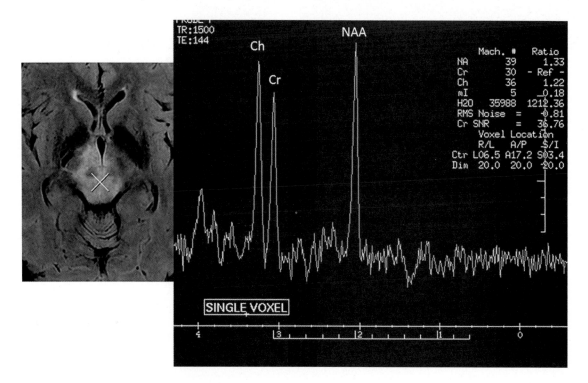

15b Which characteristic metabolic abnormality has been associated with high-grade primary CNS glioma?

    A. Marked elevation of choline peak
    B. Marked elevation of NAA peak
    C. Reduction of creatinine peak
    D. Reduction of choline peak

16 A 38-year-old woman presents with severe migrainous headaches, mild memory impairment, hearing loss, and significant constriction of peripheral visual field on visual mapping. Visual acuity is 20/25 in the right eye and 20/30 in the left eye. Key images from her MRI are shown below. Optic nerves were normal on MRI, (not shown).

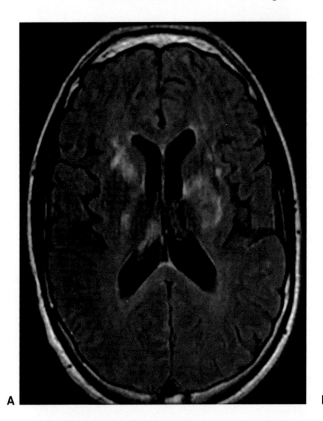 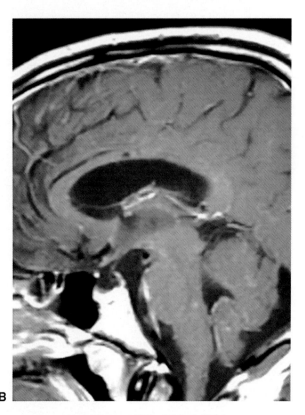

A   B

16a Based on the provided history and above key images, what is the most likely diagnosis?

    A. Lyme disease
    B. Susac syndrome
    C. Multiple sclerosis
    D. Ocular migraine

16b Which of the following tests will aid in further investigation of these findings?

    A. Contrast-enhanced Head CT
    B. MR spectroscopy
    C. Brain biopsy
    D. Fluorescein angiography of the eye

16c What is the characteristic abnormality often seen on brain MRI with the disease shown in the above figure?

    A. Deep gray matter FLAIR hyperintensities shown on image A
    B. Periventricular white matter pallor shown on image A
    C. Central corpus callosal lesion shown on image B
    D. Right medial thalamic lesion shown on image A

17 A 33-year-old woman presents with acute-onset painful unilateral visual blurring.

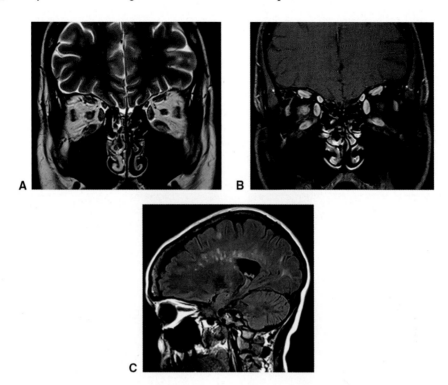

17a An LP was performed. What may be an associated CSF abnormality?

A. Neutrophil pleocytosis
B. Oligoclonal bands
C. HSV IgM
D. Cytoalbuminologic dissociation

18 A 25-year-old female presents with bilateral, painless vision deterioration for the past 2 weeks. Examination shows weakness of all 4 limbs and moderate gait ataxia. Brain MRI was otherwise essentially normal.

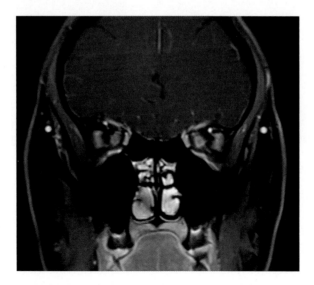

Which other imaging investigation must be performed?

A. CT abdomen to look for malignancy
B. MRA neck to evaluate status of neck vessels
C. MRI cervical spine to evaluate the cord
D. MRI lumbar spine to evaluate the cauda equina

ANSWERS AND EXPLANATIONS

1a **Answer C.**   Balo concentric sclerosis. Balo concentric sclerosis is the most appropriate diagnosis because of the classic concentric morphology of the lesion resulting from alternating rings of demyelination.

1b **Answer A.**   Lamellar demyelination with concentric morphology. Lamellar demyelination with concentric morphology is the characteristic feature for this entity. Option B, suggesting incomplete horseshoe shape enhancement, is a feature seen with many forms of demyelination including multiple sclerosis.

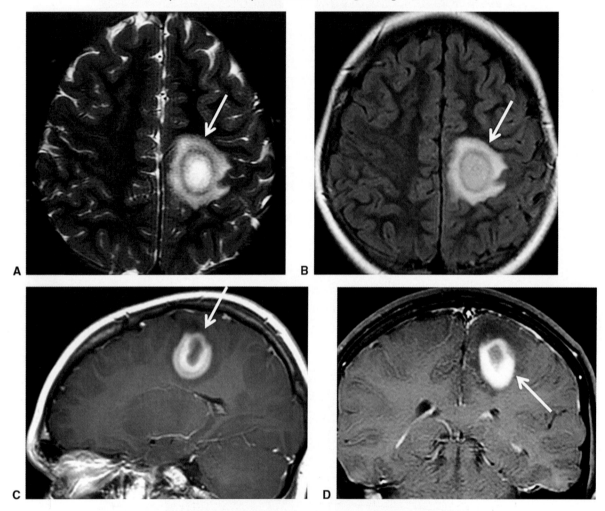

Imaging Findings: A well-defined solitary lesion in the posterior left frontal lobe centered in the precentral gyrus with alternating T2/FLAIR hyper- and hypointensities in a concentric ring-like fashion, (A and B) with intense eccentric enhancement on postcontrast T1w sequences, (C and D) consistent with Balo concentric sclerosis.

Discussion: Balo concentric sclerosis (BCS) is a rare demyelinating disease, which is considered a variant of multiple sclerosis. Its characteristic feature is concentric morphology with alternating rings of myelin preservation and myelin loss. The demyelination starts centrally in the core and then extends outward in a concentric fashion. Unlike ADEM, BCS does not necessarily have to be a monophasic condition. Clinical course can range from a single self-limiting monophasic event to MS-like relapsing, remitting, and primary progressive forms. Treatment in the acute phase is with corticosteroids with excellent response, particularly if treatment is started early.

Differential Diagnosis: Acute disseminated encephalomyelitis, multiple sclerosis, abscesses, and neoplasm. The characteristic ring-like morphology however is typical for Balo concentric sclerosis, therefore it is the most likely diagnosis in this case. Abscess may have a similar appearance but will have a different clinical presentation, and typically, DWI shows intense restricted diffusion confined to the nonenhancing necrotic center compared to BCS, which shows alternating rings of diffusion restriction similar to the morphologic appearance on T2w sequences.

References: Darke M, Bahador FM, Miller DC, et al. Baló's concentric sclerosis: imaging findings and pathological correlation. *J Radiol Case Rep* 2013;7(6):1–8.

Karaarslan E, Altintas A, Senol U, et al. Baló's concentric sclerosis: clinical and radiologic features of five cases. *AJNR Am J Neuroradiol* 2001;22(7):1362–1327.

2a **Answer A.**   Recent viral infection, fever, or immunization. Recent viral infection, fever, or immunization within past 2 to 4 weeks

2b **Answer C.**   Acute disseminated encephalomyelitis.

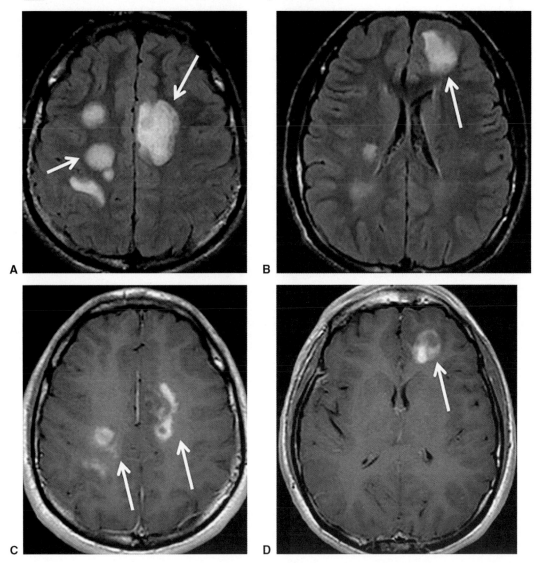

Imaging Findings: Bilateral large areas of cortical/subcortical and deep white matter FLAIR hyperintensities (A and B) with corresponding enhancement (C and D).

Discussion: Acute disseminated encephalomyelitis (ADEM) is immune-mediated multifocal inflammatory disorder of the nervous system usually preceded by viral infection. Less commonly vaccination is the triggering event, 5% to 12% of patients. Often, no history of preceding illness elicited. This can occur at any age, but more common in pediatric population with median age of about 8 years.

The precise pathogenesis is not known. "Molecular mimicry" theory proposes cross-reactivity of antibodies to antigens in pathogens with myelin antigen. Per "inflammatory cascade theory," either there is direct nervous tissue damage secondary to infection with antigens leaking into circulation or multiple cytokines/chemokines.

On imaging, there is generally widespread bilateral and asymmetric lesions. Subcortical and deep white matter are the most common sites involvement. Peripheral cortical involvement can be seen. Periventricular and callosal white matter involvement is less common, contrary to MS. Deep gray matter involvement is seen in about 50% cases. Cerebellar, brainstem, and spinal cord involvement is seen in 30% to 50% of patients. The lesion size varies from a few mm to large tumefactive nature. Enhancement is variable, and if present shows variable morphology, nodular, ring, diffuse and inhomogeneous. On CT, the lesions appear hypodense but CT is less sensitive for diagnosis. T2-weighted MR imaging is most sensitive, and the lesions are seen as ill-defined hyperintensities.

ADEM is generally monophasic. The lesions that evolve or appear within first 3 months are considered part of the initial disease. A subset of patients show recurrent or multiphasic disease. Recurrent ADEM refers to recurrence of lesions in the same location, and multiphasic disease refers to lesions occurrence at a different brain location.

Most of the patients show clinical as well as imaging resolution within months. Up to a quarter of patients can show subtle neurocognitive deficits. More aggressive variants of ADEM include acute hemorrhagic leukoencephalitis, acute hemorrhagic encephalomyelitis, and acute necrohemorrhagic leukoencephalitis.

Differential Diagnosis:

Multiple sclerosis: Generally smaller and well-defined lesions. "Black-hole" appearance of lesions on T1 images. Preferential involvement of periventricular and callosal white matter. Oligoclonal bands on CSF analysis

Vasculitis: Generally older age group. Hemorrhage is more common. Vascular imaging helps

References: Barkovich AJ, Raybaud C. *Pediatric neuroimaging*, 5th ed. Philadelphia, PA: Lippincott Williams & Wilkins, 2011.

Marin SE, Callen DJ. The magnetic resonance imaging appearance of monophasic acute disseminated encephalomyelitis. *Neuroimaging Clin N Am* 2013;23(2):245–266. doi: 10.1016/j.nic.2012.12.005.

3a   **Answer B.**   Rasmussen encephalitis. Profound atrophy in the right insulotemporal region in the setting of previous reported encephalitis is most compatible with Rasmussen encephalitis.

3b   **Answer A.**   Normal brain MRI. In the prodromal phase of illness, the MRI and CT are usually normal.

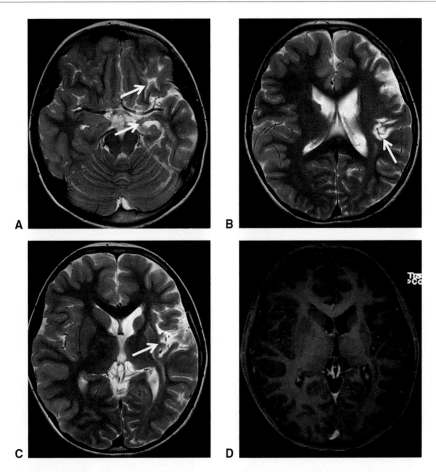

Imaging Findings: There is nonenhancing atrophy in the left hemisphere with medial temporal, orbitofrontal (A), perisylvian, (B and C) volume loss.

Discussion: Rasmussen encephalitis is progressive unilateral focal encephalitis of uncertain etiology (viral trigger of genetic predisposition to immunodysfunction is suggested) that affects patients between 1 and 15 years of age.

Three phases of the disease:

- Prodromal stage: Low seizure frequency; may exhibit mild hemiplegia. Imaging may be normal.
- Acute stage: Seizures (partial complex seizures), progressive hemiparesis, and cognitive impairment. On imaging, there is swelling of the involved parenchyma, which is usually fronto–insular–temporal and may be parietal. Cortical and subcortical CT hypodensity and MRI T2 and FLAIR cortical and white matter (WM) hyperintensity may be seen. Pial or cortical enhancement secondary to the parenchymal inflammation is occasionally seen.
- Residual or chronic stage: Stable neurologic deficits and continuing seizures refractory to medical treatment. On imaging, atrophy of the involved parenchyma may be seen

Differential Diagnosis:

- Sturge-Weber syndrome: Port-wine facial nevus and enhancement of pial angioma are the classic findings. Cortical calcifications are also seen as well as parenchymal volume loss.
- Dyke-Davidoff-Masson syndrome: There is unilateral brain atrophy, compensatory calvarial thickening, and hyperaeration of the paranasal sinuses following in utero or perinatal hemispheric infarction.

- Focal cortical dysplasia: Blurring of gray–white matter junction, subcortical WM signal abnormality, cortical thickening and signal change, and abnormal sulcal/gyral pattern. WM signal tapering from subcortical region to the ventricular margin is the classic finding.

References: Faingold R, et al. MRI appearance of Rasmussen encephalitis. *Pediatr Radiol* 2009;39(7):756.

Fiorella DJ, et al. (18)F-fluorodeoxyglucose positron emission tomography and MR imaging findings in Rasmussen encephalitis. *AJNR Am J Neuroradiol* 2001;22(7):1291–1299.

Misra UK, et al. The prognostic role of magnetic resonance imaging and single-photon emission computed tomography in viral encephalitis. *Acta Radiol* 2008;49(7):827–832.

Varadkar S, et al. Rasmussen's encephalitis: clinical features, pathobiology, and treatment advances. *Lancet Neurol* 2014;13(2):195–205.

4a **Answer D.** Autoimmune paraneoplastic limbic encephalitis. Autoimmune paraneoplastic limbic encephalitis, in view of the clinical history, is the most likely explanation for the T2/Flair hyperintensity in the bilateral medial temporal lobes (A and B) with restricted diffusion (C).

4b **Answer A.** Anti–glutamic acid decarboxylase (GAD) antibodies. Anti-glutamic acid decarboxylase antibodies have been implicated in nonneoplastic causes of autoimmune limbic encephalitis. The other antibodies mentioned in the answer choices have been associated with paraneoplastic encephalitis.

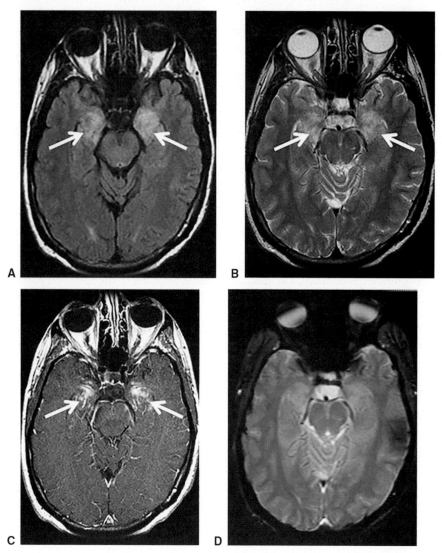

Imaging Findings: MR sequences demonstrate bilateral symmetric T2/FLAIR hyperintensity in the mesial temporal lobes (hippocampus and amygdala) (A and B) with significant enhancement (C) and no hemorrhage (D).

Discussion: Limbic encephalitis is the most common clinical paraneoplastic syndrome that is seen in patients with small cell lung cancer and is immune mediated by Anti-Hu autoantibodies (found in ~60% of patients). Other cell surface antigens such as voltage-gated potassium channels (VGKC), N-methyl-D-aspartate receptor (NMDAR), and α-amino-3-hydroxy-5-methyl-4-isoxazolepropionic acid receptor (AMPAR) may present with limbic encephalitis.

MRI is the most sensitive imaging modality (CT is usually normal) and will show T1 hypointensity, T2/FLAIR hyperintensity, no diffusion restriction, no hemorrhage, and occasional patchy enhancement in the mesial temporal lobes (hippocampus and amygdala), insula, cingulate gyrus, subfrontal cortex, and inferior frontal white matter.

FDG-PET will show increased glucose metabolism in the mesial temporal lobes. Other less common paraneoplastic syndromes:

- Brainstem encephalitis: Seen with testicular germ cell tumors, on MRI will show T2 hyperintensity in the midbrain, pons, cerebellar peduncles, and basal ganglia.
- Paraneoplastic cerebellar degeneration: Seen with breast cancer, ovarian cancer, and Hodgkin lymphoma; and on MRI will show cerebellar atrophy.

Differential Diagnosis:

- Status epilepticus: Clinical history of seizure is usually present. On MRI, there is usually unilateral abnormal T2/FLAIR single corresponding to the clinical side of the seizure. DWI restriction and cortical enhancement are typical.
- Low-grade glioma: Unilateral T2 hyperintense mass with mild mass effect. No enhancement is typical. Can be impossible to differentiate from limbic encephalitis.
- Herpes encephalitis: DWI restriction, mass effect, enhancement, and hemorrhage are common. Characterized clinically by rapid-onset and febrile illness.

References: Darnell RB, et al. Paraneoplastic syndromes affecting the nervous system. *Semin Oncol* 2006;33(3):270–298.

Khan NL, et al. Histopathology of VGKC antibody-associated limbic encephalitis. *Neurology* 2009;72(19):1703–1705.

Kotsenas AL, et al. MRI findings in autoimmune voltage-gated potassium channel complex encephalitis with seizures: one potential etiology for mesial temporal sclerosis. *AJNR Am J Neuroradiol* 2014;35(1):84–89.

Voltz R, et al. A serologic marker of paraneoplastic limbic and brain-stem encephalitis in patients with testicular cancer. *N Engl J Med* 1999;340(23):1788–1795.

5a **Answer B.** Progressive multifocal leukoencephalopathy (PML). There are nonenhancing asymmetric confluent white matter lesions with periventricular and subcortical involvement typical for PML.

5b **Answer D.** Immune reconstitution inflammatory syndrome (IRIS). Presence of enhancement in the PML lesions with worsening of FLAIR hyperintensity upon immune reconstitution is most compatible with IRIS.

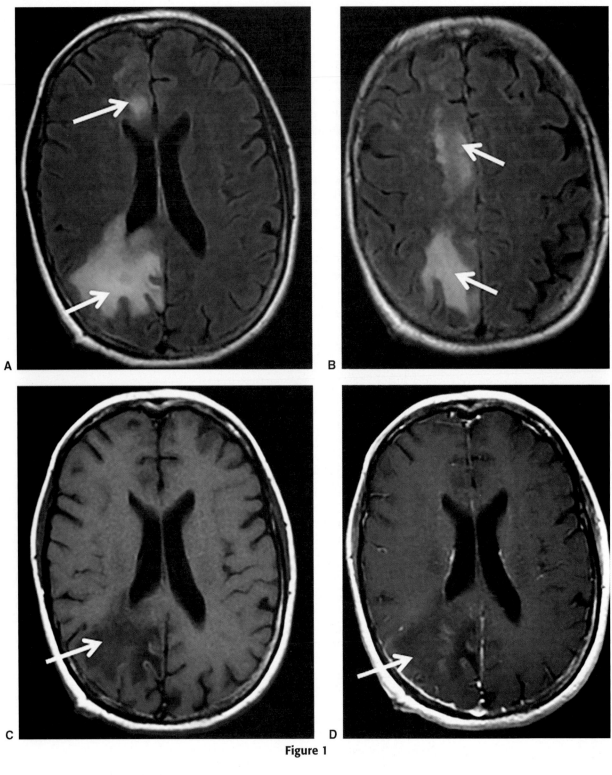

Figure 1

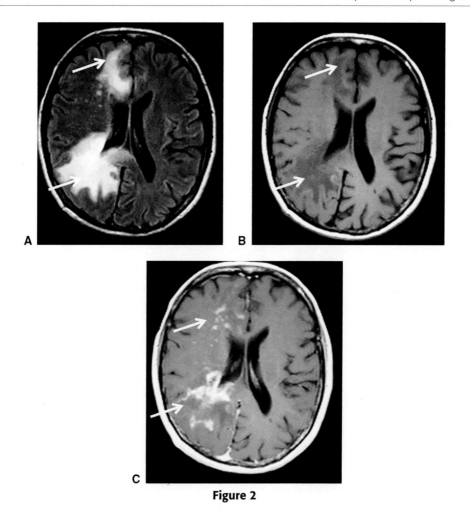

Figure 2

Imaging Findings: Figure 1. Confluent, large white matter FLAIR hyperintensities involving right frontal and parietooccipital lobes including subcortical U fiber involvement and lack of mass effect (A and B). No significant enhancement of mass effect is appreciated (C and D). In the current clinical setting, these findings most likely represent progressive multifocal leukoencephalopathy.

Figure 2. Subsequently, there is worsening of FLAIR hyperintense signal (A) and now development of intense enhancement (B and C). Findings are most compatible with immune reconstitution inflammatory syndrome (IRIS).

Discussion: Progressive multifocal leukoencephalopathy (PML) is a rapidly progressive and potentially fatal CNS infection due to reactivation of JC virus in the setting of immunosuppression. This includes severely immunosuppressed patients with HIV/AIDS, transplant recipients, or those undergoing monoclonal antibody treatment (e.g., natalizumab) such as for multiple sclerosis (MS). On imaging, these patients may present with extensive, confluent white matter changes, some of which may show restricted diffusion and hazy peripheral or nodular punctate enhancement.

Immune reconstitution inflammatory syndrome is seen with development of significant mass effect, often involvement of deep gray matter structures and more intense enhancement. PML-IRIS results after treatment with restoration of immunocompetence leading to an overwhelming inflammatory response directed against JC virus antigen. For clinical diagnosis of PML, clinical features, MRI findings, and lumbar puncture with CSF JCV PCR may be used for diagnosis.

Reference: Carruthers RL, et al. Progressive multifocal leukoencephalopathy and JC virus-related disease in modern neurology practice. *Mult Scler Relat Disord* 2014;3(4):419–430.

6a **Answer B.**   Tumefactive demyelinating lesion. The lack of restricted diffusion is atypical for abscess, and central nonenhancement is atypical for lymphoma. Low-grade astrocytoma is a differential possibility, but the age group, well-circumscribed nature, peripheral T2 hypointense ring, and thin rim of enhancement favor the diagnosis of demyelination.

6b **Answer C.**   Routine clinical follow-up and an MRI within 6 to 8 weeks. Because of diagnostic overlaps, a short interval follow-up is prudent in such cases. In addition, because these patients can relapse into clinically definite multiple sclerosis or NMO, close clinical follow-up is also warranted. FDG-PET has been reported to be less intensely positive in tumefactive demyelination compared to neoplasm, but at this stage, with response to empiric treatment, this will not be the expected course of action.

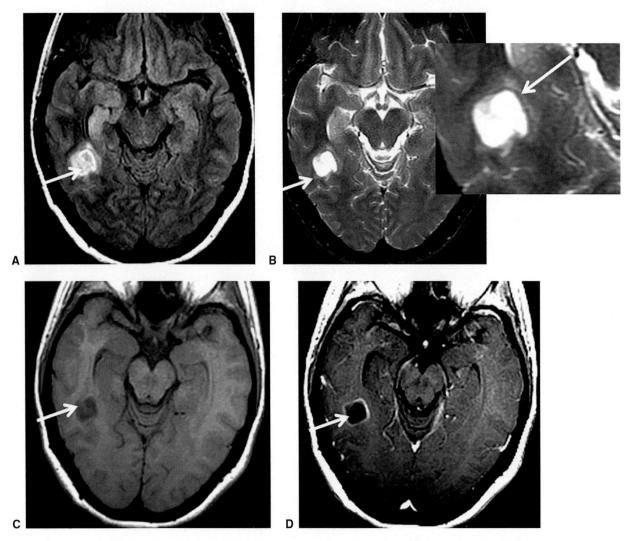

Imaging Findings: This ring-enhancing lesion without restricted diffusion and a peripheral T2 hypointense ring is most likely to represent a tumefactive demyelinating lesion.

Discussion: Tumefactive demyelination.

Tumefactive demyelinating lesions are typically larger than 2 cm in size with mass effect and/or edema. Majority of the lesions are focal and supratentorial, making diagnosis difficult particularly if the patient has no known history of demyelinating disease. Certain imaging features, such as a T2-hypointense ring surrounding the lesion, open of ring of enhancement with the open aspect pointing toward gray matter and hypodensity on CT corresponding to the areas of enhancement on MRI have been associated with demyelinating lesions more than neoplasms or infections. Restricted diffusion may be seen in the lesion core or at the lesion edge. The degree of restricted diffusion with abscess is usually more intense than seen with tumefactive MS.

In the proper clinical setting, biopsy can be deferred in favor of empirical treatment unless a diagnosis of lymphoma is strongly suspected because CNS lymphoma often responds to steroids reducing the yield on subsequent biopsy. Even on biopsy, a 31% misdiagnosis rate has been reported, and often repeat biopsy has been suggested.

Short-term management with IV steroids is typically used with excellent response. Follow-up MRI within 6 to 8 weeks should be considered, particularly if the diagnosis of tumefactive demyelination is not confirmed.

References: Frederick MC, Cameron MH. Tumefactive demyelinating lesions in multiple sclerosis and associated disorders. *Curr Neurol Neurosci Rep* 2016;16(3):26.

Pilz G, Harrer A, Wipfler P, et al. Tumefactive MS lesions under fingolimod: a case report and literature review. *Neurology* 2013;81(19):1654–1658.

7a **Answer A.** Left-sided facial paralysis.

7b **Answer C.** Tympanic segment. The proximal tympanic segment can normally enhance due to perineural venous plexus.

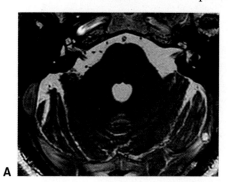 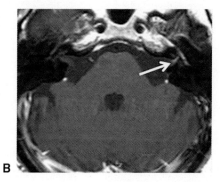 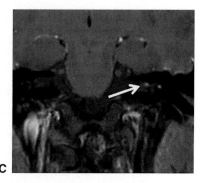

A   B   C

Imaging Findings: Enhancing meatal and labyrinthine segment of the left facial nerve is seen (B and C) without corresponding mass lesion or nodularity on the axial 3D CISS (A).

Discussion: Bell palsy is defined as acute peripheral nerve paralysis of unknown cause. Herpes simplex reactivation is the commonly proposed mechanism. Imaging is generally undertaken when the clinical presentation is unusual, to rule out other potential etiologies.

Contrast enhancement is most commonly seen at the geniculate ganglion and the proximal tympanic segment although mild enhancement has also been described in the mastoid , labyrinthine and meatal segments. This is due to the presence of a perineural venous plexus.

Distinctive imaging features of Bell palsy are abnormal enhancement of the facial nerve, commonly extending from intracanalicular through tympanic segment and at the most mild smooth enlargement of the nerve. This abnormal enhancement may persist for months after clinical improvement.

Other facial nerve neuritis can have a similar appearance. Ramsay Hunt syndrome (herpes zoster oticus) typically shows abnormal enhancement in the facial nerve, the vestibulocochlear nerve, the internal auditory canal, and often the inner ear labyrinth. Vesicles can be seen in the external ear. In cases of cranial nerve involvement with CNS Lyme disease, abnormal enhancement is seen in multiple cranial nerves, 7th nerve being the most commonly involved nerve. Unilateral involvement is more common, but bilateral involvement is characteristic.

If there is nodularity and enlargement of the nerve, alternate etiologies like metastasis, lymphoproliferative disorders, and perineural spread of malignancy should be considered.

Reference: Gebarski SS, Telian SA, Niparko JK. Enhancement along the normal facial nerve in the facial canal: MR imaging and anatomic correlation. *Radiology* 1992;183(2):391–394. doi: 10.1148/radiology.183.2.1561339.

8a **Answer D.** Neurosarcoidosis. It is the most likely diagnosis given the age group, reported chest x-ray findings, and elevated ACE levels.

8b **Answer A.** <1% of cases. Isolated CNS sarcoidosis without systemic manifestations is extremely rare, <1% of cases.

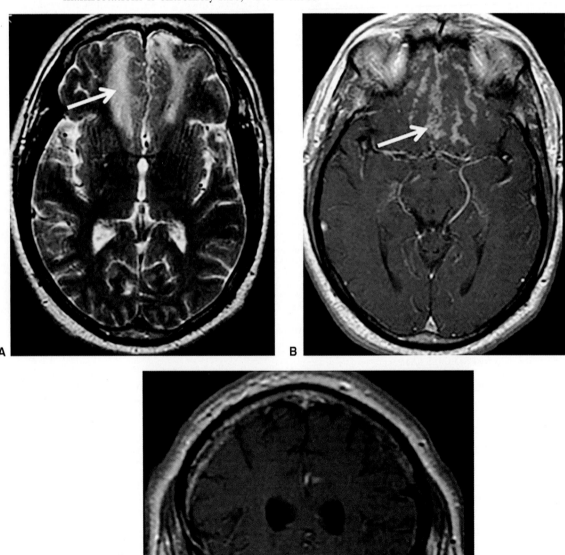

Imaging Findings: There is bilateral inferior frontal parenchymal T2 hyperintensity (A) with pial enhancement along the sulci (B and C).

Discussion: Sarcoidosis is an idiopathic systemic disorder characterized by noncaseating granulomas on pathology. Serum ACE levels have been found to be elevated during active disease and often used to diagnose and monitor the disease. Imaging features of neurosarcoidosis are nonspecific making it a challenging diagnosis in the absence of systemic disease. It has a predilection for basilar pial involvement; however, it can present with parenchymal, pial, and dural lesions anywhere in the brain. Management is not well established with steroids being the first line of treatment.

References: Smith AB, Horkanyne-Szakaly I, Schroeder JW, et al. From the radiologic pathology archives: mass lesions of the dura: beyond meningioma-radiologic-pathologic correlation. *Radiographics* 2014;34(2):295–312.

Smith JK, Matheus MG, Castillo M. Imaging manifestations of neurosarcoidosis. *AJR Am J Roentgenol* 2004;182(2):289–295.

9a **Answer C.** One or more lesion in at least two of four designated areas of CNS. One or more lesion in at least two of four designated areas of CNS (periventricular, juxtacortical, infratentorial, or spinal cord).

9b **Answer B.** Progressive multifocal leukoencephalopathy. Progressive multifocal leukoencephalopathy, due to JC virus reactivation in the setting of immunosuppression, is a potentially lethal complication of natalizumab and requires close clinical monitoring.

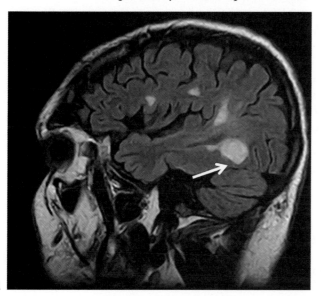 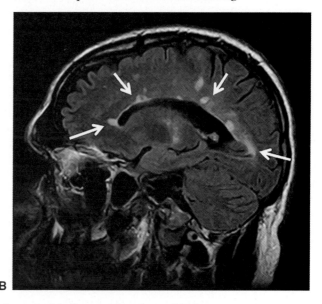

A   B

Imaging Findings: Scattered cortical/subcortical and pericallosal ovoid lesions characteristic for multiple sclerosis are seen (A and B). Note large juxtacortical lesion in the posterior temporal lobe, (arrow image A), which overlaps a part of the cortex. This image fulfills the criteria for dissemination in space with presence of both periventricular and cortical/juxtacortical lesions.

Discussion: Multiple sclerosis is a chronic demyelinating illness of the central nervous system with unclear pathogenesis. It has a female preponderance (~2:1) and is more prevalent in the Caucasian population.

There are four major clinical subtypes of multiple sclerosis.

1. Relapsing–remitting multiple sclerosis (RRMS) (about 85%).
2. Secondary progressive multiple sclerosis (SPMS). Majority of RRMS convert to this type over years.

3. Primary progressive multiple sclerosis (PPMS). This subtype is progressive from the beginning (5% to 10% of MS patients). MRI findings are less dramatic relative to clinical disability.

4. Progressive relapsing multiple sclerosis (PRMS), involves relapses within PPMS. This is the rarest form of the disease.

MRI is a key factor in diagnosis of multiple sclerosis for assessment of dissemination in space and time to establish the diagnosis of multiple sclerosis.

According to the revised 2010 McDonald criteria, the presence of one or more lesions in the designated CNS regions is defined as dissemination in space. These regions are periventricular, juxtacortical, infratentorial, and spinal cord. However, subsequently, the recent expert consensus (MAGNIMS consensus guidelines, *Lancet Neurology.* 2016) recommends further revisions to the 2010 criteria, such as three or more periventricular lesions, inclusion of the optic nerve as another designated site and inclusion of cortical lesions instead of only juxtacortical lesions. Dissemination in time is defined as a new T2w or gadolinium-enhancing lesion on a follow-up MRI irrespective of the timing of the baseline MRI or simultaneous presence of an enhancing and nonenhancing lesion at any time.

On MRI, majority of these lesions are supratentorial. Less than 10% of lesions are infratentorial. The typical location is periventricular with perivenular distribution. They tend to be oval, round, or linear with an orientation parallel to lateral ventricles ("Dawson fingers"). Alternating areas of linear hyperintensity and isointensity along the ependyma on sagittal FLAIR images, known as "ependymal dot-line sign" is an early sign. On T1-weighted images, approximately 30% of these plaques appear hypointense (black holes). The T1 hypointensity in acute stages is mostly related to the edema and the majority become isointense within 3 months. The chronic black holes represent advanced axonal loss with greater extracapsular fluid and correlate with disability. Progressive atrophy indicating irreversible tissue damage also correlates with disability. Active lesions with disruption of the blood–brain barrier exhibit contrast enhancement on MRI. Less than 30% of patients show enhancing lesions. The classic peripheral enhancement incomplete ring of enhancement (horseshoe shaped) is often seen with larger lesions. Contrast enhancement in active lesions is transient and usually disappears by 4 weeks. It is unusual for a multiple sclerosis plaque to be enhancing beyond 3 months. Diffusion restriction can be seen in the small percentage of active lesions.

References: Filippi M, Rocca MA, Ciccarelli O, et al.; MAGNIMS Study Group. MRI criteria for the diagnosis of multiple sclerosis: MAGNIMS consensus guidelines. *Lancet Neurol* 2016;15(3):292–303.

Lassmann H. The pathologic substrate of magnetic resonance alterations in multiple sclerosis. *Neuroimaging Clin N Am* 2008;18(4):563–576. doi: 10.1016/j.nic.2008.06.005.

Osborn AG. *Osborn's brain: imaging, pathology, and anatomy*, 1st ed. Salt Lake City, UT: Amirsys Publishing, 2013.

Polman CH, Reingold SC, Banwell B, et al. Diagnostic criteria for multiple sclerosis: 2010 revisions to the McDonald criteria. *Ann Neurol* 2011;69(2):292–302.

Traboulsee A, Li DK. Conventional MR imaging. *Neuroimaging Clin N Am* 2008;18(4):651–673. doi: 10.1016/j.nic.2008.07.001.

10 **Answer C.**   Marburg variant of multiple sclerosis. The confluent tumefactive lesions shown are typical for this entity. NMO typically shows mild to no brain involvement. BCS lesions show a typical lamellated appearance. Susac syndrome shows small lesions unlike this case, including characteristic central corpus callosal lesions.

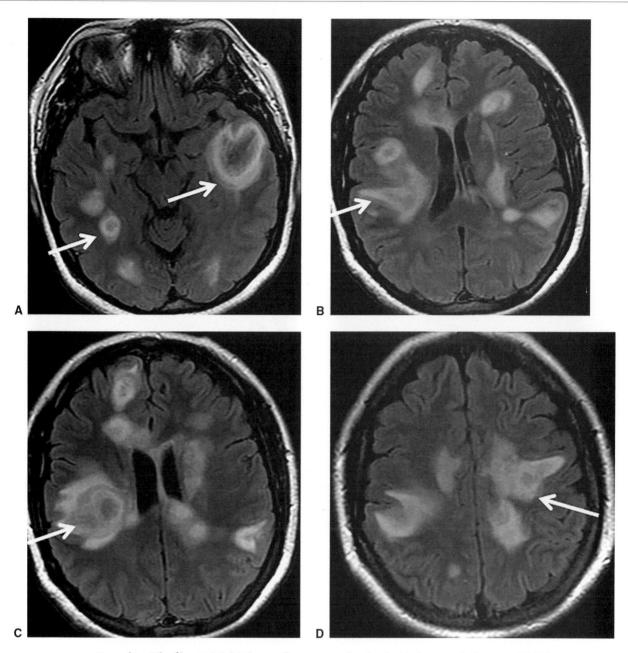

Imaging Findings: Multiple confluent tumefactive hyperintense lesions on FLAIR with profound edema and mass effect (A to D).

Discussion: Marburg variant of multiple sclerosis is a rare entity with extensive multifocal areas of tumefactive demyelination. These lesions have severe inflammation and edema with evidence of enhancement and mass effect. Severe forms of ADEM may have a very similar appearance; however, ADEM is commonly seen in younger patients. Marburg variant has a severe and often lethal clinical course. Management is challenging relying on high-dose steroids, plasma exchange, immunoglobulin, and disease-modifying agents with poor outcome, such as severe disability or death.

Reference: Sarbu N, Shih RY, Jones RV, et al. White matter diseases with radiologic-pathologic correlation. *Radiographics* 2016;36(5):1426–1447.

11a Answer A.   Restricted diffusion within the splenium of corpus callosum. There is intense DWI hyperintensity within the splenium of CC with corresponding FLAIR hyperintensity. The degree of DWI hyperintensity is likely not explained by T2 shine through (in practice, this can be confirmed on ADC map, not shown with this image).

11b **Answer D.**   Marchiafava-Bignami disease (MBD). In the provided clinical scenario, this is the most likely diagnosis. Although all the options are also associated with chronic alcoholism and cirrhosis, the imaging manifestations shown here most closely resemble MBD. It is important to note that MBD may coexist with these other entities.

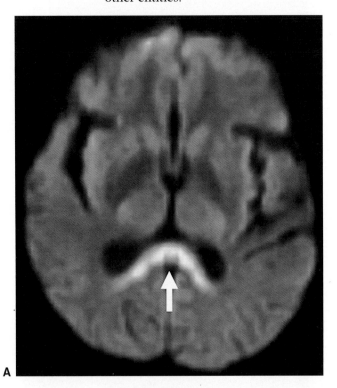
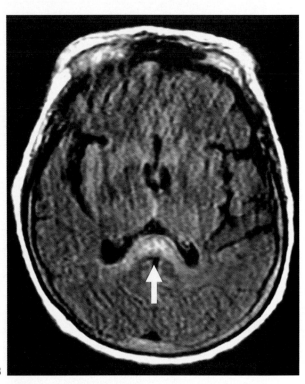

A   B

Imaging Findings: There is restricted diffusion in the splenium of corpus callosum with high signal on DWI and corresponding FLAIR hyperintensity. Note that in practice, it is essential to correlate DWI hyperintensity with corresponding low signal on ADC map (not shown here) to confirm restricted diffusion.

Discussion: Marchiafava-Bignami disease (MBD) is a rare necrotizing degeneration of corpus callosum commonly seen in chronic alcoholics. The exact pathogenesis is unclear. Chronic alcoholism and malnutrition-related deficiency of vitamin B complex are thought to be factors. Lesions typically involve the body of corpus callosum and can extend into both genu and splenium. The diagnosis is made in combination with clinical features. In the acute setting, these patients present with disorientation and confusion and may have seizures. The prognosis is variable, ranging from coma and death to near-complete recovery. Improved prognosis has been seen recently, likely related to earlier detection. Management is similar to Wernicke-Korsakoff syndrome with replacement of thiamine, folate, and vitamin B_{12} being the mainstay.

References: Arbelaez A, Pajon A, Castillo M. Acute Marchiafava-Bignami disease: MR findings in two patients. *AJNR Am J Neuroradiol* 2003;24(10):1955–1957.

Mirsattari SM, Lee DH, Jones MW, et al. Transient lesion in the splenium of the corpus callosum in an epileptic patient. *Neurology* 2003;60(11):1838–1841.

12a **Answer A.** CNS lupus. The enhancing lesions shown here involving cortical/cortical–subcortical junction in the setting of autoantibodies are most compatible with neuropsychiatric manifestation of lupus. The other options can have similar imaging manifestations, but are not associated with the autoantibodies.

12b **Answer B.** Stroke. CNS lupus is also associated with large vessel occlusive disease (LVOD) and can present with stroke. Therefore, it should be a differential consideration in a young patient with LVOD.

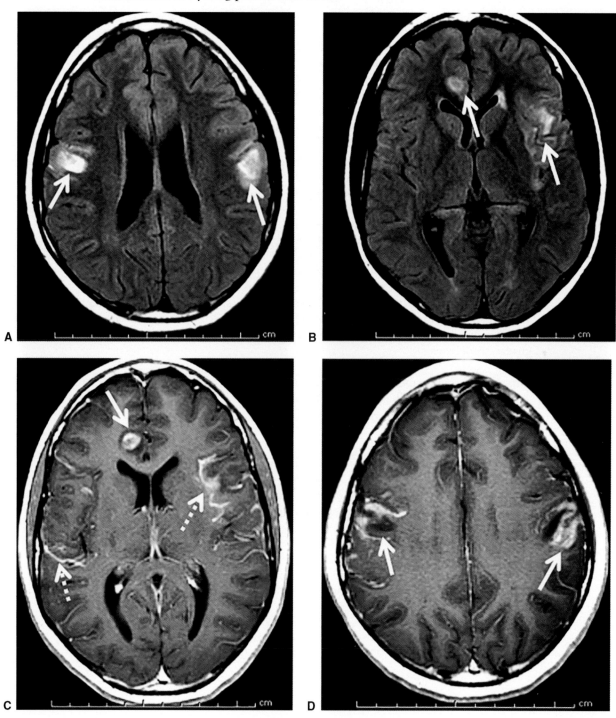

Imaging Findings: There are multiple bilateral FLAIR hyperintense cortical/subcortical lesions, (A and B) with enhancement on postcontrast T1w sequences, (C and D). Note the pial enhancement seen with some of these lesions such as shown on image C (dotted arrow).

Discussion: Systemic lupus erythematosus is a chronic systemic autoimmune disorder with multisystem involvement. This disease has a strong female preponderance (7 to 15:1 female:male ratio), particularly prevalent among women in the reproductive age group. Neuropsychiatric manifestations range from cerebrovascular, cognitive dysfunction, seizures, psychosis, and peripheral nervous system disorders. The patient can have other systemic abnormalities such as nephritis with persistent proteinuria, leukopenia, arthritis, and positive serologic markers such as positive antinuclear AB and anti-DsDNA AB. Seizures can occur, reported as one of the early events. In addition, large vessel occlusive disease or stroke due to hypercoagulable state or cardioembolic source can occur. Differential diagnosis is other forms of vasculitis, primary CNS angiitis, or neurosarcoidosis. Clinical features are key in differentiating these entities.

References: Joseph V, Anil R, Aristy S. Neuropsychiatric systemic lupus erythematosus: a diagnostic conundrum. *J Clin Med Res* 2016;8(10):757-759.

Mitsias P, Levine SR. Large cerebral vessel occlusive disease in systemic lupus erythematosus. *Neurology* 1994;44:385-393.

Pomper MG, Miller TJ, Stone JH, et al. CNS vasculitis in autoimmune disease: MR imaging findings and correlation with angiography. *AJNR Am J Neuroradiol* 1999;20(1):75-85.

13a **Answer B.** Multiple cranial neuropathies. There is enhancement of the basilar cisterns, R>L, including extension within the right Meckel cave, (image a) and right along the right 7th/8th nerve cisternal segments, predisposing the patient to cranial polyneuropathy. Cranial polyneuropathies may be seen with variety of other dura–arachnoid (pachymeningeal) or pia–arachnoid, (leptomeningeal) disease processes.

13b **Answer A.** Tuberculous meningitis. TB meningitis is commonly associated with basilar exudates and enhancement of basal meninges. The other entities, options B to D, can also have meningeal enhancement, but no specific predilection for basal meninges is reported.

13c **Answer D.** Neurosarcoidosis. This is the most appropriate choice, because as stated above, the other entities may have meningeal enhancement but no specific predilection for basal meninges. The other diagnoses associated with basal meningeal enhancement include Wegener granulomatosis and fungal infections.

14 **Answer B.** IgG4-related disease. The clinical scenario suggesting coexisting autoimmune pancreatitis and imaging findings are most likely reflective of IgG4-related hypertrophic pachymeningitis.

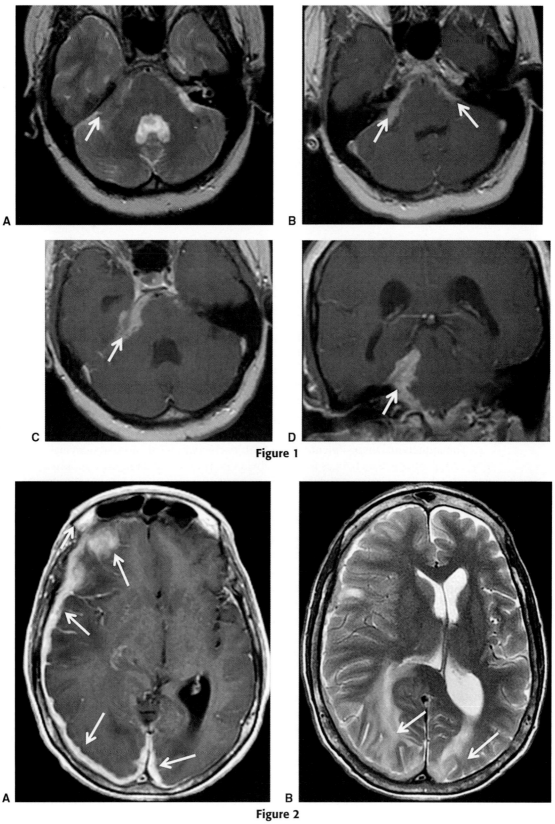

Figure 1

Figure 2

Imaging Findings: Figure 1. There is irregular enhancing soft tissue density in the prepontine cistern, CP angles, and along the course of right 7th/8th nerve complex and trigeminal nerves.

Figure 2. There is diffuse dural (also referred to as pachymeningeal) enhancement involving the right cerebral hemisphere and medial left occipital lobe, (A) with associated parenchymal T2 hyperintensity in the medial occipital lobes bilaterally (B). This appearance in the provided clinical scenario is most consistent with IgG4-related hypertrophic pachymeningitis.

Discussion: Basal cisternal exudates/meningeal enhancement as seen in this case has a wide differential diagnosis. Fungal infections and other granulomatous diseases such as sarcoid, TB, Wegener can have this appearance. It is important to note that while there is a predilection for basal meninges, these diseases can also have more diffuse meningeal or even parenchymal involvement.

The patterns of meningeal enhancement can be pachymeningeal (dural–arachnoid) as seen with meningiomas and intracranial hypotension or be leptomeningeal (pia–arachnoid) meningeal carcinomatosis or meningoencephalitis or both. Meningeal enhancement poses a risk for more diffuse CSF dissemination particularly essential to note with metastatic disease, in which early CSF sampling should be considered.

The second case shown here, IgG4-related hypertrophic pachymeningitis, is another example of dural or pachymeningeal enhancement with associated parenchymal changes. IgG4-related disease, (IgG-RD), is an immune-mediated fibroinflammatory condition that can have multisystemic involvement, including both intracranial and extracranial manifestations, such as pancreatitis, sialadenitis, dacrocystitis, lymphadenopathy, thyroiditis, cholangitis, and pulmonary manifestations.

The intracranial involvement can be both pachymeningeal and parenchymal; however, parenchymal changes may not always be present. In addition, hypophysitis and orbital inflammatory pseudotumor have been associated with IgG-RD. Of note, many of the cases previously thought to be idiopathic hypertrophic pachymeningitis might have also been IgG-RD.

Differential diagnosis: TB, sarcoid, fungal infections, Wegener granulomatosis, metastatic disease, atypical meningioma, secondary CNS lymphoma. Clinical features will be key in differentiating these entities.

References: Lu LX, Della-Torre E, Stone JH, et al. IgG4-related hypertrophic pachymeningitis: clinical features, diagnostic criteria, and treatment. *JAMA Neurol* 2014;71(6):785–793.

Smirniotopoulos JG, Murphy FM, Rushing EJ, et al. Patterns of contrast enhancement in the brain and meninges. *Radiographics* 2007;27(2):525–551.

Toyoda K, Oba H, Kutomi K, et al. MR imaging of IgG4-related disease in the head and neck and brain. *AJNR Am J Neuroradiol* 2012;33(11):2136–2139.

15a **Answer A.** Proton MR spectroscopy. Proton MR spectroscopy is the best noninvasive way of further noninvasive characterization of this abnormality because certain high-grade neoplastic abnormalities such as high-grade glioma may show a characteristic elevation of choline. Although MR perfusion may be useful, CT perfusion does not have sufficient soft tissue detail to elucidate these changes. MR angiogram and follow-up MR are not the best ways to evaluate the brainstem signal changes shown here.

15b **Answer A.** Marked elevation of choline peak. Marked elevation of choline peak and reduction in NAA are seen with neoplastic conditions due to rapid cell turnover and loss of healthy neuroglial tissue, respectively. A lipid peak may be seen with higher-grade neoplasms because of associated necrosis.

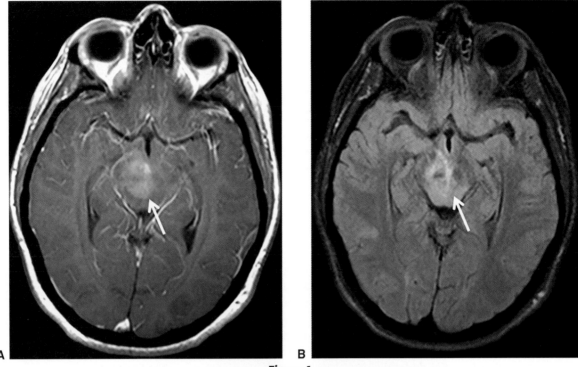

Figure 1

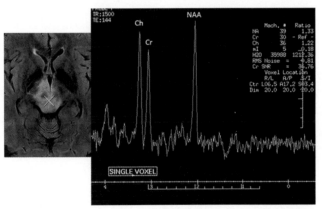

Figure 2

Imaging Findings: Figure 1. There is a heterogeneously enhancing (A) expansile infiltrative FLAIR hyperintense lesion involving the mesodiencephalic junction (MDJ) (B).

Figure 2. Single voxel spectra at TE of 144 ms, showing mild elevation of choline peak at 3.22 ppm. In a normal spectrum, the choline is slightly lower than the Cr peak at 3.03 ppm with the NAA being the highest peak at 2.01 ppm. There is no discernible lactate (inverted at this TE at 1.3 ppm) or lipid peak (at 1.2 to 1.4 ppm).

Discussion: Behçet disease is a multisystem inflammatory disorder of unknown etiology. There is variable involvement of the central nervous system most commonly involving the mesodiencephalic junction, (MDJ) as in this case, followed by the rest of the brainstem, telencephalon, cerebellum, and basal ganglia. Vasculitis is a hallmark of this disease and more commonly affects the venous system. Rarely, spinal cord involvement has been reported. Predominantly nonhemorrhagic lesions are seen; rarely, the lesions may demonstrate hemorrhage. Rarely, hemispheric lesions may be seen in the subcortical white matter. Steroids are used for first-line management in the acute phase with good response. A subset of patients present with subsequent relapses or progressive course and can be managed with disease-modifying therapies such as azathioprine.

Differential diagnosis includes an infiltrative brainstem astrocytoma, SLE or non-Behçet vasculitis, and sarcoidosis. A lower/intermediate-grade infiltrative astrocytoma cannot be excluded on imaging alone, particularly because both these entities may have mild degree of choline elevation, enhancement, and perfusion abnormalities. Sarcoidosis can show confluent periventricular WM abnormalities and meningeal enhancement, both of which are uncommon with neuro-Behçet. SLE and non-Behçet vasculitis have subcortical lesions; however, brainstem involvement is relatively uncommon.

References: Kalra S, Silman A, Akman-Demir G. et al. Diagnosis and management of Neuro-Behçet's disease: international consensus recommendations. *J Neurol* 2014;261(9):1662–1676.

Koçer N, Islak C, Siva A, et al. CNS involvement in neuro-Behçet syndrome: an MR study. *AJNR Am J Neuroradiol* 1999;20(6):1015–1024.

Yeo M, Lee HL, Cha M, et al. Neuro-Behçet disease presenting as a solitary cerebellar hemorrhagic lesion: a case report and review of the literature. *J Med Case Rep* 2016;10(1):360.

16a **Answer B.**   Susac syndrome. The triad of encephalopathy, visual field abnormalities from branch retinal arterial occlusions, and hearing loss is classic of Susac syndrome. Lyme disease and multiple sclerosis can have similar white matter changes but typically do not affect hearing. Ocular migraine causes transient monocular blindness, but bilateral visual field fixed defects are not seen. Remember that all the four listed choices can cause the shown FLAIR signal abnormalities and only history and clinical examination can further narrow the differential diagnosis.

16b **Answer D.**   Fluorescein angiography of the eye. This is the best way to assess for retinal arterial occlusions, essential for diagnosing this condition.

16c **Answer C.**   Central corpus callosal lesion shown on image B.

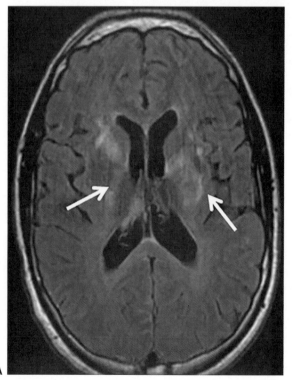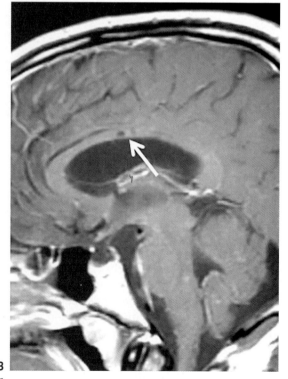

Figure 1

Imaging Findings: Figure 1. There are numerous FLAIR hyperintensities in bilateral basal ganglia, thalamic regions, (A) and mid body central corpus callosal lesion, (B), the latter being characteristic for susac syndrome in the current clinical setting, (as opposed to callmososeptal distribution of lesions seen with MS).

Discussion: Susac syndrome is a microangiopathy consisting of a triad of encephalopathy, branch retinal artery occlusions, and hearing loss. The disease is more common in women (M:F ratio 1:3) and typically presents in second to fourth decade. Etiology is unknown, but immune-mediated endotheliopathy has been implicated leading to microinfarctions from occlusion of cerebral, retinal, and cochlear arterioles. Therefore, Susac syndrome is also called SICRET syndrome—small infarctions of cochlear, retinal, and encephalic tissue.

Imaging findings closely resemble MS with multifocal white matter involvement including corpus callosum. The corpus callosum involvement is characteristically central compared to peripheral, callososeptal involvement seen with MS. The lesions may enhance during the acute phase. Leptomeningeal enhancement may be seen in 30%, whereas deep gray matter involvement (basal ganglia/thalamus) may be seen in 70%. As encephalopathy subsides, white matter lesions may become inconspicuous and atrophy becomes evident.

Common symptoms are headaches, personality/memory disturbances, dysarthria, vertigo, sensorineural hearing loss, usually low- to mid-frequency range, accompanied by tinnitus, segmental loss of vision in one or both eyes, and scotomas. Ophthalmologic evaluation with retinal fluorescein angiography is necessary to demonstrate the peripheral retinal arteriolar branch occlusion. Given relatively nonspecific imaging findings, a good clinical history/examination is key for diagnosis. It is a self-limiting disorder that may last 2 to 4 years. Treatment involves steroids, IVIG, immunosuppressive drugs, and cochlear implantation.

Differential diagnosis: Multiple sclerosis (relative sparing of deep gray matter), ADEM especially because deep gray matter involvement is common like Susac, Lyme disease, or age-related microangiopathy (no eye or cochlear involvement). In both MS and ADEM, the corpus callosal involvement is at the callososeptal interface with a characteristic central involvement seen with Susac syndrome.

References: Demir MK. Case 142: Susac syndrome. *Radiology* 2009;250(2):598–602.

Saenz R, Quan AW, Magalhaes A, et al. MRI of Susac's syndrome. *AJR Am J Roentgenol* 2005;184(5):1688–1690.

Susac JO. Susac's syndrome. *AJNR Am J Neuroradiol* 2004;25(3):351–352.

17 **Answer B.**   Oligoclonal bands. The diagnosis is right optic neuritis with MS. Oligoclonal bands may be seen in CSF. Cytoalbuminologic dissociation is seen with Guillain-Barré syndrome.

18 **Answer C.**   MRI cervical spine to evaluate the cord. In a young patient with bilateral optic nerve enhancement and limb weakness, neuromyelitis optica should be strongly suspected. Unlike MS, NMO tends to cause bilateral optic nerve involvement. NMO frequently shows long-segment spinal cord lesions, more commonly in the cervical than thoracic cord, that may or may not enhance.

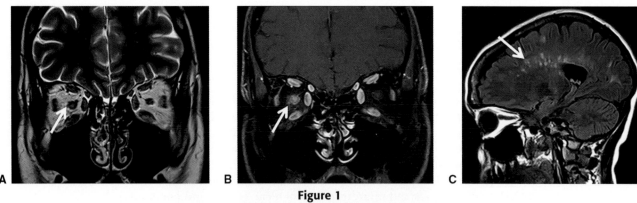

Figure 1

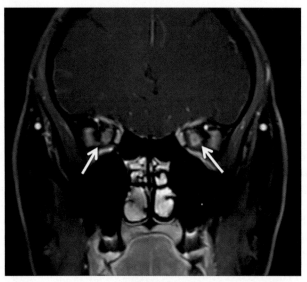

Figure 2

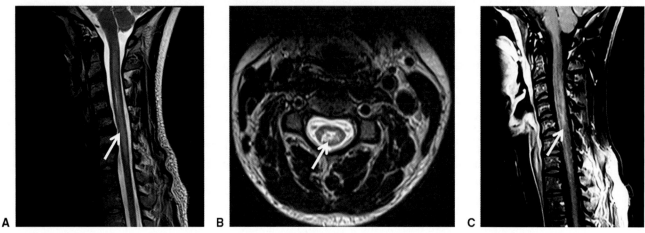

Figure 3

Imaging Findings: Figure 1. Coronal T2 and coronal fat sat postcontrast T1 images show enlargement with hyperintensity and contrast enhancement in the retrobulbar right optic nerve. Sagittal FLAIR shows multiple ovoid hyperintense lesions in the corpus callosum and centrum semiovale.

Figure 2. Coronal postcontrast T1 fat sat image shows enhancement of bilateral optic nerves (A).

Figure 3. Sagittal T2 and axial T2 images showing long-segment hyperintensity in the cervical spinal cord with mild expansion (A and B). Sagittal postcontrast T1 fast sat image shows streaky cord enhancement (C).

Discussion: Optic neuritis (ON) is inflammation of the optic nerve. Optic nerve is unique in its myelination, making it an extension of the brain itself. Unlike other cranial nerves, the optic nerve is myelinated by oligodendroglia and not by the Schwann cells, which are a hallmark of the peripheral nervous system. In addition, the optic nerve sheath is a continuation of intracranial dura matter.

ON typically consists of the classic triad of visual loss, periocular pain, and dyschromatopsia. The single most common cause of optic neuritis is multiple sclerosis (MS), and hence much of the demographics mirrors that of MS.

Other causes of ON include demyelinating lesions like neuromyelitis optica (NMO) or other less common etiologies such as autoimmune disease like sarcoidosis, systemic lupus erythematosus, infectious, and parainfectious causes like syphilis, tuberculosis, inflammatory like sinusitis, and postvaccination immunologic causes like vaccinations against measles and rubella.

MRI is investigation of choice and shows high T2, FLAIR signal in the optic nerve proper, with or without enhancement. Optic neuritis of MS is usually unilateral, whereas in NMO, it is bilateral. Inflammation of the optic nerve sheath (perineuritis) shows parallel dural enhancement in a tram-track pattern. Severe MS may have some perineuritis along with optic neuritis. Other causes that predominantly cause perineuritis are discussed under differential diagnosis.

Steroid administration is the mainstay for treatment.

Differential diagnosis: MS (usually unilateral optic neuritis, short-segment cord lesions, multiphasic, presence of brain demyelinating plaques), neuromyelitis optica (bilateral, long-segment cord lesions; brain involvement when present has a periependymal distribution), ischemia (painless, may show restricted diffusion in optic nerve), infection (usually associated with ethmoid or sphenoid infection), and optic nerve glioma (bulky, often tortuous, enhancing optic nerve, long segment, association with NF-1). Up to 75% of female patients and 35% of male patients initially presenting with optic neuritis ultimately develop MS.

References: Atkins EJ, Biousse V, Newman NJ. The natural history of optic neuritis. *Rev Neurol Dis* 2006;3(2):45–56.

Cornblath WT, Quint DJ. MRI of optic nerve enlargement in optic neuritis. *Neurology* 1997;48(4):821–825.

Kupersmith MJ, Alban T, Zeiffer B, et al. Contrast-enhanced MRI in acute optic neuritis: relationship to visual performance. *Brain* 2002;125(4):812–822.

3 Skull, Ventricles, and Developmental Abnormalities

HISHAM M. DAHMOUSH • SHYAM SABAT • SATHISH KUMAR DUNDAMADAPPA • PRACHI DUBEY

QUESTIONS

1 A 40-year-old male presents with acute-onset headache and altered mental status shortly after minor blunt trauma to the head. Key images are provided below.

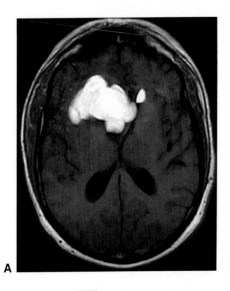
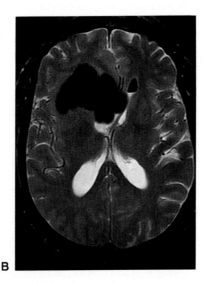
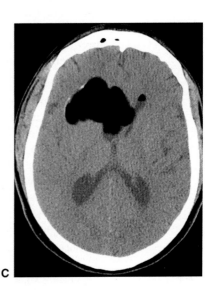

A   B   C

1a What is the most likely diagnosis?

A. Intraventricular rupture of a colloid cyst
B. Intraventricular rupture of a dermoid cyst
C. Pneumoventricle
D. Subacute intraventricular hematoma

1b What is the most likely explanation of T1 hyperintensity within this lesion on precontrast images, as shown in Image A?

A. Fat
B. Sebaceous proteinaceous contents
C. Hemorrhagic contents
D. Calcification

2   A 40-year-old male presents with chronic headaches and recently worsening nausea and vomiting. Key images from initial workup are shown below.

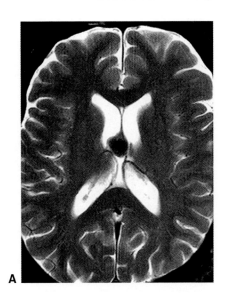
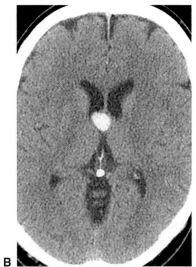
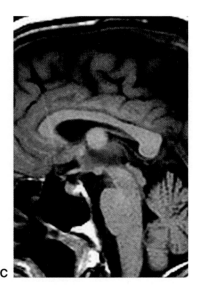

A   B   C

2a   Based on the above images, what is the most likely diagnosis?

A. Intraventricular meningioma

B. Colloid cyst

C. Subependymal giant cell astrocytoma

D. Central neurocytoma

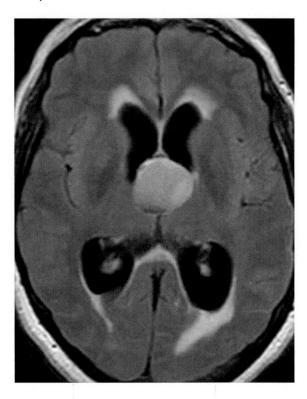

2b   What is the most likely explanation for the periventricular white matter hyperintensity on FLAIR image shown above?

A. Periventricular leukomalacia (PVL)

B. Ependymitis granularis

C. Transependymal CSF flow

D. Chronic microangiopathic change

3 A 70-year-old male with progressive cognitive decline and gait abnormality presents for further assessment of symptoms. Key images from MRI are provided below.

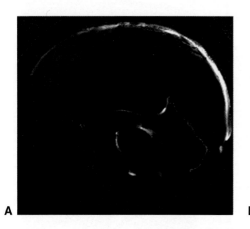

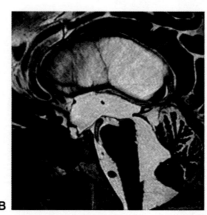

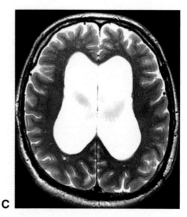

A   B   C

3a Based on the above images and clinical features, what is the most likely diagnosis?

A. Aqueductal stenosis
B. Tectal glioma
C. Idiopathic normal pressure hydrocephalus (iNPH)
D. Age-related white matter atrophy

3b Which other diagnostic tests can be performed to aid in the diagnosis of idiopathic normal pressure hydrocephalus?

A. High-volume lumbar puncture
B. CT myelogram
C. Transcranial Doppler US
D. Florbetapir amyloid imaging

4 Below are key images from a neonatal MRI performed for a congenital abnormality.

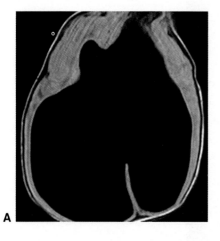

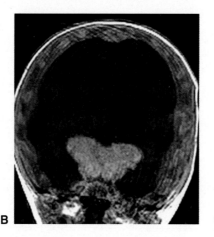

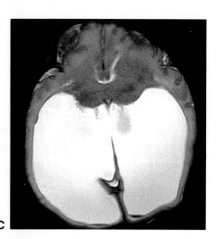

A   B   C

Based on the above images, what is the most appropriate diagnosis?

A. Microform holoprosencephaly
B. Semilobar holoprosencephaly
C. Alobar holoprosencephaly
D. Lobar holoprosencephaly

5   Severe ventricular enlargement was noted on CT. MRI was performed for better assessment. Key images are shown below.

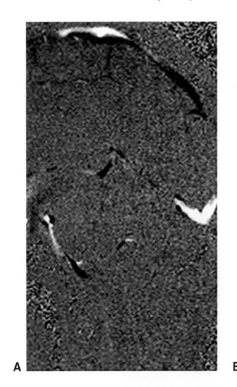

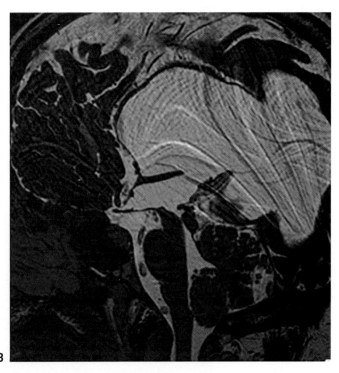

A   B

Based on the above images, what is the most likely diagnosis?

A. Idiopathic normal pressure hydrocephalus
B. Aqueductal stenosis
C. Communicating hydrocephalus
D. Corpus callosal dysgenesis

6   An infant presents with recurrent apneic spells thought to be seizures. Further workup reveals abnormal brain MRI. Key images are shown below.

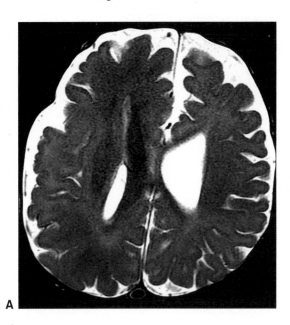

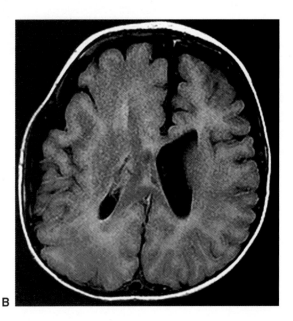

A   B

6a What is the most likely diagnosis?

    A. Lissencephaly
    B. Hemimegalencephaly
    C. Schizencephaly
    D. Dyke-Davidoff-Masson syndrome

6b What is the characteristic abnormality in the above disorder?

    A. Cerebral hemiatrophy
    B. Hamartomatous overgrowth
    C. Absence of cortical gyration
    D. Small ipsilateral ventricle

7 An MRI was performed for characterization of a congenital abnormality. Key image is shown below.

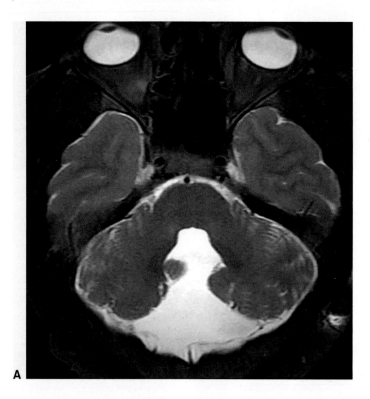

A

7a The congenital abnormality in the above image is a result of which of the following embryologic malformations?

    A. Aplasia or hypoplasia of the cerebellar vermis
    B. Partial fusion of the cerebellar hemispheres
    C. Formation of a cerebellar cleft
    D. Formation of a retrocerebellar cyst

7b Which of the following clinical features is highly prevalent with this condition?

    A. Micrognathia
    B. Microcephaly
    C. Craniofacial anomalies
    D. Macrocephaly

8 Key images from an MRI performed for evaluation of refractory seizures are shown.

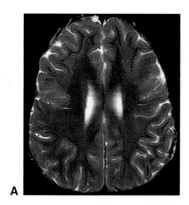
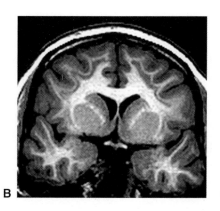
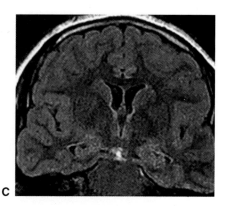

A   B   C

What is the most striking abnormality on MRI in this patient who also had an abnormal EEG?

A. Subependymal nodular heterotopia
B. Subcortical dysmyelination
C. Subcortical band heterotopia
D. Bifrontal focal cortical dysplasia

9 Based on the following image, what is the most likely diagnosis?

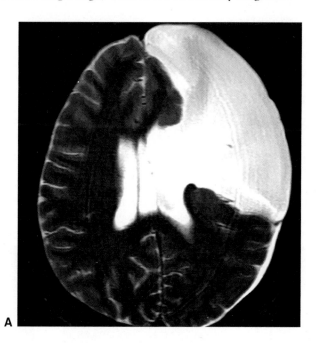

A

9a What is the most likely diagnosis?

A. Porencephalic cyst
B. Open-lip schizencephaly
C. Closed-lip schizencephaly
D. Cystic encephalomalacia

9b Which of the following is a key feature of this diagnosis?

A. Cleft lined by gray matter
B. Cleft lined by white matter
C. Cleft without ependymal communication
D. Presence of a cyst wall

10

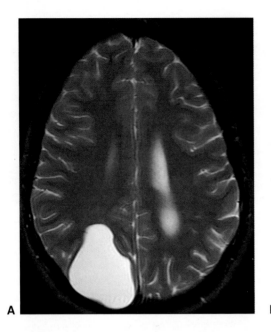
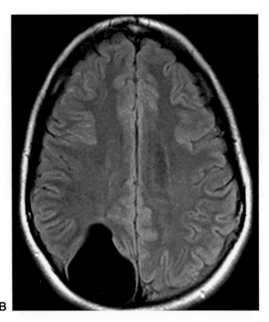

A

B

10a What is the key finding seen on this image that distinguishes this entity from other morphologically similar conditions?

    A. Peripheral cortical location
    B. Contact with the pial surface
    C. White matter lining the cyst wall
    D. Scalloping of the calvarium

10b What is the most likely diagnosis?

    A. Porencephalic cyst
    B. Open-lip schizencephaly
    C. Closed-lip schizencephaly
    D. Hydranencephaly

11 A 35-year-old female presented with post-LP headache and photophobia. Key images from an MRI are shown below.

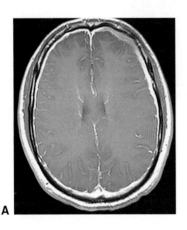
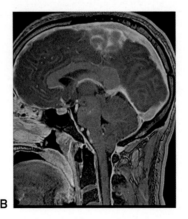
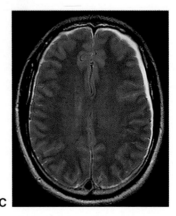

A

B

C

11a What is the most likely diagnosis in the current clinical setting?

    A. Meningoencephalitis
    B. Bifrontal subdural empyema
    C. Chiari 1 malformation
    D. Intracranial hypotension

11b What is the most likely explanation for the pachymeningeal enhancement seen with this entity?

  A. Congenital developmental anomaly
  B. Dural venous engorgement
  C. Infection related to nonsterile puncture technique
  D. Reactive because of chronic subdural hematoma

12 Key images from an MRI of a child with cerebral palsy born preterm with congenital heart disease are provided below.

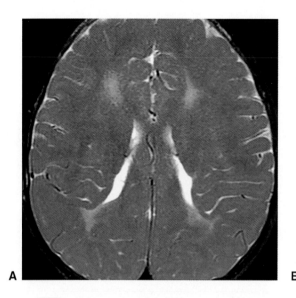
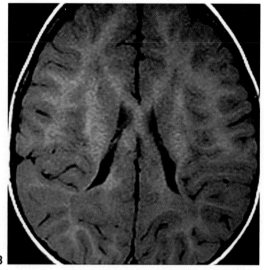

A   B

12a What is the most likely diagnosis?

  A. No abnormality is noted.
  B. Periventricular leukomalacia
  C. Colpocephaly
  D. Tuberous sclerosis

12b What is the most likely etiologic factor for this appearance in the provided clinical setting?

  A. Hypoxic–ischemic white matter injury
  B. Congenital neuronal migration abnormality
  C. Antenatal CMV exposure
  D. Gestational diabetes

13 A 19-year-old male presents with seizures.

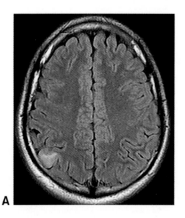
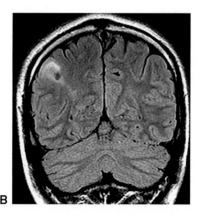
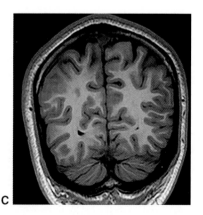

A   B   C

13a What is the most likely diagnosis?

    A. Polymicrogyria
    B. Ependymoma
    C. Focal cortical dysplasia
    D. Gray matter heterotopia

13b Which of the following is a characteristic imaging feature for this entity?

    A. Blurring of the gray–white matter junction
    B. Gray matter signal intensity on all pulse sequences
    C. Mass effect and vasogenic edema
    D. Cortical thinning

14 A 75-year-old male presented to the ER after fall. A head CT was performed and showed an incidental finding. Key images are provided below.

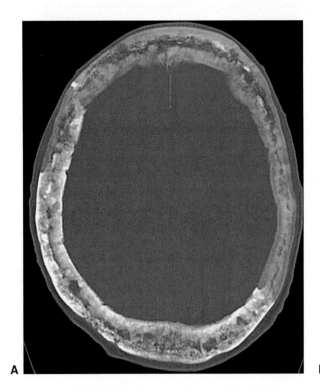 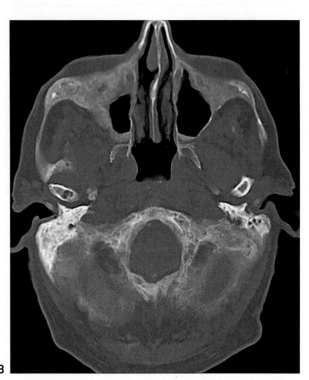

A   B

14a What can be potential neurologic complications associated with this disease process?

    A. Gait impairment
    B. Progressive cognitive decline
    C. Multiple cranial neuropathies
    D. Refractory seizures

14b What percentage of patients may have a sarcomatous transformation complicating the above disease process?

    A. <10%
    B. 30% to 40%
    C. >90%
    D. None

15 A 19 year-old female with profound learning disability presents for initial evaluation. An MRI was performed. Key images are shown below.

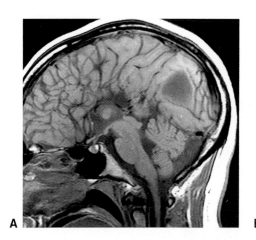
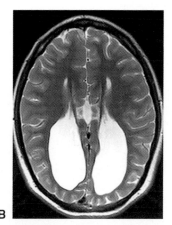
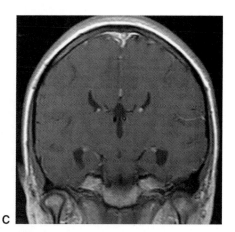

A   B   C

15a What is the most likely diagnosis?

  A. Porencephaly

  B. Holoprosencephaly

  C. Agenesis of the corpus callosum

  D. Communicating hydrocephalus

15b The above condition is

  A. Highly associated with other CNS anomalies.

  B. Not associated with genetic mutations.

  C. Easily diagnosed with prenatal US.

  D. Accurately diagnosed with fetal MRI at 17 weeks of gestation.

16 A 33-year-old woman with chronic headaches and an abnormal MRI.

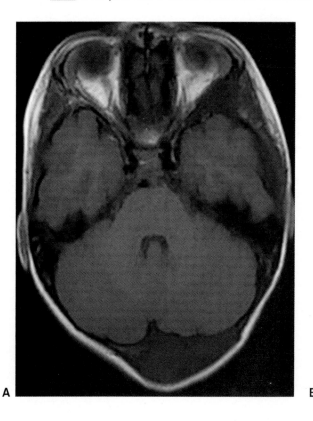
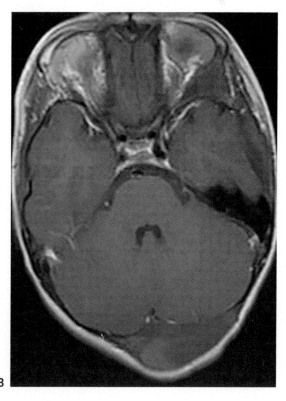

A   B

16a What is the most appropriate next step?

    A. A follow-up MRI with gadolinium
    B. A CT head without contrast
    C. Recommend a bone scan.
    D. Recommend an FDG-PET.

A follow-up evaluation with a noncontrast CT was performed.

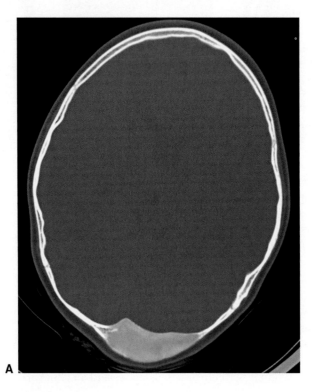

A

16b What is the most likely diagnosis?

    A. Paget disease
    B. Sphenoid bone metastasis
    C. Fibrous dysplasia
    D. Plasmacytoma

17 Two different patients present with the same diagnosis. Patient 1 (A and B) is a 19-month-old boy with hypotonia, developmental delay, and abnormal eye movements, whereas patient 2 (C) is a 13-year-old girl with ataxia, hypotonia, and hyperreflexia.

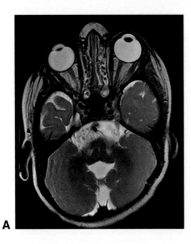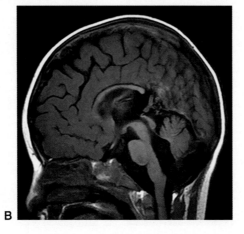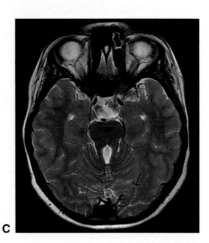

A   B   C

17a What is the most likely diagnosis?

    A. Dandy-Walker malformation
    B. Pontine tegmental cap dysplasia
    C. Rhombencephalosynapsis
    D. Joubert syndrome

17b Which of the following statements best describes the "molar tooth" appearance?

    A. A sign specific for Joubert syndrome
    B. A sign predictive of hypotonia, ataxia, and developmental delay
    C. Results from lack of decussation of inferior cerebellar peduncles
    D. Describes the morphology of the cerebellar vermis

18 Patient 1 (A) is a 1-day-old girl with abnormal prenatal MRI. Patient 2 (B) is a 9-year-old boy with history of congenital hydrocephalus and poor feeding.

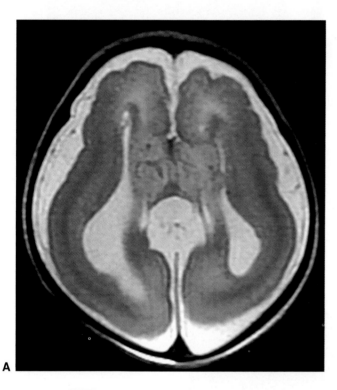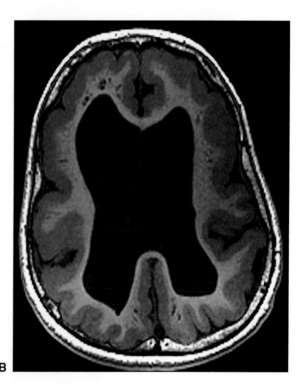

A   B

18a What is the most likely diagnosis?

    A. Normal premature brain
    B. Lissencephaly
    C. Focal cortical dysplasia
    D. Subcortical gray matter heterotopia

18b What is the most helpful finding in predicting the underlying genetic mutation?

    A. The degree of cortical thickness
    B. The predilection for lobes involved
    C. The other associated anomalies
    D. The severity of clinical phenotype

19 A 25-year-old woman with headache and blurred vision. Key images from an MRI are shown below.

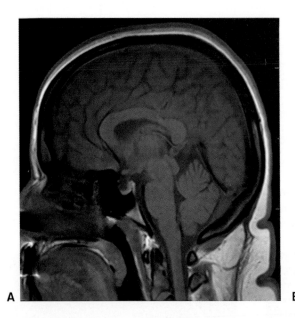

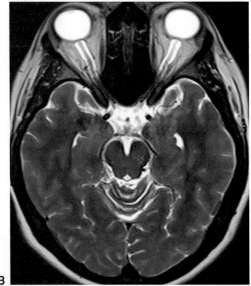

A   B

19a What is the most likely diagnosis in the current clinical setting?

A. CSF hypotension
B. Pseudotumor cerebri
C. Morning glory syndrome with bilateral optic nerve colobomas
D. Overshunting

19b What imaging would you recommend to further increase your diagnostic probability?

A. Color Doppler
B. Ultrasound B scan of the eyes
C. MR venogram
D. CT venogram

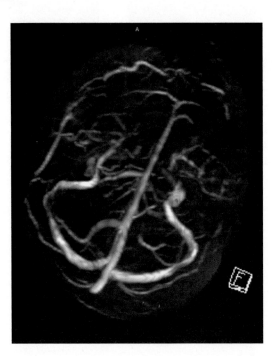

19c An MRV was performed and key image is shown. What can be considered as the next step?

- A. Catheter cerebral angiogram
- B. Nuclear cisternogram
- C. Lumbar puncture
- D. CT myelogram

20 A 9-month-old male with nystagmus and abnormal eye exam. Key images from an MRI are shown below.

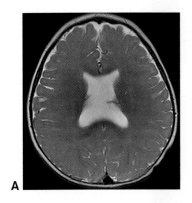
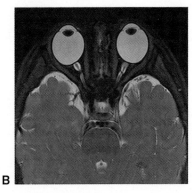
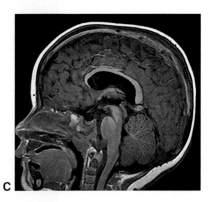

A B C

20a What is the most likely diagnosis?

- A. Hydrocephalus
- B. Agenesis of the corpus callosum
- C. Septooptic dysplasia
- D. Pituitary stalk interruption syndrome

20b What is the most common malformation associated with this entity?

- A. Focal cortical dysplasia
- B. Brain tumors
- C. Schizencephaly
- D. Polymicrogyria

21 A 5-week-old girl presents with abnormal head shape. Key image from a CT head is shown below.

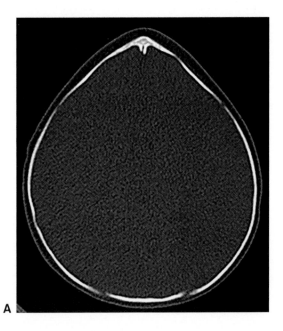

A

21a Which suture has undergone premature synostosis?

A. Sagittal suture
B. Lambdoid suture
C. Coronal suture
D. Metopic suture

A 2-year-old girl presents with abnormal head shape and syndactyly. A volume-rendered 3D reconstruction from a CT head was generated, shown below.

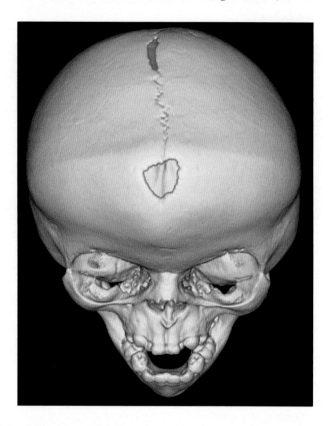

21b Which of the following terms best describes the resulting skull morphology from the above shown premature synostosis?

A. Brachycephaly
B. Scaphocephaly
C. Trigonocephaly
D. Cloverleaf skull

ANSWERS AND EXPLANATIONS

1a **Answer B.** Intraventricular rupture of a dermoid cyst.

1b **Answer A.** Fat. Protein, calcification, and hemorrhage will show varying degree of hyperattenuation on CT unlike this case.

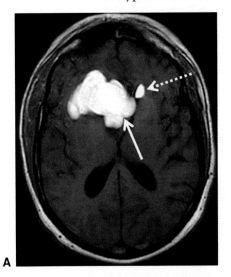
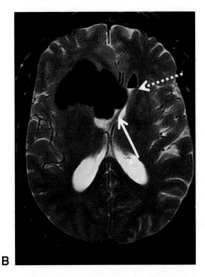
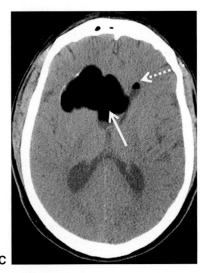

A   B   C

Imaging Findings: Lobulated T1 hyperintense intraventricular mass (A), which is hypointense on fat saturation T2 (B) and hypoattenuating on CT, most compatible with fat. Note a fat fluid level is seen anteriorly in the frontal horn of the left lateral ventricle. These features are most compatible with intraventricular rupture of a fatty lesion, such as dermoid cyst.

Discussion: Ruptured dermoid with intraventricular fat fluid level. Dermoid cysts are rare congenital inclusion cysts, resulting from inclusion of embryonic ectoderm into neural tube during 3rd to 5th weeks of embryonic life. They tend to occur in the midline, commonly sellar region, frontonasal region, and in the posterior fossa. The cyst wall is characterized by a stratified squamous epithelium capsule that contains dermal elements including sebaceous glands, sweat glands, and hair follicles. The contents of cyst include desquamated epithelium, sebaceous gland secretions, fat, and hair. Calcification and rarely teeth can be seen.

Unruptured lesions are mostly asymptomatic; the symptoms depend on location and size and mostly related to the mass effect. The dermoid cysts can grow, related to increase of internal contents by desquamation of epithelium and secretion of adnexal glands. Rupture of dermoid is rare, but well documented. The rupture is usually spontaneous but has also been reported after closed head trauma. It is hypothesized that increases in glandular secretions, possibly related to age-related hormonal changes mainly lead to rapid enlargement and subsequent rupture. On rupture, patients present with various symptoms including headache, seizures, focal neurologic deficits, aseptic meningitis, hydrocephalus, vasospasm, and cerebral ischemia. Aseptic meningeal inflammation by ruptured contents and aqueductal occlusion are felt to be the etiology for these symptoms.

On imaging, these are mostly fatty lesions, secondary to liquid cholesterol. On CT scans, the lesions show fat density. On MRI, the lesions are hyperintense on T1-weighted images and shows variable intensity in T2-weighted images. They can be heterogeneous, related to the calcification. They show no enhancement following contrast administration. On rupture, fat density/intensity droplets will be seen in subarachnoid spaces and also within the ventricular system. Pial enhancement can be seen from chemical meningitis in cases of rupture.

Differential diagnosis:

Epidermoid cyst: This is another inclusion cyst and shows a near CSF signal and not fat signal.

Lipoma: Homogenous fat attenuation.

References: Koh YC, Choi JW, Moon WJ, et al. Intracranial dermoid cyst ruptured into the membranous labyrinth causing sudden sensorineural hearing loss: CT and MR imaging findings. *Am J Neuroradiol* 2012;33(5):E69–E71. doi: 10.3174/ajnr.A2627.

Liu JK, Gottfried ON, Salzman KL, et al. Ruptured intracranial dermoid cysts: clinical, radiographic, and surgical features. *Neurosurgery* 2008;62(2):377–384; discussion 384. doi: 10.1227/01.neu.0000316004.88517.29.

Osborn AG, Preece MT. Intracranial cysts: radiologic-pathologic correlation and imaging approach. *Radiology* 2006;239(3):650–664. doi: 10.1148/radiol.2393050823.

2a **Answer B.** Colloid cyst.

2b **Answer C.** Transependymal CSF flow. This is the most likely explanation given the confluent periventricular FLAIR hyperintensity in the setting of hydrocephalus due to a large colloid cyst obstructing the foramen of Monro. Ependymitis granularis is a normal variant, smaller triangular foci of FLAIR hyperintense signal seen abutting the frontal horns of lateral ventricles. Chronic microangiopathic change is unlikely given no other deep or subcortical white matter changes are seen. PVL is seen in children because of prematurity-related white matter injury resulting in necrosis and cyst formation, unlike this case.

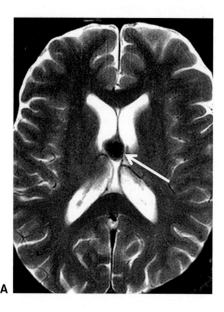
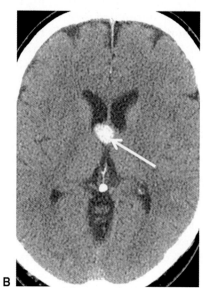
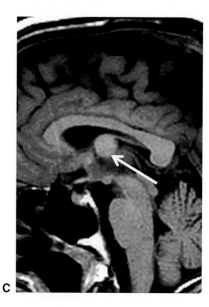

A B C

Figure 1

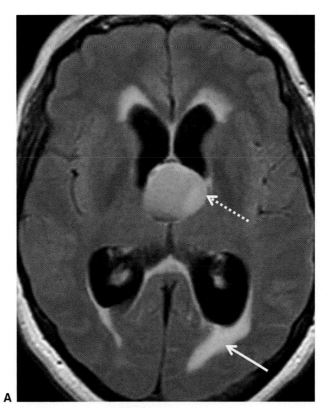

Figure 2

Imaging Findings: Figure 1. There is a rounded hypointense structure on T2w sequence at the foramen of Monro (A), that is, hyperdense on CT (B) and isointense to white matter on Sag T1w (C).

Figure 2. There is periventricular FLAIR hyperintensity in the setting of obstructive hydrocephalus due to a colloid cyst obstructing the foramen of Monro.

Discussion: Colloid cysts are rare anterior third ventricular lesions, typically draped by fornices. Location other than anterior third ventricle (other ventricles or even outside the ventricular system) has been reported, but very rare. These are spherical smooth-walled cysts and vary in size from a few millimeters to several centimeters.

The cyst is lined by simple to pseudostratified epithelial lining with interspersed goblet cells and ciliated cells. The cyst content is likely derived from secretions and breakdown products from the epithelium.

They are typically seen in adults in third to fifth decade of life with headache being the most common presenting symptom. On CT, about two-thirds of the lesions are hyperdense and about one-third isodense and rarely hypodense. The appearance on MRI is more variable. On T1 images, 50% of lesions are hyperintense and the rest hypointense or isointense. On T2-weighted images, most are hypointense. Hemorrhage and fluid–fluid levels can occasionally be seen. Following contrast administration, the lesions either do not enhance or only show thin peripheral enhancement. The smaller lesions are often better seen on CT and can occasionally be not apparent on MRI because of their signal characteristics and also related to thicker slices. Biventricular hydrocephalus is the dreaded complication of colloid cysts, secondary to obstruction at the foramen of Monro. They may have pendulous attachment to third ventricular roof and can cause intermittent hydrocephalus. Acute hydrocephalus and sudden death are known to occur with these lesions. But in our clinical experience, these are rare with smaller lesions. These are generally surgically treated. Hypodense appearance on CT and iso- to hyperintensity on T2 images suggest less viscous and more fluid-like content and may correlate with easier stereotactic aspiration. Recurrence rate is about 10% with incomplete resection of the wall.

References: Armao D, Castillo M, Chen H, et al. Colloid cyst of the third ventricle: imaging-pathologic correlation. *Am J Neuroradiol* 2000;21(8):1470–1477.

Marshman LA, Chawda SJ, David KM. Change in CT radiodensity of a colloid cyst of the third ventricle: case report and literature review. *Neuroradiology* 2004;46(12):984–987. doi: 10.1007/s00234-004-1303-2.

3a **Answer C.** Idiopathic normal pressure hydrocephalus (iNPH). This is most likely given the clinical features of cognitive dysfunction and gait abnormality in the setting of profound ventriculomegaly out of proportion to sulcal enlargement is seen. Image A shows prominent flow through the aqueduct on the phase contrast CSF flow study and Image B shows wide patency of the aqueduct, arguing against the diagnosis of aqueductal stenosis. Tectal glioma also causes obstruction at the aqueductal level, not seen in this case. The lack of sulcal enlargement is atypical for age-related atrophy.

3b **Answer A.** High-volume lumbar puncture. Pre-LP and post-LP functional testing can be performed with withdrawal of 30 to 40 mL of CSF as an additional diagnostic tool for idiopathic NPH. The other choices are not appropriate tools for assessment of iNPH.

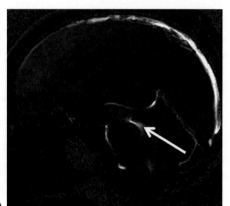
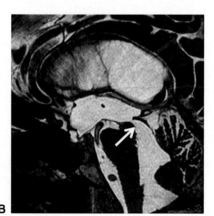
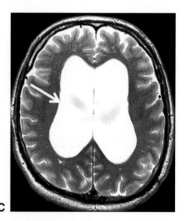

A   B   C

Imaging Findings: Sagittal phase contrast CSF flow MRI showing hyperdynamic flow through the cerebral aqueduct (A). Sagittal 3D CISS showing a patent cerebral aqueduct with prominent dilation of lateral, third, and fourth ventricle (B). Axial T2w image showing dilated lateral ventricles out of proportion to sulcal enlargement. There is no evidence of periventricular transependymal CSF flow (C). These features in the current clinical setting are most compatible with normal pressure hydrocephalus.

Discussion: Idiopathic normal pressure hydrocephalus (iNPH) is a syndrome of ventricular enlargement associated with the clinical Hakim-Adams triad of urinary incontinence, dementia, and gait abnormalities without an obstructive cause.

It is thought to be related to nonobstructive impairment of CSF reabsorption. Ventriculosulcal disproportion is present in the form of widening of the ventricles and sylvian fissure with narrowing of suprasylvian and medial hemispheric subarachnoid spaces.

Evans index is used as an estimate of ventricular enlargement, measured as a ratio between the maximal diameter of the frontal horns and the inner diameter of the skull, with a ratio of >0.3 considered abnormal. Recent study shows, however, that more than one-fifth of the population-based sample had an EI > 0.3 and an EI ≥ 0.3 was average for men 80 years or older in age. This suggests that diagnosis of iNPH cannot be made based on EI alone, and clinical features as well as data from other diagnostic test should be factored into consideration.

A phase contrast MRI with measurement of aqueductal CSF stroke volume, high-volume LP (drainage of 30 to 40 cc of CSF, with pre-LP and post-LP functional status assessment), and nuclear cisternogram are other diagnostic test that can be utilized for iNPH diagnosis.

Management can be conservative or surgical using VP shunting or recently endoscopic third ventriculostomy. Hyperdynamic CSF flow through the aqueduct has been associated with good response to shunting. Phase contrast MRI can be used to quantify the aqueductal stroke volume, with iNPH patients who have twice the aqueductal stroke volume compared to age-matched controls, being most responsive to shunting.

References: Bradley WG Jr. Magnetic resonance imaging of normal pressure hydrocephalus. *Semin Ultrasound CT MR* 2016;37(2):120–128.

Jaraj D, Rabiei K, Marlow T, et al. Estimated ventricle size using Evans index: reference values from a population-based sample. *Eur J Neurol* 2017;24(3):468–474.

Tudor KI, Tudor M, McCleery J, et al. Endoscopic third ventriculostomy (ETV) for idiopathic normal pressure hydrocephalus (iNPH). *Cochrane Database Syst Rev* 2015;(7):CD010033.

4 **Answer B.** Semilobar holoprosencephaly. The interhemispheric fissure is seen posteriorly with partial fusion of the thalami. The septum pellucidum is absent and >50% of frontal lobes are not separated.

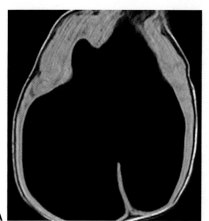
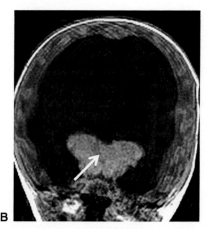
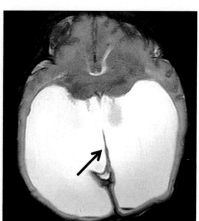

A   B   C

Imaging Findings: A large ventricle with absent septum pellucidum (A), presence of partially fused thalami (arrow B), and posteriorly seen interhemispheric fissure (A and C) are present. Findings are suggestive of semilobar holoprosencephaly.

Discussion: Holoprosencephaly (HPE) is the most common developmental malformation of the CNS. It has a multifactorial etiology with chromosomal/genetic causes, syndromic associations, exposure to teratogens, maternal diabetes, alcohol, and smoking. It can vary from minimal or microform subtypes with no to minimal anatomic defects on MRI to alobar, the most severe and lethal variant. Primary morphologic subtypes of HPE are as follows:

1. Alobar HPE: complete lack of hemispheric cleavage, characterized by a primitive monoventricle, fused thalami.

2. Semilobar HPE: partial cleavage with presence of falx or interhemispheric fissure posteriorly, >50% fusion of the frontal lobes and partial fusion of thalami. Anterior mantle of continuous brain parenchyma may be seen.
3. Lobar HPE: The interhemispheric fissure is nearly completely present with complete or near-complete cleavage of the thalami. The third ventricle and splenium/posterior body corpus callosum may also be present. Septum pellucidum is absent, and inferior frontal lobes may be fused.
4. Middle interhemispheric HPE: lack of cleavage of posterior frontal and parietal regions, characteristic of vertically oriented sylvian fissures

A dorsal cyst is commonly seen with the alobar form. Differentiation between semilobar and lobar forms may often be difficult, and presence of a rudimentary frontal horn and third ventricle may point toward the latter. Prognosis with this condition is poor. The severity along the spectrum of HPE determines survival with most severe forms being lethal in early childhood/infancy, and milder forms can survive longer, however, with significant developmental delays and morbidity.

Differential Diagnosis: Differential diagnosis is severe hydrocephalus and hydranencephaly. Evaluation of thalamic and hemispheric separation and presence of septum pellucidum can help distinguish from HPE.

Reference: Winter TC, Kennedy AM, Woodward PJ. Holoprosencephaly: a survey of the entity, with embryology and fetal imaging. *Radiographics* 2015;35(1):275–290.

5 **Answer B.** Aqueductal stenosis. Marked hydrocephalus most severely involving the lateral ventricle with relative sparing of the fourth ventricle is seen. Based on the lack of flow through the cerebral aqueduct on Image A and anatomic obstruction seen within the aqueduct on B, the most appropriate diagnosis is aqueductal stenosis.

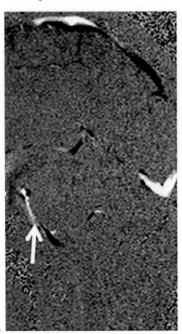
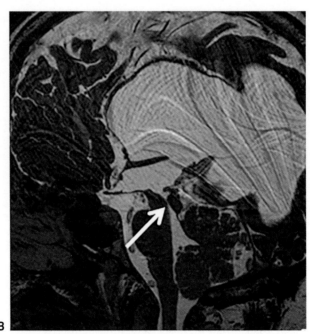

A   B

Imaging Findings: Sagittal phase contrast CSF flow study shows lack of flow through the aqueduct (A) in the setting of prominent enlargement of the third and lateral ventricles (B). There is a soft tissue focus within the aqueduct seen on the sagittal 3D CISS (B).

Discussion: Aqueductal stenosis (AS) is one of the causes of noncommunicating hydrocephalus. It is a triventricular hydrocephalus with dilation of lateral and third ventricle with relative sparing of the fourth ventricle. It can be caused by congenital or acquired obstruction at the level of aqueduct of Sylvius.

Congenital causes:

1. Aqueductal stenosis: Narrowing is generally focal and can be proximal or distal, more commonly proximal at the level of superior colliculi or intercollicular sulcus. Diffuse narrowing can also be seen (aqueduct atresia). In many cases of narrowing, the aqueduct can be divided into ventral and dorsal columns with several ductules within the dorsal column, known as "forking."
2. Aqueductal web/membrane
3. Aqueductal gliosis: postinflammatory, secondary to perinatal hemorrhage or infection

Acquired causes:

1. Intrinsic obstruction: adhesion due to hemorrhage, meningitis, ventriculitis
2. Extrinsic compression: tectal plate glioma, pineal tumor

Imaging features include triventricular dilatation—dilatation of lateral and third ventricles and relatively small/normal-sized fourth ventricle. Relatively small/occluded aqueduct seen on thin/3D fluid-sensitive sequences. Sagittal 3D steady state sequence (FIESTA/CISS) is commonly used for this purpose. There is visible CSF obstruction in the aqueduct (lack of CSF flow–related artifact on T2-weighted images). Cardiac-gated phase contrast CSF flow studies are helpful. Periaqueductal mass may also be seen on MRI, because CT can be insensitive to tectal masses. Periventricular edema is variable, generally present in symptomatic patients.

Differential Diagnosis: Differential diagnosis includes normal pressure hydrocephalus, because it is not uncommon for the fourth ventricle to be smaller in size in NPH. CSF flow studies are helpful in demonstrating presence of flow across the aqueduct in difficult cases.

Endoscopic third ventriculostomy and VP shunting are the treatment options for the hydrocephalus.

References: Aqueduct Stenosis | Radiology Reference Article | Radiopaedia.org. Available at http://radiopaedia.org/articles/aqueduct-stenosis. Accessed on June 10, 2016.

Barkovich AJ, Raybaud C. *Pediatric neuroimaging*, 5th ed. Philadelphia, PA: Lippincott Williams & Wilkins, 2011.

Harrison MJ, Robert CM, Uttley D. Benign aqueduct stenosis in adults. *J Neurol Neurosurg Psychiatry* 1974;37(12):1322–1328.

Rumboldt Z, ed. *Brain imaging with MRI and CT: an image pattern approach.* Cambridge, UK: Cambridge University Press, 2012.

Stoquart-El Sankari S, Lehmann P, Gondry-Jouet C, et al. Phase-contrast MR imaging support for the diagnosis of aqueductal stenosis. *AJNR Am J Neuroradiol* 2009;30(1):209–214. doi: 10.3174/ajnr.A1308.

6a **Answer B.** Hemimegalencephaly. There is enlargement of the right cerebral hemisphere with a dysmorphic right lateral ventricle and areas of abnormal cortical thickening and gyral pattern.

6b **Answer B.** Hamartomatous overgrowth. Hamartomatous overgrowth of one hemisphere or part of it with associated neuronal migration anomalies are characteristic abnormalities seen with this disorder. Cerebral hemiatrophy is seen with Dyke-Davidoff-Masson syndrome. Absence of cortical gyration is seen with lissencephaly (smooth cortical surface). This disorder can have enlargement of ipsilateral ventricle; however, some cases may show smaller ipsilateral ventricle.

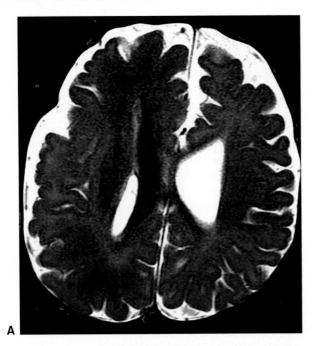
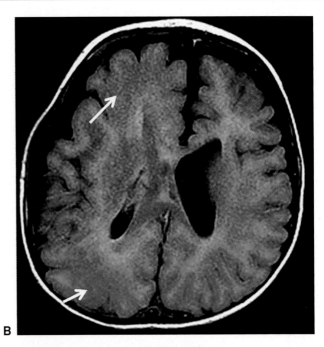

A   B

Imaging Findings: There is enlargement of the right cerebral hemisphere with dysmorphic appearance of the right lateral ventricle. Broadening of gyri with thickened cortical mantle is also noted in the right frontal and parietooccipital cortices (arrows B). These findings are most consistent with hemimegalencephaly.

Discussion: Hemimegalencephaly is a congenital developmental condition characterized by hamartomatous overgrowth of one or part of a hemisphere with associated neuronal migrational anomalies as is evident in the form of pachygyria-polymicrogyria along with unilateral hemispheric enlargement.

There is no gender predilection. The disease can be isolated or part of a syndrome such as tuberous sclerosis, or NF type 1. Typically hemispheric, rarely, total hemimegalencephaly can involve unilateral hemisphere, with ipsilateral brainstem and cerebellum. There may be characteristic enlargement of the frontal horn of the lateral ventricle although the ipsilateral ventricle enlargement is less pronounced compared to the rest of the involved hemisphere. Some patients may even have smaller ipsilateral ventricle. Agyria, pachygyria, and polymicrogyria may be associated with this condition.

Clinically, patients have severe developmental delay, refractory seizures, and hemiplegia/hemianopia. Prognosis is poor because of significant neurologic dysfunction. Primary goal of management is seizure control for which antiepilepsy drugs are used. In patients with refractory epilepsy anatomic or functional hemispherectomy can be performed.

Reference: Broumandi DD, Hayward UM, Benzian JM, et al. Best cases from the AFIP: hemimegalencephaly. *Radiographics* 2004;24(3):843–848.

7a **Answer A.** Aplasia or hypoplasia of the cerebellar vermis. This image shows wide opening of the fourth ventricle and absence of a cerebellar vermis. This appearance is characteristic of Dandy-Walker malformation.

7b **Answer D.** Macrocephaly. Macrocephaly is the most common clinical feature associated with Dandy-Walker malformation present in >90% of infants with this condition.

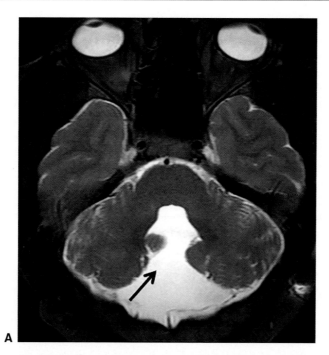

A

Imaging Findings: Wide opening of the fourth ventricle seen along the posterior edge continuous with a posterior fossa cystic space. No vermis is identified. The cerebellar hemispheres are maintained without evidence of hypoplasia or fusion. This appearance is characteristic of Dandy-Walker malformation.

Discussion: Dandy-Walker malformation shown here is characterized by abnormal vermian development. The vermis is either absent or profoundly hypoplastic. There is associated dilation of the fourth ventricle with a large opening into a cystic posterior fossa space as shown here. The tentorium may be elevated because of a large posterior fossa. These patients may have associated hydrocephalus that can benefit from early shunting. Developmental delay, seizures, mental retardation, and macrocephaly are common clinical manifestations. Macrocephaly is the most common clinical manifestation association with this condition and can be seen early in infancy.

Reference: Abdel Razek AA, Castillo M. Magnetic resonance imaging of malformations of midbrain-hindbrain. *J Comput Assist Tomogr* 2016;40(1):14–25.

8   Answer C.   Subcortical band heterotopia.

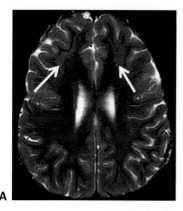

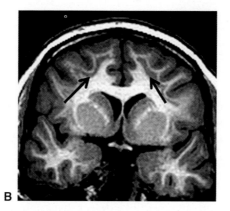

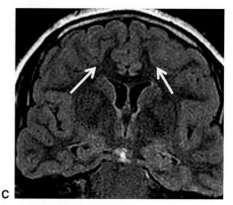

A   **B**   **C**

Imaging Findings: There is curvilinear subcortical band of abnormal signal that is isointense to gray matter on all sequences, most compatible with subcortical laminar heterotopia.

Discussion: Subcortical band heterotopia (SBH), also referred to as "double cortex," is a congenital neuronal migration disorder associated with abnormal gray matter settling underneath the cortex separated from the cortex by a thin layer of white matter. The thickness of the abnormal subcortical gray matter can vary from thin curvilinear to a thick band of tissue. Subcortical band heterotopia (SBH) is classified with lissencephaly complex (agyria–pachygyria) and not with the other heterotopias. SBH may result from less severe mutations of DSX or LIS1 gene, in addition, a genetic defect on X chromosome in the gene that codes for doublecortin is implicated in some of the cases. Based on the extent of abnormality on the spectrum, the patient can be asymptomatic or have seizures and intellectual impairment.

The most common form of heterotopias is subependymal or periventricular heterotopia, typically the nodular form. These heterotopias due to abnormal neuronal migration can be classified as follows:

- Subependymal (periventricular) heterotopia
- Subcortical nodular heterotopia (not the band type; note that SBH is classified with lissencephaly as a part of the classic lissencephaly spectrum)
- Marginal glioneuronal heterotopia (or sometimes referred to as leptomeningeal heterotopias). This is a rare entity, with glioneuronal proliferations overlying the cortex and protruding into the subarachnoid spaces.

References: Barkovich AJ, Kuzniecky RI, Jackson GD, et al. Classification system for malformations of cortical development: update 2001. *Neurology* 2001;57(12):2168–2178.

Guerrini R, Parrini E. Neuronal migration disorders. *Neurobiol Dis* 2010;38:154–166.

Nalbantoglu M, Erturk-Cetin O, Gozubatik-Celik G, et al. The diagnosis of band heterotopia. *Pediatr Neurol* 2014;51(1):178–180.

9a **Answer B.** Open-lip schizencephaly.

9b **Answer A.** Cleft lined by gray matter. It is a key feature for diagnosis.

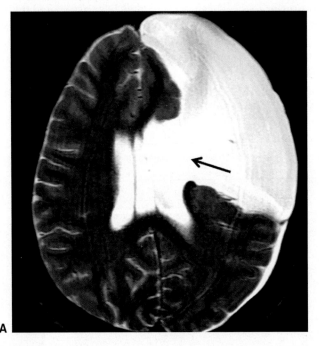

A

Imaging Findings: A large open cleft-like defect that communicates with the ventricle (arrow) and pial surface and is lined by gray matter. This is most compatible with open-lip schizencephaly. If the loss of brain tissue is minimal and the cleft walls are apposed, it is termed as closed-lip schizencephaly.

Discussion: Schizencephaly is a disorder of cortical malformation characterized by a gray matter–lined cleft that communicates with pial and ependymal lining. Depending on the amount of loss of neural tissue, the cleft can be wide as in this case, referred to as open-lip schizencephaly or minimal with apposed walls, namely, closed-lip schizencephaly. In the latter, the demonstration of ependymal communication may be challenging, and usually, an outward dimple is noted in the ventricle wall. This can be associated with subependymal heterotopia usually adjacent to the ependymal continuation and juxtaposed dysplastic cortical gyri. These are usually unilateral; however, one-third of the cases are bilateral. These are most common in the frontal or frontoparietal lobes. This is a rare abnormality and often found in conjunction with polymicrogyria. Depending on the severity of defect, the patients may be neurologically intact to profound neurologic defects, mental retardation, and developmental delay. Nearly all patients have epilepsy.

References: Barkovich AJ, Guerrini R, Kuzniecky RI, et al. A developmental and genetic classification for malformations of cortical development: update 2012. *Brain* 2012;135(Pt 5):1348-1369. doi: 10.1093/brain/aws019.

Barkovich AJ, Raybaud CA. Neuroimaging in disorders of cortical development. *Neuroimaging Clin N Am* 2004;14(2):231-254.

Hayashi N, Tsutsumi Y, Barkovich AJ. Morphological features and associated anomalies of schizencephaly in the clinical population: detailed analysis of MR images. *Neuroradiology* 2002;44(5):418-427.

10a Answer C. White matter lining the cyst wall. The white matter lining is typically seen with porencephalic cyst as in this case, distinguishing it from schizencephaly.

10b Answer A. Porencephalic cyst. The lack of gray matter lining the cyst wall differentiates this from schizencephaly. Hydranencephaly on the other hand is much more severe with profound loss of brain tissue and a large fluid-filled cavity.

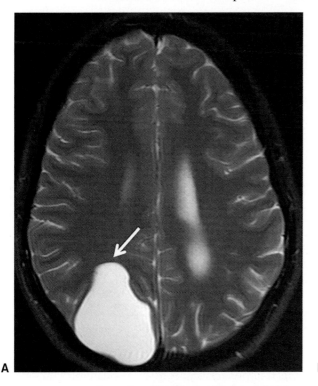 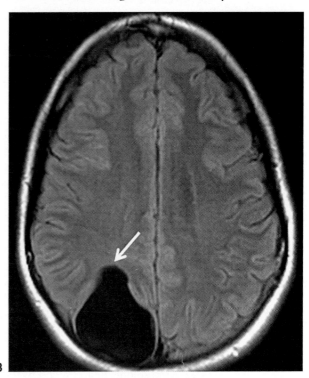

A B

Imaging Findings: Right parietal parasagittal cystic cavity without any septations or internal complexity. It is lined by nongliotic white matter (arrow) with thinning of the overlying cortex.

Discussion: Porencephaly refers to CSF-containing cavity that replaces normal brain parenchyma.

Porencephaly, multicystic encephalomalacia, and hydranencephaly are related entities, with differences in age of the patient at the time of insult and also the degree of insult. Rarely, a familial form is seen because of COL4A1 mutation encoding type IV collagen, basement membrane component, resulting in porencephalic cyst, intracranial hemorrhages, and aneurysms.

The typical porencephalic cyst, also known as an encephaloclastic porencephaly or type I porencephaly, results from insult after late second trimester. These are smooth-walled cavities with no or only minimal surrounding gliosis.

Hydranencephaly refers to an extreme form of bilateral porencephaly and is due to disruption of the fetal anterior circulation and destruction of the developing cerebral hemispheres. Each cerebral hemisphere is replaced by a large fluid-filled sac covered by thin meninges.

When the insult occurs late in gestation or at/after birth, there is generally more pronounced astroglial reaction and CSF-filled cavities are multiple with shaggy walls and septations. This is referred to as multicystic encephalomalacia.

The porencephalic cyst typically results from vascular insult or is infectious in etiology. Acquired cysts can also happen from injury late in life and are usually secondary to trauma, surgery, ischemia, or infarction. Most common etiology is felt to be periventricular hemorrhagic infarction, either arterial or venous. The location of the lesion varies with the nature of the insult. If it is secondary to vascular insult, the lesion is seen in vascular distribution. Injury resulting from mild to moderate hypotension tends to be in watershed areas. With severe hypotension, only the immediate periventricular white matter may be spared. If hypoglycemia is the inciting event, lesions tend to be in parietal and occipital lobes. With infection, the site is nonspecific, reflecting the region of brain involvement by infection.

On imaging, cystic degeneration develops 7 to 30 days after the insult. The cavities can be unilateral or bilateral and cortical or subcortical and usually, although not invariably, communicate directly with the ventricular system. The wall is smooth with no or only minimal surrounding gliosis. The content of cyst is isointense to CSF on all MR sequences. Wallerian degeneration can be evident in distant white matter tracts.

Differential Diagnosis: Differential diagnosis includes arachnoid cyst (extra-axial in location; no changes in the adjacent brain parenchyma), ependymal cyst (intraventricular; no changes in the adjacent brain parenchyma), and neuroglial cyst (intra-axial; typically, no changes in the adjacent brain parenchyma, no evidence for distant wallerian degeneration, and does not communicate with the ventricular system). Occasionally, it may be difficult to differentiate a small porencephalic cyst from this entity.

References: Barkovich AJ, Raybaud C. *Pediatric neuroimaging*, 5th ed. Philadelphia, PA: Lippincott Williams & Wilkins, 2011.

Durrani-Kolarik S, Manickam K, Chen B. COL4A1 mutation in a neonate with intrauterine stroke and anterior segment dysgenesis. *Pediatr Neurol* 2017;66:100–103.

Naidich TP, ed. *Imaging of the brain. Expert radiology series.* Philadelphia, PA: Saunders/Elsevier, 2013.

Osborn AG, Preece MT. Intracranial cysts: radiologic-pathologic correlation and imaging approach. *Radiology* 2006;239(3):650–664. doi: 10.1148/radiol.2393050823.

11a Answer D.   Intracranial hypotension. Diffuse pachymeningeal enhancement is seen throughout the brain and partially imaged upper cervical cord. Note bilateral L>R subdural effusions and presence of mild downward displacement of the cerebellar tonsils, depression of the floor of third ventricle, and narrowed appearance of the fourth ventricle. In the provided clinical setting, these findings are compatible with intracranial hypotension.

11b **Answer B.**   Dural venous engorgement. The dural enhancement seen in these patients is thought to have resulted from venous engorgement and not infection, trauma, or any congenital abnormality.

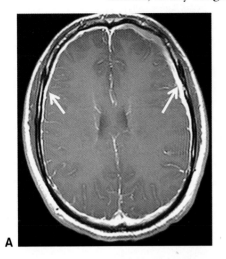 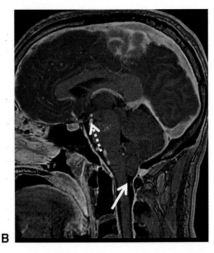 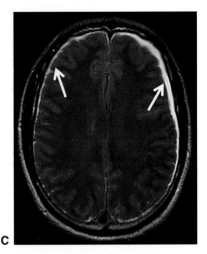

A   B   C

Imaging Findings: Diffuse pachymeningeal enhancement is seen (arrows A) on axial postcontrast T1w image. On sagittal T1w, there is depression of the floor of third ventricle (dotted arrow, B) and mild tonsillar descent (arrow B). Bilateral L>R, subdural effusions are also seen on T2w axial image (C). These findings in the current clinical setting are consistent with intracranial hypotension.

Discussion: Intracranial hypotension (ICH) can be spontaneous or acquired, the common causes being a lumbar puncture, surgery, and trauma. It typically presents as orthostatic headache, although nonpositional and exertional headaches have been reported. In addition to headaches, symptoms include neck stiffness, tinnitus, hyperacusis, photophobia, and nausea, as well as a wide variety of cranial nerve symptoms. Rarely, symptoms can be severe, even resulting in coma.

The etiology for spontaneous ICH is commonly CSF leak in the spine, cervicothoracic spine being the most common location. Perineural cyst/dural diverticula are the common sites of the leak. Connective tissue disorders can also predispose to spontaneous CSF leak.

CSF opening pressure of <6 cm of water is considered low pressure. However, opening pressures are not always obtained and are not completely reliable in patients with intracranial hypotension. Given the lack of baseline, pressures can also be within the normal range in patients. Imaging is the mainstay for diagnosis.

Many of the imaging features can be explained by the Monro-Kelly hypothesis, which states that the volume in intracranial compartment is constant and a fall in CSF volume results in compensatory enlargement of venous and arterial structures and formation of subdural collections. Each of the various imaging features by themselves is nonspecific and can be seen in other intracranial pathologies. However, a combination of findings is reliable for the diagnosis of intracranial hypotension. Imaging may be negative in a small percentage.

Findings on the unenhanced CT scan can be subtle, with subdural fluid collections being the most prominent feature, and effacement of basal cisterns, small sulci, and ventricles can be seen.

MRI is the investigation of choice for the diagnosis of ICH. Diffuse pachymeningeal thickening with intense enhancement is the most common feature, seen in over 80% of patients. This is secondary to venous engorgement in the dura. Engorged vertebral venous plexus in the cervical spinal canal is also a common finding. Subdural fluid collections (commonly hygromas, rarely hematomas) can be seen and are commonly bilateral. Distended dural venous sinuses and pituitary engorgement are commonly present. In more severe cases, sagging brainstem is seen, with midbrain displaced below the level of the dorsum sella, reduced pontomamillary distance, and flattening of the pons against the clivus. Tonsillar displacement can also be seen, which can mimic the appearance of Chiari malformation. Optic chiasm and hypothalamus can be seen stretched and draped over the sella.

Additional imaging to identify the actual site of leak can be undertaken, especially in patients not improving on conservative treatment (fluid replacement, bed rest, epidural blood patch). Contrast-enhanced MRI of the entire spine and dynamic CT myelogram are the commonly performed tests for this purpose.

References: Cauley KA, Fulwadhva U, Dundmadappa SK. Apparent diffusion coefficient measurements to support a diagnosis of intracranial hypotension. *Br J Radiol* 2014;87(1040):20140131. doi: 10.1259/bjr.20140131.

Osborn AG. *Osborn's brain: imaging, pathology, and anatomy*, 1st ed. Salt Lake City, UT: Amirsys Pub, 2013.

Rumboldt Z, ed. *Brain imaging with MRI and CT: an image pattern approach*. Cambridge, UK: Cambridge University Press, 2012.

12a **Answer B.** Periventricular leukomalacia.

12b **Answer A.** Hypoxic–ischemic white matter injury.

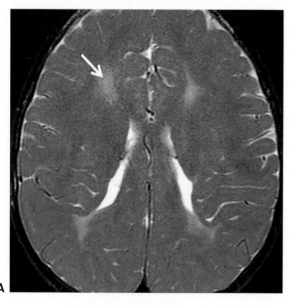 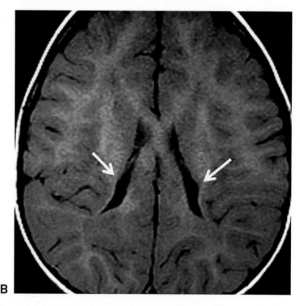

A   B

Imaging Findings: There is periventricular white matter volume loss and signal changes on FLAIR and T1 suggestive of gliosis with wavy margin of the lateral margin. Findings are compatible with periventricular leukomalacia in the current clinical setting.

Discussion: Periventricular leukomalacia refers to a pattern of white matter injury as a result of mild to moderate hypoxic–ischemic injury usually in the premature brain.

This is thought to be because of increased vulnerability of the oligodendrocyte precursor cells to oxidative stress from hypoxic–ischemic injury. Low cerebral vascularity has been shown in the affected periventricular regions. Motor and visual impairment are typical clinical manifestations.

Early in the course of disease, there is periventricular restricted diffusion, followed later in disease by T2 hyperintensity and subsequently by cavitation, necrosis, and cyst formation and ultimately by volume loss. There is also ventricular enlargement, with wavy contours of the lateral ventricle. These changes are most commonly present abutting the lateral ventricle in the peritrigonal region and in the region of the foramen of Monro. This causes an overlap with terminal zone of myelination (TZM); however, TZM T2 hyperintensity is separated from the ependymal margin by a thin band of T2 low signal unlike PVL that extends up to the ventricular ependymal.

On US, four stages of PVL are seen (stage 1, globular areas of increased echogenicity within 48 hours followed by transient normalization seen between 2nd and 4th weeks). Periventricular cyst formation occurs at 3 to 6 months and finally end stage with resolution of cysts, periventricular volume loss, and ventricular enlargement.

MRI shows periventricular white matter foci T1 hyperintensity surrounded by T2 hyperintensity at 3 to 4 days. Subsequently, there is T2 hypointensity with some cases showing foci of hemorrhage. End-stage PVL shows volume loss in the periventricular white matter and centrum semiovale and dilation of the trigones with an irregular ventricular outline. Thinning of corpus callosum posterior body and splenium may also be present.

References: Back SA. Perinatal white matter injury: the changing spectrum of pathology and emerging insights into pathogenetic mechanisms. *Ment Retard Dev Disabil Res Rev* 2006;12(2):129–140.

Chao CP, Zaleski CG, Patton AC. Neonatal hypoxic-ischemic encephalopathy: multimodality imaging findings. *Radiographics* 2006;26(Suppl 1):S159–S172.

de Vries LS, Benders MJ, Groenendaal F. Progress in neonatal neurology with a focus on neuroimaging in the preterm infant. *Neuropediatrics* 2015;46(4):234–241.

Huang BY, Castillo M. Hypoxic-ischemic brain injury: imaging findings from birth to adulthood. *Radiographics* 2008;28(2):417–439.

Varghese B, Xavier R, Manoj VC, et al. Magnetic resonance imaging spectrum of perinatal hypoxic-ischemic brain injury. *Indian J Radiol Imaging* 2016;26(3):316–327.

13a **Answer C.**   Focal cortical dysplasia. The images demonstrate findings most consistent with focal cortical dysplasia (FCD) type IIB.

13b **Answer A.**   Blurring of the gray–white matter junction. Blurring of gray and white matter junction is seen with this entity.

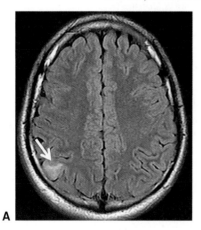
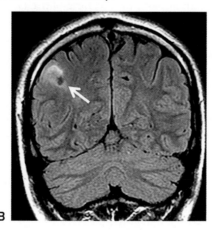
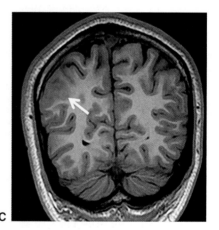

A   B   C

Imaging Findings: Axial (A) and coronal (B) FLAIR images and coronal T1-weighted image (C) are shown. FLAIR images demonstrate focal high-signal abnormality in the cortex and subjacent white matter of the right parietal lobe with a funnel-shaped configuration toward the ventricular margin. T1-weighted image highlights the focal loss of sharp gray–white matter junction in the right parietal lobe with blurring of this junction.

Discussion: Focal cortical dysplasias (FCD) are a heterogeneous group of abnormalities related to neuronal disorganization. The etiology is multifactorial and likely a result of in utero insults involving the fifth layer of the cerebral cortex. Patients typically present with intractable seizures with onset in childhood or early adulthood. Histologically, there may be heterotopic neurons in the white matter, deranged cortical lamination, giant and dysmorphic neurons, and balloon cells (large cells containing a large cytoplasm).

A classification is proposed by the Diagnostic Method Commission of the International League against Epilepsy (ILAE). FCD type I is characterized by abnormal cortical lamination, whereas FCD type II is characterized by dysmorphic neurons without (IIA) or with (IIB) balloon cells. FCD type III is associated with a principal lesion such as hippocampal sclerosis (IIIA), glial or glioneuronal tumor (IIIB), vascular malformation (IIIC), or sequela of trauma, ischemia, and infection (IIID).

Imaging studies of affected patients with FCD with balloon cells (FCD IIB) are characteristic. The region involved is usually small. The key findings are focal cortical thickening, T2 signal increase in the cortex, focal loss of the gyral architecture, excessive depth of a sulcus as compared with its contralateral homolog, blurring of the cortical–white matter junction, and T2 prolongation of the underlying white matter. In many patients, a linear, curvilinear, or funnel-shaped focus of abnormal signal intensity can be identified extending from the cortical–white matter junction to the superolateral margin of the lateral ventricular surface ("transmantle dysplasia"), which is practically pathognomonic of FCD type IIB.

The transmantle dysplasia characteristic of type IIB FCD is never found in FCD type I. The brain may appear normal in 20% to 25% of FCD type I and FCD type IIA; therefore, it is important to recognize that a normal brain MRI does not exclude an FCD. Other imaging studies, such as interictal and ictal single photon emission computed tomography (SPECT), positron emission tomography (PET), or magnetoencephalography (MEG), may be helpful in detecting the seizure focus when MRI is negative.

Differential Diagnosis: Differential diagnosis includes polymicrogyria, a disorder of cortical organization characterized by irregular cortical contour; shallow anomalous sulci; normal or apparent thickening of the cortex that is isointense to normal cortex; and irregular nodular gray–white matter junction. Slowly growing indolent cortically based neoplasms such as gangliomas and dysembryoplastic neuroepithelial tumors (DNET) also present with seizures and can appear similar to or can be associated with FCD. Gray matter heterotopias are collections of gray matter nodules outside the cortex and deep gray matter structures, are associated with seizures, and are isointense to gray matter on all pulse sequences.

References: Blümcke I, et al. The clinicopathologic spectrum of focal cortical dysplasias: a consensus classification proposed by an ad hoc Task Force of the ILAE Diagnostic Methods Commission. *Epilepsia* 2011;52(1):158-174.

Colombo N, et al. Focal cortical dysplasias: MR imaging, histopathologic, and clinical correlations in surgically treated patients with epilepsy. *AJNR Am J Neuroradiol* 2003;24(4):724-733.

14a **Answer C.** Multiple cranial neuropathies. This is a case of Paget disease of the skull. Calvarial enlargement in these patients can result in multiple cranial nerve compressions simultaneously.

14b **Answer A.** <10%. Sarcomatous transformation is rare but can be seen in <10% of patients. The risk is higher in patients with extensive skeletal involvement (5% to 10%) and <1% in patients with limited skeletal involvement.

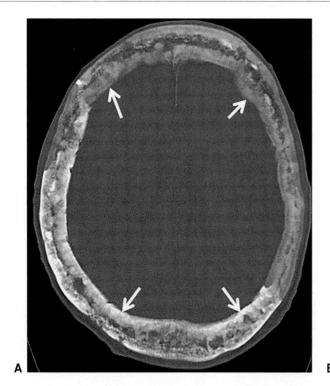
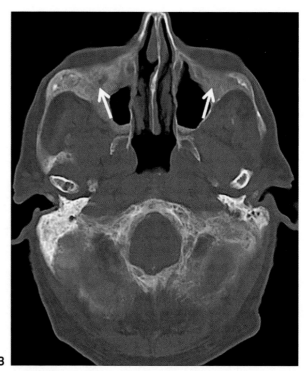

A   B

Imaging Findings: Axial CT on bone windows shows thickening and enlargement of the skull present diffusely with heterogeneous areas of sclerosis. The term "cotton wool" appearance has been used for this morphology on radiographs. This appearance is most compatible with Paget disease.

Discussion: Paget disease is a chronic skeletal disorder of unknown etiology commonly seen in the elderly. It results from progressive osseous resorption and abnormal remodeling, with three phases of disease process. First is osteoclastic and predominantly lytic (incipient phase); second is mixed phase, which is lytic and blastic (active phase); and last is blastic phase (late inactive phase). The mixed phase is typically manifested in the form of typical imaging features seen with this entity, such as cortical thickening, trabecular coarsening, osseous expansion, and areas of osteolysis. The late inactive phase is dominated by osseous sclerosis.

It can involve any bone but commonly involves the lumbar spine and pelvis. The sacrum, long bones, and cranium can also be involved. The disease is commonly polyostotic; however, rarely, monostotic types may be seen. Clinically, the cranium involvement can present with multiple cranial neuropathies, increasing head size, and leontiasis ossea (a facial deformity due to mandibular/facial involvement). These patients can also have basilar invagination, craniocervical compression, and hydrocephalus. In the skull, the osteolysis can appear as large areas of radiolucency on radiograph, termed as "osteoporosis circumscripta." Biochemically, these patients can have an elevated serum alkaline phosphatase, which can be used to monitor disease activity. Rarely, neoplastic involvement is seen with Paget disease such as due to sarcomatous transformation and giant cell tumor.

Differential diagnosis:

- Fibrous dysplasia, usually ground glass and characteristically involving the facial bones
- Diffuse osteoblastic metastasis, difficult to differentiate; both may show high radionuclide uptake on bone scan. A history of a primary malignancy such as prostate cancer is helpful.
- Myelofibrosis, associated bone marrow changes, hepatosplenomegaly
- Renal osteodystrophy, clinical history, and presence of subperiosteal bone resorption

Current management relies upon second-generation bisphosphonates and calcitonin, which are inhibitors of bone resorption. The prognosis has improved recently with the use of second-generation bisphosphonates.

Reference: Theodorou DJ, Theodorou SJ, Kakitsubata Y. Imaging of Paget disease of bone and its musculoskeletal complications: review. *AJR Am J Roentgenol* 2011;196(6 Suppl):S64–S75.

15a **Answer C.** Agenesis of the corpus callosum. The images demonstrate classic imaging findings of agenesis of the corpus callosum (ACC).

15b **Answer A.** Highly associated with other CNS anomalies.

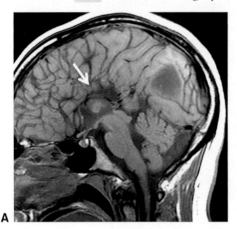 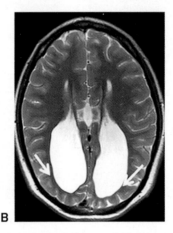 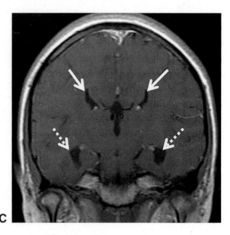

A   B   C

Imaging Findings: Sagittal T1-weighted, axial T2-weighted, and coronal postcontrast T1-weighted images are shown. Midline sagittal image (A) shows absence of the corpus callosum with radiating medial sulci and absent cingulate gyrus. Axial T2w image also demonstrates parallel orientation of the lateral ventricles with enlarged atria and occipital horns, known as colpocephaly (B). Coronal T1w image shows the characteristic appearance of the frontal horns and temporal horns.

Discussion: Complete agenesis and partial agenesis (hypogenesis) of the corpus callosum can result from various genetic, infectious, vascular, or toxic causes. Isolated agenesis of the corpus callosum without clinical symptoms is very rare. The more frequent manifestations of ACC include seizures, macrocephaly, delayed development, learning disability, and hypothalamic dysfunction.

Callosal anomalies are highly associated with other CNS anomalies such as anterior and hippocampal commissure anomalies, Chiari 2 malformation, Dandy-Walker malformation, malformations of cortical development, X-linked hydrocephalus, cephaloceles, and midline facial anomalies. Callosal anomalies are also associated with specific syndromes. The most common of these syndromes is Aicardi syndrome (ACC plus periventricular or subcortical gray matter heterotopia, polymicrogyria, cerebellar hypoplasia, posterior fossa cysts, and microphthalmia), which occurs exclusively in girls.

The normal corpus callosum anatomical division includes the rostrum, genu, body, isthmus, and splenium (from anterior to posterior). It is sequentially formed, starting with the posterior genu, anterior body, posterior body and anterior genu, the splenium, and finally the rostrum. A deviation from this pattern may indicate the presence of holoprosencephaly (only the posterior CC is formed).

Prenatal sonographic findings that raise the possibility of corpus callosum agenesis are absence of the cavum septum pellucidum, enlarged atria and occipital horns of the lateral ventricles, and a high-riding third ventricle. Direct visualization of the entire corpus callosum on a midline sagittal sonographic image is difficult. Fetal MRI is useful in the evaluation of suspected callosal anomalies after 20 weeks.

MRI findings of ACC include lateral ventricles, which are oriented parallel to each other, colpocephaly (disproportionate dilatation of trigones and occipital horns of the lateral ventricles due to deficient white matter), high-riding third ventricle, and atypical fiber bundles (Probst bundles), which run in an anteroposterior direction just lateral to the interhemispheric fissure. Sagittal images are the best sequence for the evaluation of the extent of the abnormality of the corpus callosum. Complete agenesis of the corpus callosum is accompanied by an absent cingulate gyrus and sulcus with a resultant radiating or "sunburst" configuration of the cerebral sulci. On coronal images, crescent-shaped lateral ventricles (because of impression on the medial walls of the ventricles by the medially positioned bundles of Probst), abnormal configuration of the frontal horns of the lateral ventricles that have a "steer's horns" appearance, incomplete inversion of the hippocampi, and medial extension of the temporal lobes due to poorly formed white matter in the ventral cingulum are well seen.

Differential diagnosis is limited because the imaging appearance of agenesis of the corpus callosum is characteristic.

References: Hetts SW, et al. Anomalies of the corpus callosum: an MR analysis of the phenotypic spectrum of associated malformations. *AJR Am J Roentgenol* 2006;187(5):1343–1348.

Schell-Apacik CC, et al. Agenesis and dysgenesis of the corpus callosum: clinical, genetic and neuroimaging findings in a series of 41 patients. *Am J Med Genet A* 2008;146A(19):2501–2511.

Tang PH, et al. Agenesis of the corpus callosum: an MR imaging analysis of associated abnormalities in the fetus. *AJNR Am J Neuroradiol* 2009;30(2):257–263.

16a **Answer B.** A CT head without contrast. Often, the best modality to evaluate a bony abnormality on MRI is a plain radiograph or CT. These are more sensitive to osseous detail compared to an MR. In this case, although the MRI appearance was relatively nonspecific, the CT appearance was classic for the diagnosis of fibrous dysplasia.

16b **Answer C.** Fibrous dysplasia.

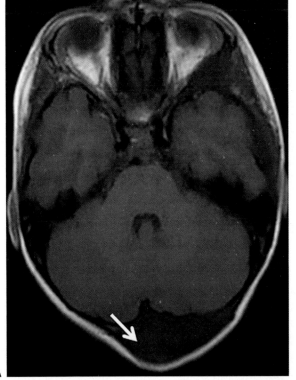

A   B

Figure 1

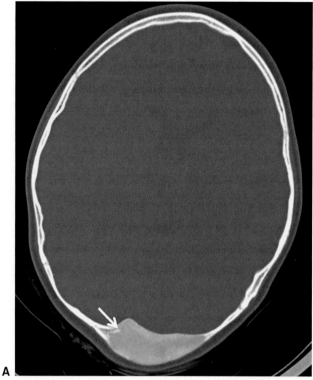

A

Figure 2

Imaging Findings: Figure 1. Pre- and postcontrast T1-weighted axial MR sequences (A and B) demonstrate an expansile mildly enhancing mass centered in the occipital bone.

Figure 2. Subsequent CT bone window demonstrates ground-glass attenuation and expansion of the occipital bone without associated soft tissue components or evidence of osteolysis. These imaging features are most consistent with fibrous dysplasia.

Discussion: Fibrous dysplasia is a congenital, nonhereditary, gradually progressive disorder where normal bone is progressively replaced by immature woven bone and fibrous tissue. The etiology of this disorder remains uncertain. Abnormalities in mesenchymal differentiation, osteoblastic hyperplasia, and premature arrest of osteogenesis at immature woven stage with disturbance of cancellous bone maintenance are some of the proposed etiologic considerations.

Commonly monostotic and asymptomatic, it is typically diagnosed in the third decade of life. It may be polyostotic with craniofacial osseous involvement. Polyostotic subtypes may have an earlier age of onset and be associated with more severe skeletal deformities. Extensive polyostotic craniofacial fibrous dysplasia may be physically deforming (leontiasis ossea, "lion-like facies") and symptomatic because of mass effect from osseous expansion, neurovascular compression, and dental malocclusions. Polyostotic fibrous dysplasia may be associated with endocrinopathies and cafe au lait skin macules, triad seen in McCune-Albright syndrome. The initial features of this entity may be lucent lesions and thinning of cortex with gradually increasing attenuation with disease progression. Based on the stage of the disease, the bone may have a predominantly lucent, mottled, or ground-glass sclerosis. Typical disease course is benign, although rarely malignant transformation to osteosarcoma, fibrosarcoma, and malignant fibrous histiocytoma may occur.

References: Chong VF. Fibrous dysplasia involving the base of the skull. *AJR Am J Roentgenol* 2002;178(3):717–720.

Lustig L. Fibrous dysplasia involving the skull base and temporal bone. *Arch Otolaryngol Head Neck Surg* 2001;127(10):1239–1247.

17a **Answer D.** Joubert syndrome. The images demonstrate classic imaging findings of Joubert syndrome and related disorders.

17b **Answer B.** A sign predictive of hypotonia, ataxia, and developmental delay. The imaging finding is characteristic of Joubert syndrome but can also be seen with other disorders such as oral–facial–digital syndrome type VI, COACH syndrome, and Dekaban-Arima syndrome; therefore, it is not specific. Patients typically present with hypotonia, ataxia, and developmental delay. The molar tooth appearance results from absence of decussation of the superior cerebellar peduncles. The cerebellar vermis is hypoplastic.

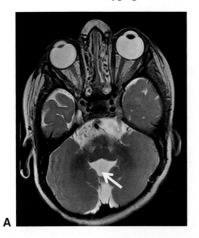
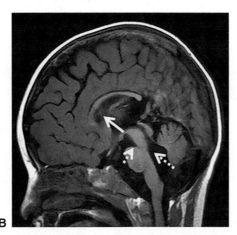
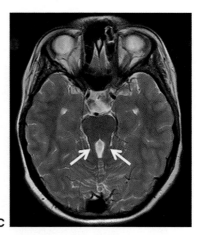

A   B   C

Imaging Findings: Axial T2-weighted and sagittal T1-weighted images from patient 1 (A, B) and axial T2-weighted image (C) from patient 2 are shown. Figure (A) shows the bat-wing configuration of the fourth ventricle, and Figure (B) demonstrates the hypoplastic inferior cerebellar vermis, thinning at the junction of the pons and midbrain and of the dorsal pons (dashed arrow), and the associated thinning of the corpus callosum (solid arrow). Figure (C) highlights the typical appearance of molar tooth malformation with thickened, elongated, and horizontally oriented superior cerebellar peduncles.

Discussion: Molar tooth malformations were first described by Joubert and colleagues in 1969 in four siblings. Joubert syndrome is an autosomal recessive disorder characterized by episodic hyperpnea, ataxia, abnormal eye movements, and intellectual disability. Although molar tooth malformation is the imaging hallmark of Joubert syndrome, it can be seen with other disorders, which as a group are referred to as Joubert syndrome and related disorders. Almost all patients with the molar tooth malformation have hypotonia, ataxia, developmental delay, and oculomotor apraxia. Renal disease (nephronophthisis or multicystic dysplastic kidney), hepatic fibrosis and cysts, and ocular anomalies (coloboma, retinal dysplasia) can be associated.

The molar tooth sign (MTS) refers to the abnormal shape of the midhindbrain, which resembles a molar tooth on axial imaging. Enlarged elongated horizontally oriented superior cerebellar peduncles due to lack of decussation of superior cerebellar peduncles results in this morphology. There is a deep interpeduncular fossa and absence of decussation of the corticospinal tract. The absent decussation of the superior cerebellar peduncles can also be identified on diffusion tensor imaging (DTI). The cerebellar vermis is hypoplastic to varying degrees ranging from a thin cleft to a large defect with wide separations of the cerebellar hemispheres that resembles a Dandy-Walker cyst. The fourth ventricle is higher in position and has a bat-wing appearance superiorly and triangular appearance in the midportion on axial images. The pons may be small with thinning of the junction of the pons and midbrain (pontomesencephalic isthmus) on sagittal images. Midline cleft in the superior cerebellar vermis is best identified on coronal images. Callosal dysgenesis, callosal thinning, and migration anomalies are also associated with molar tooth malformation.

References: Poretti A, et al. Joubert syndrome and related disorders: spectrum of neuroimaging findings in 75 patients. *AJNR Am J Neuroradiol* 2011;32(8):1459–1463.

Poretti A, et al. Joubert syndrome: neuroimaging findings in 110 patients in correlation with cognitive function and genetic cause. *J Med Genet* 2017. [Epub ahead of print].

18a **Answer B.** Lissencephaly. Smooth thick cortex is the typical imaging appearance for lissencephaly.

18b **Answer B.** The predilection for lobes involved.

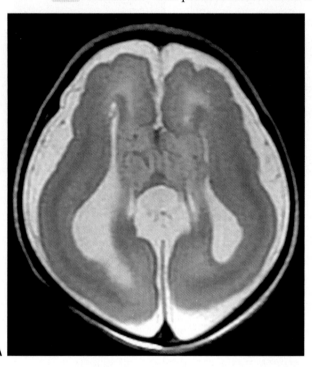
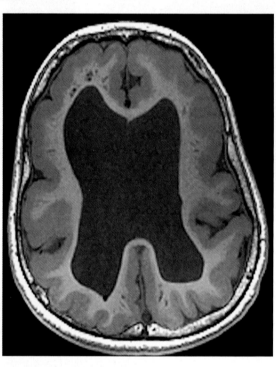

Imaging Findings: Axial T2-weighted (A) and axial T1-weighted (B) images from two different patients are shown. (A) shows agyria of the brain posteriorly with thick smooth cortex (thin dark outer cortical layer, hyperintense cell sparse zone, and thick inner cortical layer) and pachygyria in the frontal lobes. (B) demonstrates pachygyria predominantly in the frontal lobes with relative sparing posteriorly. Also note enlarged ventricles because of long-standing shunted hydrocephalus.

Discussion: Lissencephaly refers to a smooth appearance of the brain surface. Agyria is defined as complete absence of gyri (complete lissencephaly), whereas pachygyria has a few broad and flat gyri (incomplete lissencephaly); both agyria and pachygyria have thick cortex. Lissencephaly is traditionally divided into two subtypes: classic (type 1) and cobblestone (type 2). Classic lissencephaly results from an arrest of neuronal migration and a four-layered cortex, whereas cobblestone lissencephaly develops from overmigration of neurons beyond the pial surface and onto the overlying subarachnoid tissue. Cobblestone lissencephaly is most commonly associated with congenital muscular dystrophies and will not be discussed further.

Children with classic lissencephaly present with poor feeding, hypotonia, opisthotonos, delayed developmental milestones, and epilepsy; the time of onset depends on the severity of the malformation. Although many genes can be involved, 40% to 80% of cases arise from LIS1 or DCX (XLIS) mutations. In the LIS1 lissencephaly, the abnormalities are more prominent in the posterior portion of the cerebral hemispheres. On the contrary, the abnormal cortex is more prominent in the frontal lobes in cases of DCX lissencephaly. DCX mutations also result in band heterotopia in girls.

Imaging of agyria–pachygyria demonstrates a thick cortex with a thin outer cortical layer, a cell-sparse zone, and a thick inner cortical layer in addition to shallow vertical sylvian fissures, which gives the brain its "figure-of-eight" or "hour-glass" configuration. The cell sparse zone has abnormal low T1 and high T2 signal. The gray–white matter junction is smooth. In band heterotopia (double cortex), there is bilateral and symmetric band of heterotopic gray matter, which is clearly separate from the cortical ribbon; the overlying cortex is not smooth and is typically not as thin as the outer cortical layer in agyria–pachygyria.

Caution: Smooth agyric appearance of the brain is normal up to 26 weeks of gestation, so this diagnosis should be used with caution in fetal MRIs and in extreme prematurity.

Differential Diagnosis: Differential diagnosis is polymicrogyria, which may simulate pachygyria as apparent thickening of the cortex can be identified on MRI; however, the gray–white matter interface is irregular in polymicrogyria and smooth in lissencephaly. Furthermore, the shallow sulci in polymicrogyria are anomalous, whereas the shallow sulci in lissencephaly are anatomically recognized sulci. Subcortical gray matter heterotopia presents as a swirling mass of gray matter signal intensity within the white matter that may cause deformity of the ventricular system. Focal cortical dysplasia can have thick cortex, but the region involved is usually small and the gray–white matter is blurred.

References: Barkovich AJ, et al. Malformations of cortical development. *Neuroimaging Clin N Am* 2004;14(3):401–423.

Gaitanis JN, et al. Genetics of disorders of cortical development. *Neuroimaging Clin N Am* 2004;14(2):219–229.

19a **Answer B.** Pseudotumor cerebri. Pseudotumor cerebri (or idiopathic intracranial hypertension, IIH). Partially empty sella may be a normal finding in elderly patients but should raise a red flag in a young patient, especially a female, whose pituitary is supposed to be very hormonally active.

19b **Answer C.** MR venogram. MR venogram shows bilateral transverse sinus stenosis in outer thirds of the sinuses in 90% of the cases.

19c **Answer C.** Lumbar puncture. Lumbar puncture, bedside or image guided, is performed to measure the elevated CSF pressure and confirm the diagnosis. It may also be used as a temporary therapeutic measure prior to lumboperitoneal shunt.

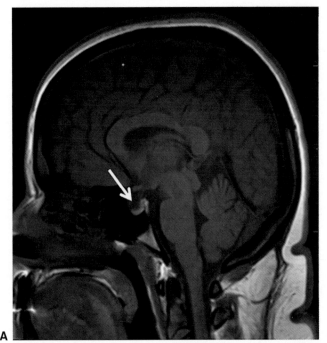
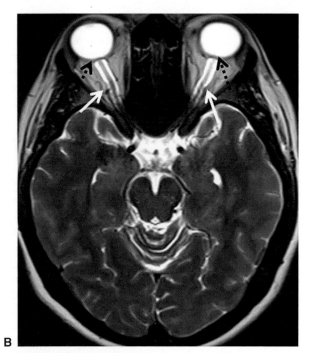

Figure 1

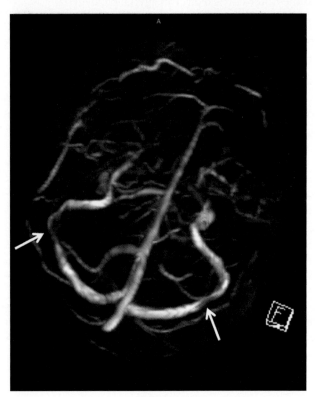

Figure 2

Imaging Findings: Figure 1. Sagittal T1 (A) and axial T2 images (B) show a partially empty sella (A) and markedly distended CSF space around bilateral optic nerves (*solid arrow*, B) with flattening of posterior sclera and convexity of optic nerve heads into the globe (*dotted arrow*, B).

Figure 2. TOF MR venogram without contrast-rotated MIP shows bilateral transverse sinus stenosis seen along the lateral aspect of the transverse venous sinus.

Discussion: Pseudotumor cerebri (idiopathic intracranial hypertension, IIH) is a clinical syndrome of raised intracranial pressure without any intracranial mass or hydrocephalus. It typically affects obese women of childbearing age. Etiology is poorly understood.

Typical clinical presentation is with headaches, transient or gradual visual loss, photopsia, horizontal diplopia, and pulse synchronous tinnitus. If untreated, it may result in permanent visual loss. Papilledema is often present but may be unilateral. Clinical diagnosis is supported by high opening pressures on lumbar puncture (mean about 25 mm of H_2O).

Imaging findings include partially empty sella, prominent subarachnoid space around the optic nerves, tortuosity of the optic nerves, papilledema manifested by flattening of the posterior sclera, intraocular convexity of optic nerve head, and enhancement of intraocular optic nerve. Other evidence of enlarged arachnoid outpouchings may be seen as enlarged Meckel caves and arachnoid pits/meningoceles over temporal bones and sphenoid wing. The latter may cause CSF leaks presenting as CSF rhinorrhea or otorrhea and even CSF hypotension. Bilateral transverse sinus stenosis, usually at the lateral ends of the sinuses, is seen in around 90%.

Management relies upon use of acetazolamide, therapeutic lumbar punctures, lumboperitoneal shunt, and optic nerve fenestration, based on specific clinical scenario.

References: Ahmed RM, Wilkinson M, Parker GD, et al. Transverse sinus stenting for idiopathic intracranial hypertension: a review of 52 patients and of model predictions. *AJNR Am J Neuroradiol* 2011;32(8):1408–1414.

Degnan AJ, Levy LM. Pseudotumor cerebri: brief review of clinical syndrome and imaging findings. *AJNR Am J Neuroradiol* 2011;32:1986–1993.

Leach J, Fortuna R, Jones B, et al. Imaging of cerebral venous thrombosis: current techniques, spectrum of findings, and diagnostic pitfalls. *Radiographics* 2006;26(Suppl 1):S19–S41.

Scoffings DJ, Pickard JD, Higgins JN. Resolution of transverse sinus stenoses immediately after CSF withdrawal in idiopathic intracranial hypertension. *J Neurol Neurosurg Psychiatry* 2007;78:8:911–912.

20a **Answer C.** Septooptic dysplasia. The images demonstrate findings of septooptic dysplasia (SOD).

20b **Answer C.** Schizencephaly.

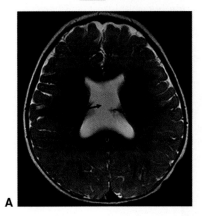 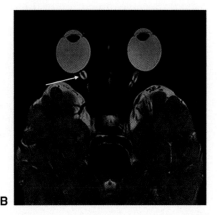 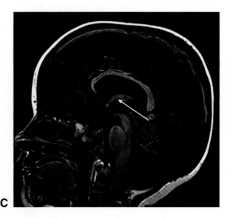

A   B   C

Imaging Findings: Axial (A and B) T2-weighted images and sagittal T1-weighted image (C) are shown. (A) shows absent septum pellucidum with prominent lateral ventricles, and (B) shows the small size of the optic nerves bilaterally. (C) shows low position of the fornix (white arrow), small visual pathways, and a normal-appearing prepubertal pituitary gland.

Discussion: Septooptic dysplasia was first described by de Morsier in 1956 (de Morsier syndrome). Although the presentation is variable, the diagnosis of septooptic dysplasia is defined by two or more of the following features: (1) midline brain abnormalities (including absence of the septum pellucidum and/or corpus callosum);

(2) hypoplasia of the optic nerves, which is usually bilateral; and (3) hypothalamic–pituitary dysfunction. Most cases are sporadic, but a familial occurrence has been described. Absence of a homeobox gene, Hesx1, is associated with SOD. Some consider it to be a mild form of lobar holoprosencephaly, although embryologically, it may be more appropriately categorized as a disorder of midline development.

The frontal horns have a box-like squared appearance on coronal images, which is similar to findings of holoprosencephaly. The fornix is low lying on sagittal images adjoining the corpus callosum only at the level of the inferior surface of the splenium, and the anterior columns of the fornix may be fused in the midline. Septooptic dysplasia is associated with malformations of cortical development. Of these, schizencephaly is the most consistent, seen in 50% of patients and classically presenting with seizures. The olfactory bulbs may be hypoplastic.

It is prudent to scrutinize the brain, pituitary, and optic pathway for subtle abnormalities once absence of the septum pellucidum is recognized. It is also important to recognize that a normal-appearing optic pathway on MRI does not exclude mild optic nerve hypoplasia; and therefore, ophthalmologic examination should be undertaken in every patient.

Differential diagnosis: The lateral ventricles are usually prominent in septooptic dysplasia; however, this is due to the underlying developmental abnormality and is not because of hydrocephalus. Anomalies of the corpus callosum can also be associated with absence of the septum pellucidum and these conditions can coexist. Pituitary stalk interruption is a developmental abnormality with ectopic bright spot of the posterior pituitary on T1-weighted images and thinning of the pituitary stalk; these features can also be seen with SOD.

References: Barkovich J, et al. Absence of the septum pellucidum: a useful sign in the diagnosis of congenital brain malformations. *AJR Am J Roentgenol* 1989;152(2):353–360.

Kuban KC, et al. Septo-optic-dysplasia-schizencephaly. Radiographic and clinical features. *Pediatr Radiol* 1989;19(3):145–150.

21a Answer D. Metopic suture. The image demonstrates keel-like appearance or trigonocephaly. This is the classic appearance for metopic synostosis.

21b Answer A. Brachycephaly. The image shows bicoronal suture synostosis. This typically results in increased transverse dimension of the skull (brachycephaly).

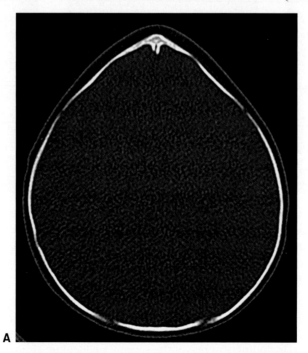

A

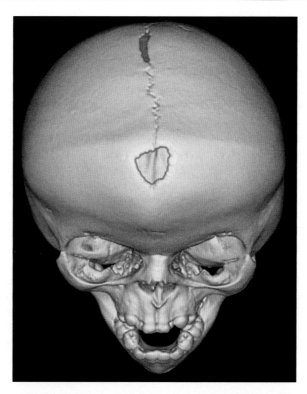

Imaging Findings: Axial bone window head CT (A) shows triangular configuration of the skull, which is pointed in the midline frontally consistent with trigonocephaly, features pathognomonic for premature metopic synostosis. 3D surface rendered reformations of the skull (B) in a patient with Apert syndrome showing bicoronal synostosis and flattening of both frontal regions. This deformity is associated with increased transverse dimension of the skull (brachycephaly).

Discussion: Craniosynostosis is the premature fusion of one or more skull sutures. Normal closure times for the cranial sutures are variable.

The metopic suture starts closing as early as 3 months and is usually closed by 9 months, but it may persist into adulthood. The sagittal, coronal, and lambdoid sutures should not be closed within the first year of life. The majority of craniosynostoses are nonsyndromic (85%) affecting one suture, and the remainder are associated with other anomalies and are syndromic (15%) typically affecting two or more sutures. Sagittal synostosis is the most common followed by coronal and metopic sutures; lambdoid synostoses are the least common. Apert (craniosynostosis, syndactyly, midface hypoplasia, and cleft palate) and Crouzon syndromes (craniosynostosis, midface hypoplasia, proptosis) are the most common syndromic craniosynostosis, and bicoronal synostosis is the most commonly fused suture in these syndromes. Genetic mutations of FGFR family of genes are the most commonly recognizable cause of craniosynostosis, although mutations of TWIST and MSX2 gene have also been implicated.

Characteristic skull shapes are seen with specific sutural craniosynostoses. As a general rule, there is growth inhibition perpendicular to the affected suture with compensatory exaggeration of growth at the open sutures. This results in elongation of the AP dimension of the skull (scaphocephaly or dolichocephaly) in sagittal synostosis and elongation of the transverse diameter of the skull (brachycephaly) in bicoronal synostosis. Metopic synostosis results in triangular appearance of the forehead (trigonocephaly).

Plagiocephaly is defined as asymmetric flattening of the skull, which can be due to unilateral coronal or lambdoid synostosis or can be deformational or positional because of children lying down on their back with the head preferentially looking to one side. Positional plagiocephaly is the most common of abnormal skull shape in infants and is characterized by a parallelogram configuration on axial images reflecting the combination of ipsilateral frontal bossing and unilateral lambdoid flattening. Other indirect features of craniosynostosis include hypotelorism (decreased distance between the globes) in metopic synostosis, hypertelorism (increased distance between the globes) in bicoronal synostosis, harlequin eye due to elevation of the lesser wing of the sphenoid bone with resultant shallow bony orbits and proptosis (exorbitism) in coronal synostosis, anterior frontal flattening in unicoronal synostosis, and unilateral occipital flattening in unilambdoid synostosis.

The diagnosis of craniosynostosis is based on clinical features including ridging of the skull along the fused suture; however, CT with 3D reconstructions play a crucial role in the confirmation of the diagnosis, defining the extent of craniosynostosis, to evaluate for underlying brain anomalies and for surgical planning. The role of plain radiography in evaluating craniosynostosis in the modern imaging era is very limited.

Imaging is also important in assessing complications resulting from craniosynostosis or associated with syndromic craniosynostosis. Developmental anomalies of the skull base and craniocervical junction, narrowing of the jugular fossa with excessive venous collaterals, and hydrocephalus can be present. Chiari 1 malformation can be identified, which is thought to be acquired because of decreased cranial volume. Fusion and segmentation anomalies of the cervical spine can be also seen.

References: Blaser S. Abnormal skull shape. *Pediatr Radiol* 2008;38(Suppl 3):S488–S496.

Blaser S, et al. Skull base development and craniosynostosis. *Pediatr Radiol* 2015;45(Suppl 3): S485–S496.

Caruso PA, et al. CT imaging of craniofacial malformations. *Neuroimaging Clin N Am* 2003;13(3):541–572.

4 Trauma

SATHISH KUMAR DUNDAMADAPPA • DAVID CHOI • ALY H. ABAYAZEED • SHYAM SABAT • PRACHI DUBEY

QUESTIONS

1   A 45-year-old male, unrestrained passenger brought to the ER after a high-speed motor vehicle accident.

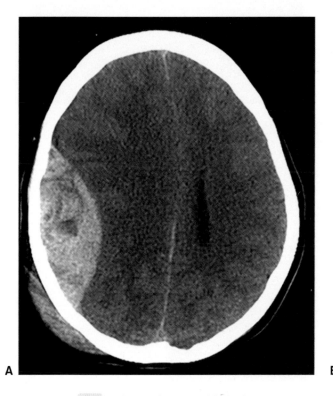

A

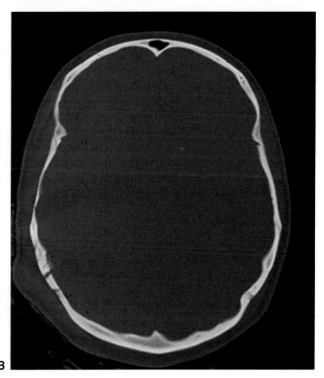

B

1a   What is the most likely diagnosis?

    A. Subdural hematoma

    B. Subdural empyema

    C. Epidural hematoma

    D. Epidural metastasis

1b Venous epidural hematomas are commonly associated with injury to what structure?

A. Dural venous sinus
B. Middle meningeal vein
C. Deep cerebral veins
D. Emissary veins

2 A 38-year-old male presents to the ER after MVA. She has fractured bilateral pterygoid plates on CT.

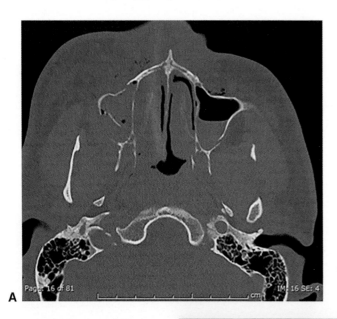

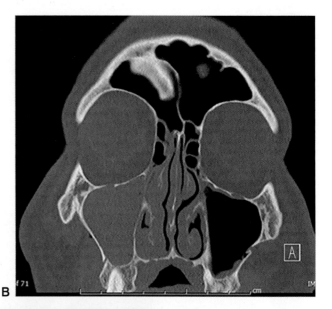

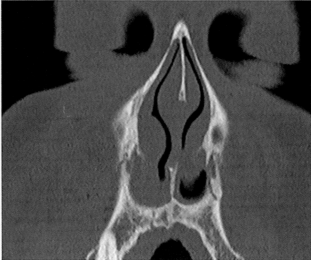

Based on the above appearance, which of the following best classifies this pattern of injury?

A. Le Fort I
B. Le Fort II
C. Le Fort III
D. Le Fort VI

3 Based on the progressive CT scan appearance shown below in a recently postoperative patient, what is the most likely diagnosis?

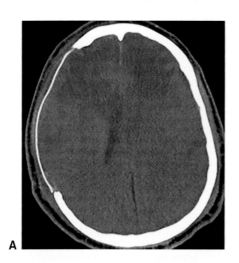
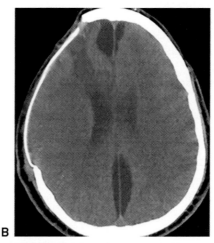
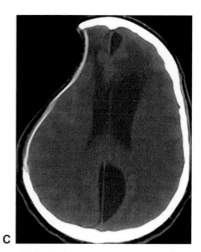

A. Extracranial herniation postcraniectomy
B. Sinking skin flap syndrome
C. Progressive postoperative encephalomalacia
D. Tension pneumocephalus

4 A 4-year-old female with right ICA dissection, following a reported fall. Head CT and MRI were performed as a part of the workup. Key images are shown below.

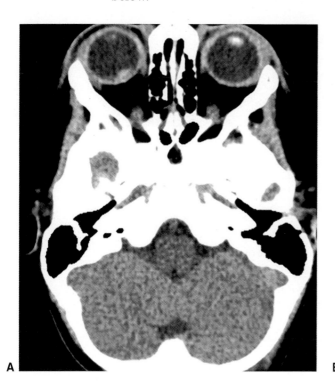
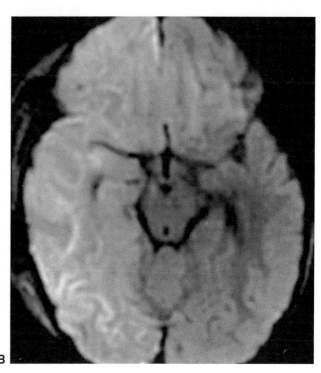

4a   Additional radiographs are being performed as a part of the workup. Based on this study, what additional evaluation should be recommended?

A. Indirect ophthalmoscopy with dilated pupils

B. 24-hour EEG monitoring

C. Muscle biopsy for mitochondrial disorders

D. MRI brain with contrast

4b   What is the reported probability of abuse in a child with head trauma and retinal hemorrhages?

A. 90%

B. 10% to 15%

C. 30%

D. <10%

5   Key images from an MRI performed for evaluation of an abnormal head CT are shown below.

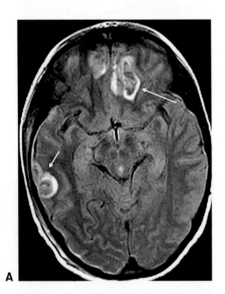
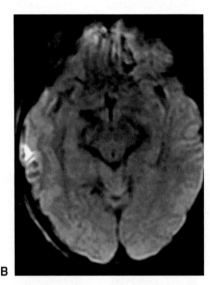
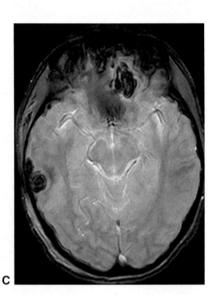

A   B   C

5a   What are the lesions indicated by arrows in image A?

A. Metastatic lesions

B. Hemorrhagic contusions

C. Multifocal embolic infarcts

D. Septic emboli with abscess

5b   Which of the following statements is accurate regarding traumatic brain contusions?

A. Commonly enlarge over first 2 days following causative event.

B. Consistently seen on immediate posttrauma imaging.

C. Caused by shear injury.

D. CT is more sensitive than MRI for detection of these abnormalities.

5c A key image from T2 FLAIR sequence obtained in the same patient is shown below.

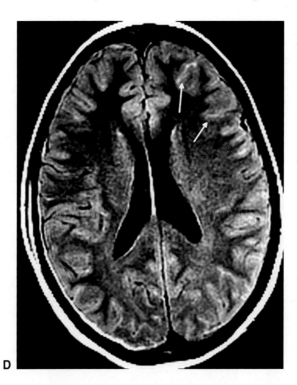

D

Which of the following abnormality is indicated by arrows in the above image?

A. Subarachnoid hemorrhage
B. Pial collateral vessels, indicating vascular occlusion
C. Leptomeningeal carcinomatosis
D. Superficial cortical veins, normal finding

6 A 40-year-old patient sustained blunt trauma to the face. Key images from CT are shown below.

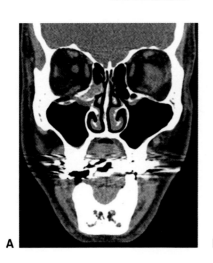

A

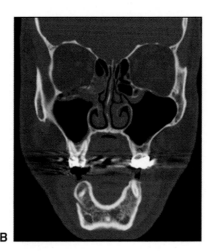

B

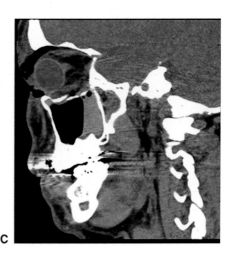

C

What is the most likely diagnosis?

A. Le Fort type III fracture
B. Zygomaticomaxillary complex fracture
C. Orbital blowout fracture
D. Nasoorbitoethmoidal fracture

7   A 30-year-old male was brought to the ER after motor vehicle accident. Key CT and MR images are shown below.

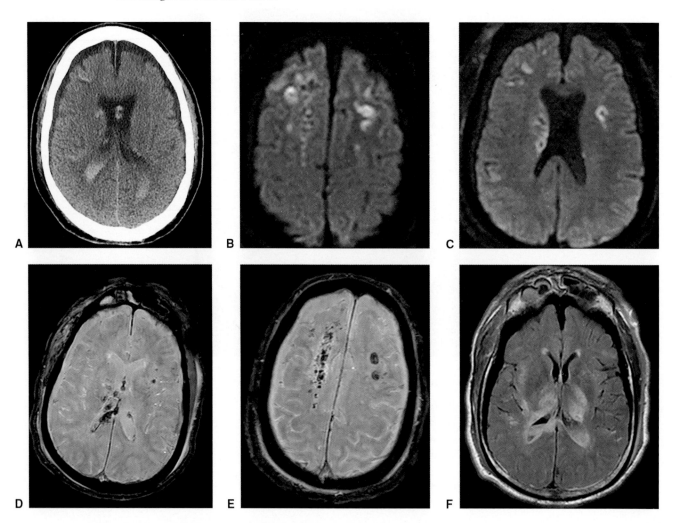

7a   What is the most likely diagnosis?

A. Hypoxic ischemic encephalopathy
B. Diffuse axonal injury
C. Multifocal embolic infarcts because of fat embolism
D. Hypertensive hemorrhages

7b   A common location of microhemorrhages in mild forms of DAI is:

A. Gray–white interface
B. Choroid plexus
C. Thalamus
D. Dorsolateral brainstem

8 Patient presents with acute headache and confusion. Noncontrast head CT was performed. Key images are shown below.

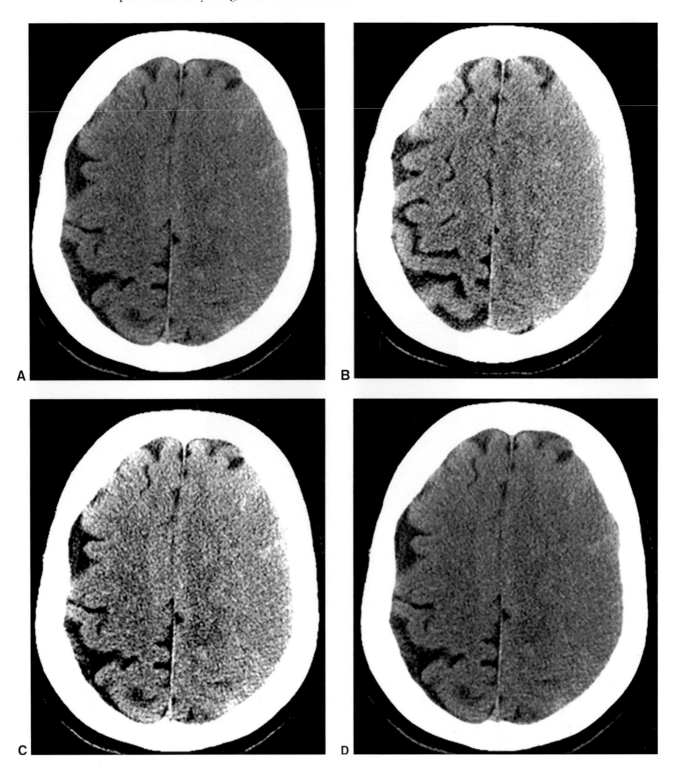

What is the most likely diagnosis?

A. No abnormality shown on provided images
B. Venous epidural hematoma
C. Idiopathic intracranial hypertension
D. Subdural hematoma

9 Patient sustained blunt trauma to the face.

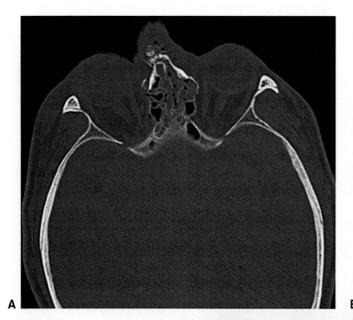

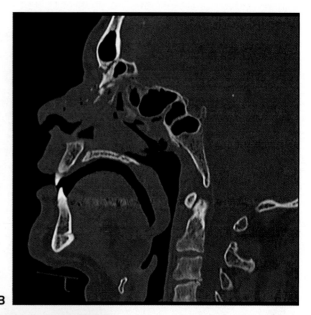

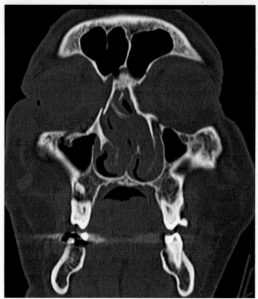

9a What is the most likely diagnosis?

    A. Comminuted nasal fracture

    B. Nasoorbitoethmoidal (NOE) fracture

    C. Le Fort type III (transfacial) fracture

    D. Bilateral medial orbital blowout fractures

9b What clinical sign would distinguish this fracture pattern from bilateral medial orbital blowout fractures?

    A. Hyphema

    B. Monocular loss of vision

    C. Telecanthus

    D. Periorbital crepitus

10 Patient sustained blunt trauma to the face.

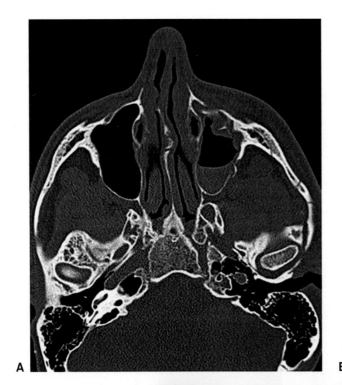

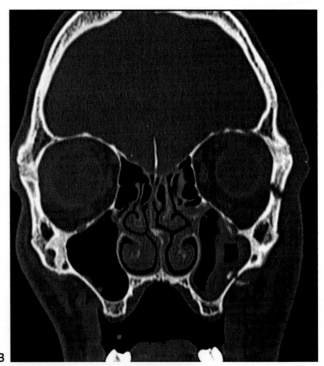

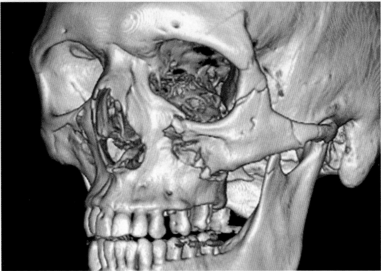

10a What is the most likely diagnosis?

    A. Zygomatic arch fracture

    B. Orbital floor blowout fracture

    C. Le Fort type II fracture

    D. Zygomaticomaxillary complex fracture

10b What neurologic sign is most specifically associated with this fracture pattern?

    A. Diplopia

    B. Anesthesia cheek/upper lip

    C. Monocular visual loss

    D. Ipsilateral sensorineural hearing loss

11 Motor vehicle accident with jaw soft tissue swelling.

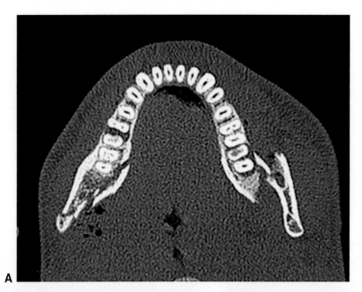

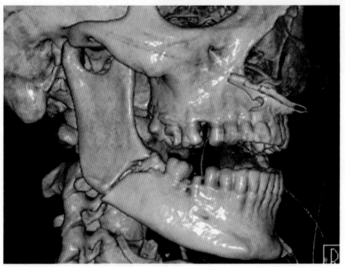

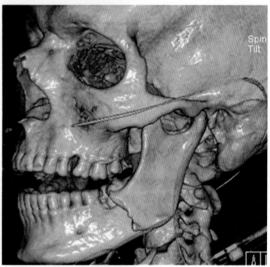

11a Which of the following statements is most accurate regarding mandibular fractures?

A. This is a "ring structure," breaks in more than one place in more than 90% of cases.

B. Mandible is the most common site of facial fracture.

C. Optimal assessment includes multiplanar reformats and 3-D volume rendering.

D. Flail mandible refers to fracture displacement of condylar process.

11b Which of the following types of mandible fracture poses the greatest risk of inferior alveolar nerve injury?

A. Angle

B. Symphysis menti

C. Coronoid process

D. Condyle

12 A young child presenting with the scalp swelling. An MRI was performed, and key images are shown below.

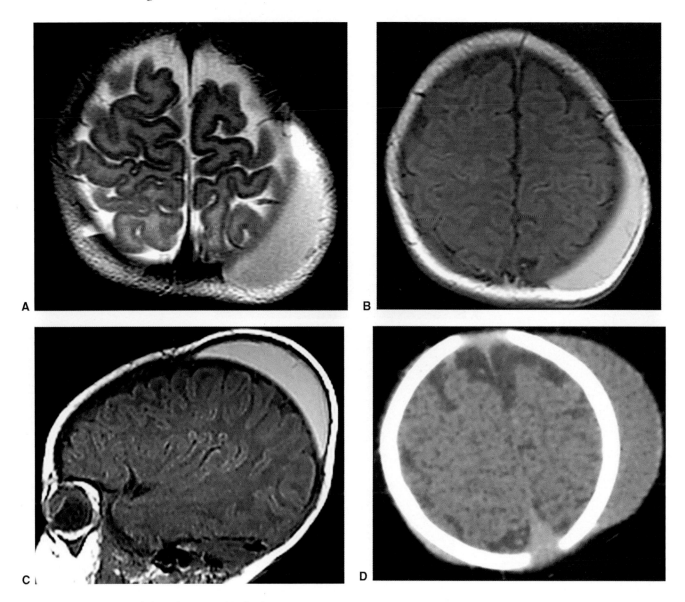

What is the most likely diagnosis?

A. Meningocele
B. Epidural hematoma
C. Cephalohematoma
D. Sinus pericranii

13 Fall on left side of face with soft tissue swelling and pain.

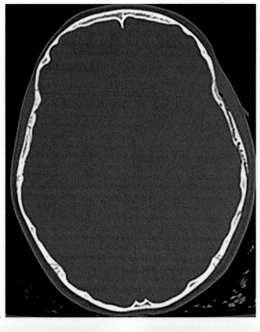

A

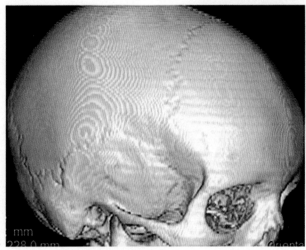

B

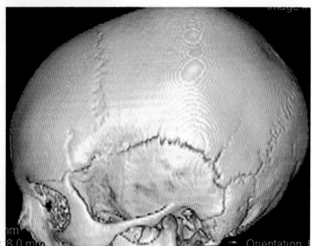

C

13a What is the diagnosis?

    A. Right squamosal sutural synostosis

    B. Left squamosal sutural diastases

    C. Normal variant

    D. Leptomeningeal cyst

13b Which of the following complications may be seen with traumatic sutural diastasis in adults?

    A. High risk of venous thrombosis

    B. Subarachnoid hemorrhage

    C. Leptomeningeal cyst

    D. Intracranial hypotension

14 Image A is from a scan obtained immediately following trauma. Image B is from follow-up study obtained 3 days later.

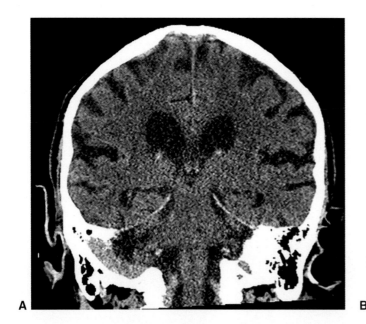
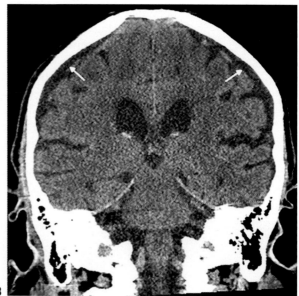

Which of the following abnormalities is indicated by arrows shown in image B?

A. Chronic subdural hematomas
B. Posttraumatic subdural hygromas
C. Acute subdural hematomas
D. Cortical atrophy

15 A young adult male was brought to the ER after a motor vehicle accident. A noncontrast CT was performed. Key images are shown below. The patient had a prior head CT 2 months ago, which was normal.

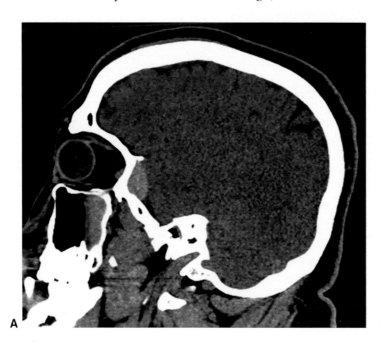
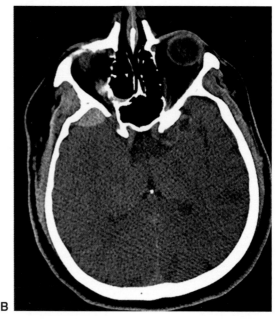

15a Based on the location and morphology of this abnormality, which of the following entities is a likely consideration?

  A. Epidural hematoma
  B. Sphenoid wing subdural hematoma
  C. Sphenoid wing meningioma
  D. Hemorrhagic contusion

15b Which of the following is the next best step in management?

  A. Short interval follow-up CT because of risk of rapid expansion
  B. Immediate surgical decompression because of risk of herniation
  C. Conservative management because of typically a benign course
  D. CT angiogram for assessment of active extravasation

16 A 10-year-old female involved in a high-speed motor vehicle accident. Key images from CT and MRI are shown below.

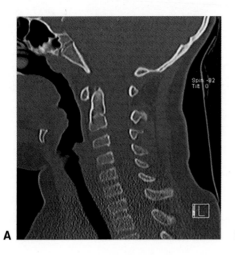 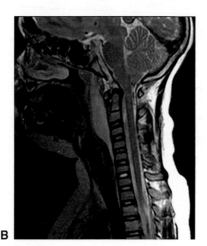 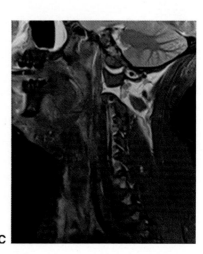

A   B   C

What is the most likely diagnosis?

  A. Craniocervical dissociation
  B. Clivus fracture
  C. Flexion teardrop fracture
  D. Hangman fracture

ANSWERS AND EXPLANATIONS

1a **Answer C.** Epidural hematoma.

1b **Answer A.** Dural venous sinus.

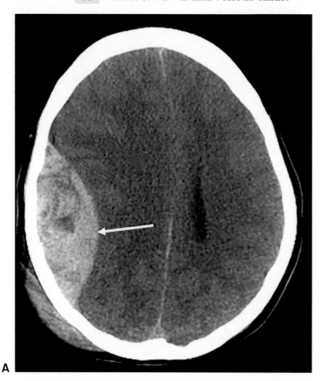

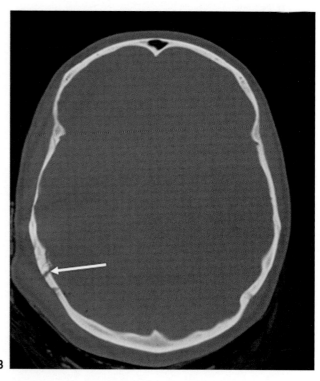

A   B

Imaging Findings: A lenticular predominantly hyperattenuating extra-axial collection with swirling intermixed iso- to hypoattenuating components. On bone windows, there is a nondisplaced fracture of the right parietal bone coursing anterior to the lambdoid suture. Findings are compatible with an acute epidural hematoma.

Discussion: Epidural hematomas are most commonly from arterial origin, resulting from injury to the meningeal arteries, typically the middle meningeal artery. These are bounded by dural attachments at the sutures and majority of these (>80%) are associated with skull fractures. Rarely, these may be seen without a fracture, usually in pediatric age group because of shearing or stretching of meningeal vessels. Venous epidural hematomas are relatively rare and typically seen with injury to dural venous sinuses.

Reference: Atlas SW. Head Trauma. In: *Magnetic resonance imaging of the brain and spine*, 4th ed. Vol. 1. Chap. 17. Lippincott Williams & Wilkins, 917–918.

2 **Answer A.** Le Fort I.

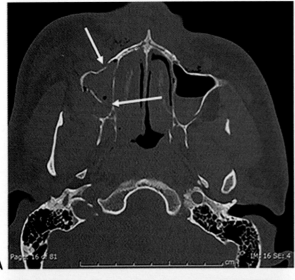

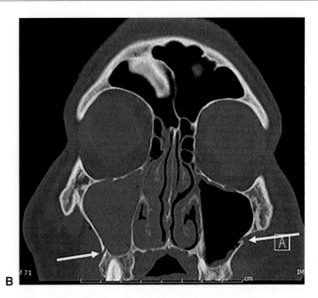

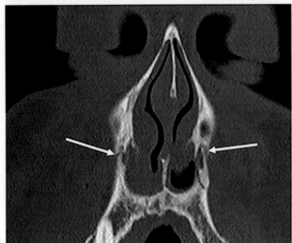

Imaging Findings: Axial and coronal noncontrast CT demonstrates fractures involving the pterygomaxillary junction and plates and fracture of inferior medial and lateral maxillary buttress.

Discussion: Le Fort 1 fracture. Multidetector computed tomography (CT) is the modality of choice for the evaluation of facial trauma because it helps accurately identify and characterize fractures. In particular, CT clearly depicts clinically relevant fractures in the eight osseous struts or buttresses that provide a scaffold for facial structures. Analyses of specific facial buttresses in a complex fracture aid determining the type of fracture and associated soft tissue injuries that may require urgent care or surgery.

Le Fort fractures are complex facial fractures that result from a high-force impact on the midface and are characterized by a variable degree of craniofacial dissociation spanning multiple facial buttresses. These fractures were first described in early 20th century by French surgeon René Le Fort, who conducted experiments applying blunt force to midface of cadavers.

Le Fort type I fracture, also known as "floating palate," results in separation of the hard palate (fracture of the medial and lateral horizontal maxillary buttresses and separation of the lower transverse maxillary buttress) from the remainder of the face and the skull base. This fracture pattern is horizontally oriented and spans the anterior, lateral, and medial maxillary walls, transecting the inferior margin of the piriform aperture and nasal septum and extending posteriorly through the pterygoid plates. The fractures are usually best depicted on coronal and three-dimensional images.

Long-term complications of Le Fort type I fracture may include malocclusion, mastication problems, facial deformity, and breathing difficulty, among others.

References: Chung KJ, et al. Treatment of complex facial fractures: clinical experience of different timing and order. *J Craniofac Surg* 2013;24(1):216–220.

Lo Casto A, et al. Imaging evaluation of facial complex strut fractures. *Semin Ultrasound CT MR* 2012;33(5):396–409.

Winegar BA, et al. Spectrum of critical imaging findings in complex facial skeletal trauma. *Radiographics* 2003;33(1):3–19.

3 **Answer B.** Sinking skin flap syndrome. There is a right-sided craniectomy with the skin flap collapsing inward in a paradoxical fashion. No evidence of postop encephalomalacia or tension pneumocephalus seen on these images.

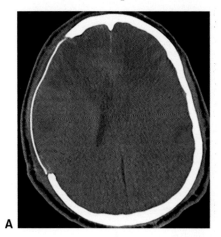 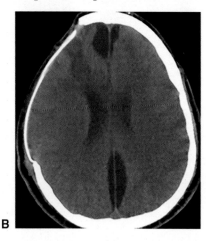 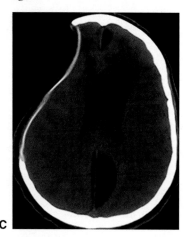

A   B   C

Imaging Findings: Right-sided craniectomy (A) with progressively sinking flap (B and C) and compression of right lateral ventricle (C).

Discussion: Sinking skin flap syndrome or trephined syndrome. It is a rare delayed complication after craniectomy associated with neurologic deterioration that resolves after a cranioplasty. Instead of extracranial herniation as intended by the decompression craniectomy to decompress the central structures, there is "paradoxical" herniation as a consequence of atmospheric pressure exceeding intracranial pressure. The underlying etiology is unclear and could be related to alteration in CSF physiology.

Radiologically, there can be presence of sunken skin flap, shift of midline structures, and lower 3rd ventricle and relative intracranial CSF volumes. Clinically, these patients may have headache, fatigability, tinnitus, discomfort at the site of the defect, depression, intolerance to vibration, and cognitive impairment. The presence of sunken skin flap itself, as shown in this case, is the most common radiologic sign associated with the clinical syndrome of trephined but is not a prerequisite for developing this condition. The second most common sign is paradoxical herniation, that is, shift of midline structures away from the craniectomy defect. Timely recognition of this entity is critical for early intervention that can significantly enhance patient outcomes.

References: Annan M, De Toffol B, Hommet C, et al. Sinking skin flap syndrome (or syndrome of the trephined): a review. *Br J Neurosurg* 2015;29(3):314–318.

Vasung L, Hamard M, Soto MC, et al. Radiological signs of the syndrome of the trephined. *Neuroradiology* 2016;58(6):557–568.

4a **Answer A.** Indirect ophthalmoscopy with dilated pupils. There is right hemispheric infarction and presence of high density abutting the retina in the right globe suggesting hemorrhage. This raises concern for nonaccidental injury and dedicated ophthalmoscopy for detailed assessment of retinal hemorrhages, pattern, and extent should be performed for both eyes. Note lower sensitivity of CT for retinal hemorrhage; therefore, careful evaluation of the left eye is also necessary despite no obvious abnormality on CT. Most instances of nonaccidental injury have bilateral involvement, which is more extensive and has foci that extend to the periphery.

4b **Answer A.** 90%. Based on a published review, 91% probability of abuse has been reported in patients with head trauma and retinal hemorrhage (Maguire et al., 2013, reference below). Others report this range can be from 50% to 100%, so of the available choices the best answer would be A.

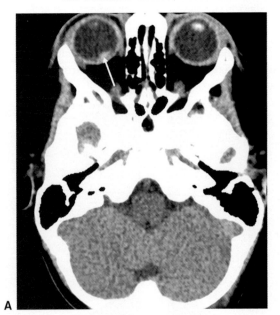 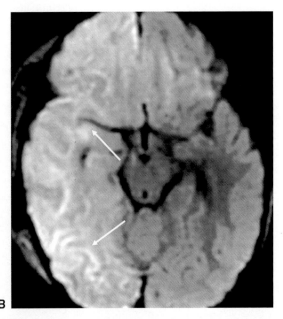

Imaging Findings: Presence of high-density focus abutting the retina in the right eye, suspicious for retinal hemorrhage (A) with right hemispheric restricted diffusion compatible with right ICA infarction in the setting of right ICA dissection.

Discussion: Retinal hemorrhage (RH) is a major factor associated with nonaccidental injury (NAI). The probability of abuse in children with head injury and RH has found to be as high as 91%. A thorough ophthalmologic evaluation with a dilated pupil is necessary for better assessment whenever abuse is suspected. RH in NAI is usually bilateral, multilayered, and extensive with peripheral involvement. Other noninflicted entities such as severe crush injuries or high-altitude fall can rarely have an overlapping appearance; therefore, careful assessment of history, clinical features, and other signs of inflicted injury in consultation with multidisciplinary specialists is necessary.

Differential possibilities, such as elevated intracranial pressure, result in relatively superficial intraretinal hemorrhage. Terson syndrome, which is associated with subarachnoid hemorrhage such as from an aneurysmal rupture, is characterized by preretinal and vitreous hemorrhage, unlike NAI, which has intraretinal hemorrhages.

References: Binenbaum G, Forbes BJ. The eye in child abuse: key points on retinal hemorrhages and abusive head trauma. *Pediatr Radiol* 2014;44(Suppl 4):S571–S577.

Maguire SA, Watts PO, Shaw AD, et al. Retinal haemorrhages and related findings in abusive and non-abusive head trauma: a systematic review. *Eye (Lond)* 2013;27(1):28–36.

5a **Answer B.** Hemorrhagic contusions. Location (anteroinferior frontal lobes and lateral temporal lobe) and associated hemorrhage are typical for traumatic hemorrhagic contusions.

5b **Answer A.** Commonly enlarge over first 2 days following causative event. Though contusions are considered primary injury, increase in number and size is commonly seen within first 48 hours following trauma. These are "brain bruises" resulting from impact of the moving brain against fixed bones/dura. MRI is much more sensitive than CT, especially for small lesions.

5c **Answer A.** Subarachnoid hemorrhage. The other choices are differential considerations for signal abnormality in subarachnoid space on FLAIR images. But given the presence of contusions, the appearance likely represents subarachnoid hemorrhage.

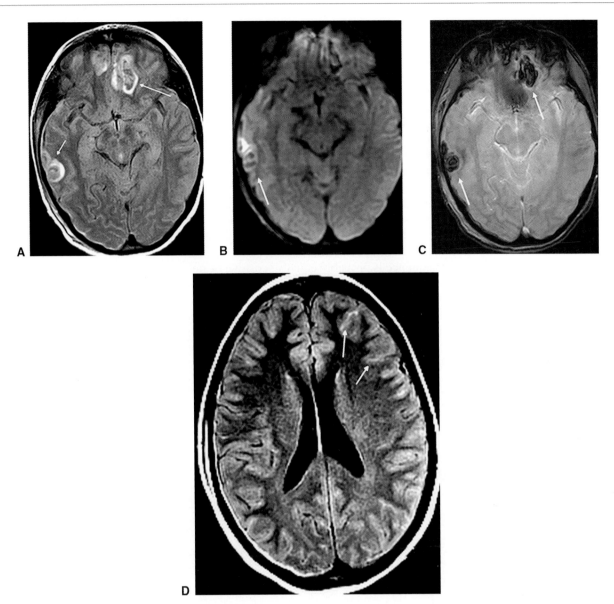

Imaging Findings: Hemorrhagic lesions showing some diffusion restriction present in inferior medial frontal lobes and lateral right temporal lobe, consistent with hemorrhagic contusions (A, B, and C). Scattered FLAIR hyperintense signal in subarachnoid spaces, left more than right, consistent with subarachnoid hemorrhage (D).

Discussion: Traumatic contusions and subarachnoid hemorrhage
Contusions:

Contusions are the most common parenchymal injury with head trauma.

Based on the mechanism, they can be classified as coup contusions (at the site of direct impact) and contrecoup contusions (injury distant to the area of direct impact).

Parasagittal contusions are known as "gliding contusions" caused by angular acceleration with impact of the brain against falx and bone occurring over parasagittal convexity. Less common, "fracture contusions" are due to direct injury to brain parenchyma from fracture fragments.

Given the mechanism, they tend to occur in typical locations—inferomedial frontal lobes, frontal tips, anterior temporal lobes, lateral temporal lobes, and parasagittal convexity. They are often bilateral. Though this is a primary injury, nearly half of the patients reveal contusions on imaging over first 48 hours.

On CT scans, contusions are seen as hyperdense hemorrhages and surrounding edema. Immediately following trauma, smaller contusions may not be well seen on CT. A characteristic "salt-and-pepper" appearance is more apparent in follow-up scans with hyperdense hemorrhages and increasing surrounding edema.

MRI is more sensitive for contusions than CT. Hemorrhages bloom on gradient- or susceptibility-weighted images and surrounding edema is easily seen on FLAIR-/T2-weighted images. Edema associated with contusions can increase up to a week. Occasionally, contusions can be nonhemorrhagic.

Subarachnoid hemorrhage:

Subarachnoid hemorrhage is the most common extra-axial hemorrhage following trauma.

CT, which is in the modality of choice for evaluation of trauma, is highly sensitive of subarachnoid hemorrhage in acute setting. If the SAH is very small, it may quickly become less apparent on CT because of dilution and distribution. CT is not very sensitive for SAH in subacute state.

MRI FLAIR sequence is probably equally sensitive or perhaps more sensitive than CT for subarachnoid hemorrhage in acute setting. However, it is nonspecific. Other etiologies for FLAIR hyperintensity along the sulci need to be excluded. In subacute phase, FLAIR- and susceptibility-weighted imagings are much more sensitive than CT. In chronic stage, hemosiderin staining of meningitis is demonstrated on gradient- or susceptibility-weighted images.

References: Gean AD, Fischbein NJ. Head trauma. *Neuroimaging Clin N Am* 2010;20(4):527–556.

Naidich TP, ed. *Imaging of the brain*. Expert Radiology Series. Philadelphia, PA: Saunders/Elsevier, 2013.

van Gijn J, Kerr RS, Rinkel GJ. Subarachnoid haemorrhage. *Lancet* 2007;369(9558):306–318.

6 **Answer C.** Orbital blowout fracture.

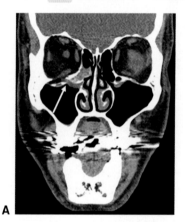 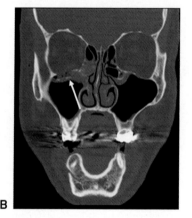 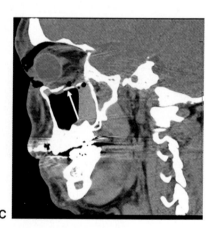

A   B   C

Imaging Findings: There is an isolated fracture fragment of the orbital floor displaced into the maxillary sinus with herniation of orbital contents, consistent with orbital floor blowout fracture.

Discussion: The orbital blowout fracture, typically of the orbital floor or medial wall, is caused by a sudden increase in intraorbital pressure from a blunt force such as a fist. Le Fort fractures disconnect portions of the face from the cranium, with pterygoid plate disruption the common denominator for all Le Fort fractures. Zygomaticomaxillary fractures disrupt the zygomaticofrontal, zygomaticomaxillary, zygomaticosphenoidal, and zygomaticotemporal sutures. The nasoorbitoethmoidal fracture comprises depressed fractures of the nasal bones, medial maxillary buttresses including the medial orbital walls, and ethmoid sinuses.

Although entrapment of the extraocular muscles can be suspected based on imaging, entrapment must be confirmed by clinical testing. Entrapment is a clinical, not an imaging diagnosis.

References: Oppenheimer AJ, Monson LA, Buchman SR. Pediatric orbital fractures. *Craniomaxillofac Trauma Reconstr* 2013;6(1):9–20.

Winegar BA, Murillo H, Tantiwongkosi B. Spectrum of critical imaging findings in complex facial skeletal trauma. *Radiographics* 2013;33(1):3–19.

7a **Answer B.**   Diffuse axonal injury.

7b **Answer A.**   Gray-white interface.

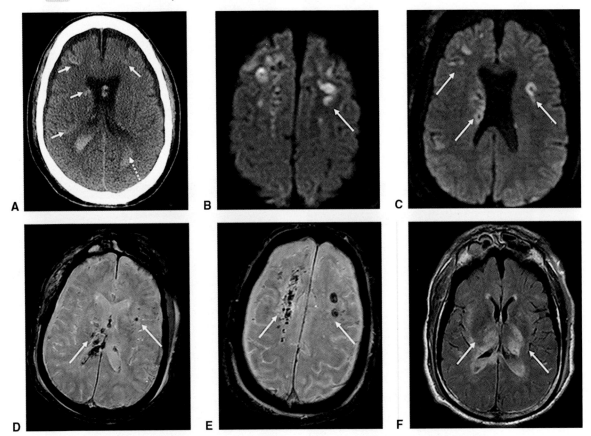

Imaging Findings: CT, FLAIR and susceptibility-weighted MR images show intraventricular hemorrhage (dotted arrow, A) and multiple small foci of parenchymal hemorrhage and edema, distributed in subcortical and deep white matter, basal ganglia, and corpus callosum (arrows D, E and F). There are foci of petechial hemorrhage, many associated with bright signal on the DWI images (arrows B and C). The constellation of findings is most consistent with diffuse axonal injury.

Discussion: Diffuse axonal injury reflects predominantly shear injury to axons, most of which is beyond the resolution of conventional MR imaging. With mild cases of diffuse axonal injury, the most commonly affected sites are at gray-white interfaces. Deeper brain structures are increasingly involved with more severe injury, including basal ganglia, thalamus, brainstem, within ventricles, and choroid plexus.

References: Koerte IK, Hufschmidt J, Muehlmann M, et al. Advanced neuroimaging of mild traumatic brain injury. In: Laskowitz D, Grant G. (eds). *Translational research in traumatic brain injury*. Boca Raton, FL: CRC Press/Taylor and Francis Group, 2016. Chapter 13. Frontiers in Neuroscience.

Provenzale JM. Imaging of traumatic brain injury: a review of the recent medical literature. *AJR Am J Roentgenol* 2010;194(1):16–19.

8 **Answer D.** Subdural hematoma. There is a left hemispheric subdural hematoma that is nearly isoattenuating to gray matter.

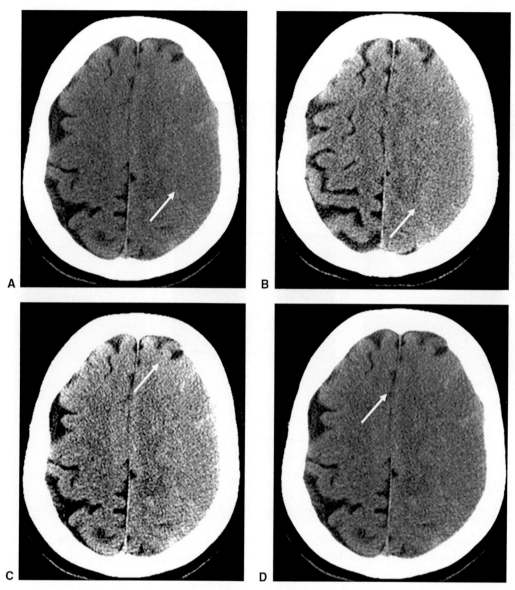

Imaging Findings: There is effacement of sulci of the left cerebral hemisphere. Closer inspection reveals a large crescentic extra-axial abnormality, nearly isodense to brain parenchyma in the left frontal and parietal regions. The abnormality crosses the expected location of the coronal suture. The findings most likely reflect an isodense subdural hematoma.

Discussion: The density of subdural hematoma may be diffusely isodense relative to brain parenchyma in several circumstances, including the subacute stage, from blood mixed with CSF, during anemia, and disseminated intravascular coagulation.

In the early subacute stage, subdural hematoma largely comprises intracellular methemoglobin, which has both T1 shortening and T2 shortening effects, which can lead to hyperintense signal on T1-weighted images, hypointense signal on T2-weighted images, and hypointense signal on FLAIR images. In the late subacute stage, lysis of the RBC leads to extracellular methemoglobin, which prolongs T2 and shortens T1, with resultant hyperintense signal on T1-weighted images, T2-weighted images, and FLAIR images.

Acute subdural hematoma is typically hyperdense but may be isodense in anemia, DIC, or hemorrhage mixed with CSF. Mixed density acute subdural hematoma may occur in setting of active bleeding (hyperacute hemorrhage is isointense), CSF mixing with hemorrhage, and retraction of clot.

References: Gandhoke GS, Kaif M, Choi L, et al. Histopathological features of the outer membrane of chronic subdural hematoma and correlation with clinical and radiological features. *J Clin Neurosci* 2013;20(10):1398–1401.

Wilms G, Marchal G, Geusens E, et al. Isodense subdural haematomas on CT: MRI findings. *Neuroradiology* 1992;34(6):497–499.

9a **Answer B.** Nasoorbitoethmoidal (NOE) fracture.

9b **Answer C.** Telecanthus.

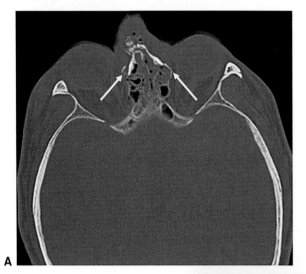

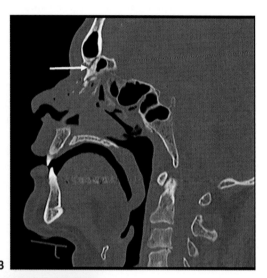

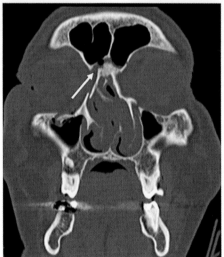

Imaging Findings: There is a comminuted depressed fracture through the nasal bones and underlying ethmoid air cells, with disruption of the superior aspect of the medial maxillary buttresses bilaterally, including the medial orbital walls, characteristic of nasoorbitoethmoidal fractures.

Discussion: In nasoorbitoethmoidal fractures, the attachment of the medial canthal ligaments is often disrupted, leading to telecanthus.

Other potential complications include epiphora from nasolacrimal apparatus injury, ocular injury with blindness, disruption of frontal sinus drainage, CSF leak, meningitis, and meningoencephalocele. The disruption of the medial orbital walls and ethmoids distinguishes this fracture pattern from isolated nasal bone fractures.

The Le Fort type III fracture, or craniofacial dissociation, involves the lateral maxillary and upper horizontal maxillary buttresses and zygomatic arches in addition to the medial maxillary buttresses. Isolated orbital blowout fractures typically involve the orbital floor or lamina papyracea.

Isolated orbital blowout fractures do not involve the orbital rim and thus would unlikely disrupt the medial canthal tendon. Hyphema, monocular loss of vision, and oculocardiac reflex (bradycardia induced by traction on extraocular muscles or pressure on the globes) may occur in both NOE and orbital blowout fractures. Periorbital crepitus typically from the sinonasal region fractures are also not specific to either fracture pattern.

Nasoorbitoethmoidal fractures may disrupt the cribriform plate or the frontal sinuses, posing risk of CSF leak, meningitis, and meningoencephalocele.

References: Hopper RA, Salemy S, Sze RW. Diagnosis of midface fractures with CT: what the surgeon needs to know. *Radiographics* 2006;26(3):783-793.

Winegar BA, Murillo H, Tantiwongkosi B. Spectrum of critical imaging findings in complex facial skeletal trauma. *Radiographics* 2013;33(1):3-19.

10a **Answer D.**   Zygomaticomaxillary complex fracture.

10b **Answer B.**   Anesthesia cheek/upper lip.

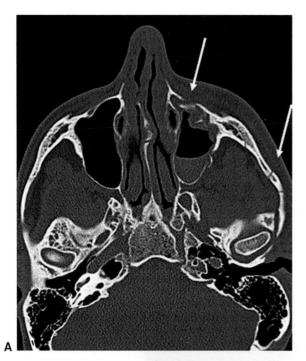

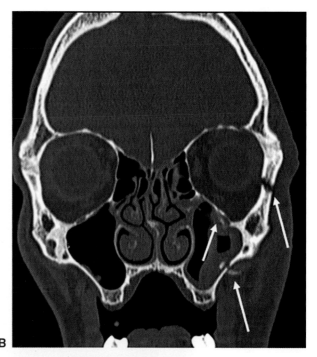

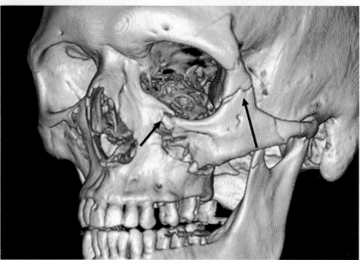

Imaging Findings: Fractures of anterior maxillary wall, zygomatic arch, lateral orbital wall, and orbital floor are shown above (A, B, C). Fractures in this case disrupt the zygomaticofrontal, zygomaticomaxillary, zygomaticosphenoidal, and zygomaticotemporal sutures. This pattern is characteristic of zygomaticomaxillary complex fractures.

Discussion: Tripod fracture (more accurately, tetrapod or quadripod fracture) is generally caused by a direct blow to the cheek. It is also known as zygomaticomaxillary complex fracture, which is generally the preferred terminology.

Zygomatic bone forms lateral orbital rim inferior to zygomatic process of the frontal bone, the lateral orbital wall anterior to the sphenoid, the anterior and lateral maxillary sinus walls superior to the hard palate, and the zygomatic arch anterior to temporal bone. It is connected to rest of the facial skeleton and calvarium by four sutures—zygomaticofrontal suture, zygomaticomaxillary suture, zygomaticotemporal suture, and zygomaticosphenoid suture.

Zygomaticomaxillary complex fracture refers to fractures involving anterior and posterolateral maxillary sinus walls, orbital floor, lateral orbital wall, and zygomatic arch, fracture lines coursing through or near the abovementioned four sutures with resultant separation of the zygoma from the calvarium and remainder of the facial skeleton. In radiographs, the zygomaticosphenoid suture fracture is not well demonstrated and only fractures through the other three sutures can be demonstrated and hence the older terminology "tripod fracture." Rotational forces by masseter muscle can displace the fractured zygoma.

References: Hopper RA, Salemy S, Sze RW. Diagnosis of midface fractures with CT: what the surgeon needs to know. *Radiographics* 2006;26(3):783–793.

Winegar BA, Murillo H, Tantiwongkosi B. Spectrum of critical imaging findings in complex facial skeletal trauma. *Radiographics* 2013;33(1):3–19.

11a Answer C. Optimal assessment includes multiplanar reformats and 3-D volume rendering. Both multiplanar reformats and 3-D images are extremely useful for detection of fractures, characterization, as well as surgical planning. Though mandible shows a tendency to break in multiple places, nearly 50% of fractures are unifocal. Flail mandible refers to fractured free anterior mandibular segment.

11b Answer A. Angle. Inferior alveolar nerve enters the mandibular canal at the lingula and exits through the mental foramen, which is at the level of second premolar. Hence, fractures of the angle and posterior body carry higher risk of injury.

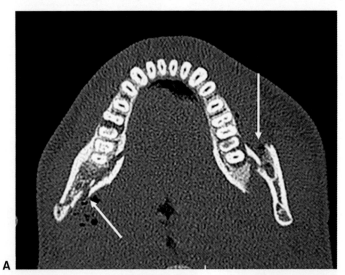

A

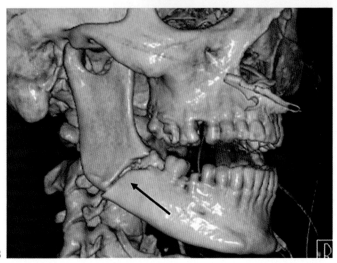

B

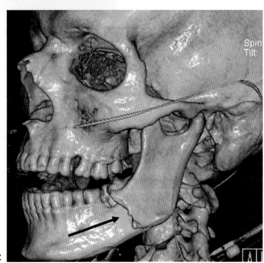

C

Imaging Findings: Fracture through bilateral mandibular angles. Given the involvement of mandibular canals (especially on the left, where the displacement of fracture fragments is more than 5 mm), there is risk of inferior alveolar nerve injury.

Discussion: Mandible is the only mobile bone in the face and the second most common site of facial fracture after the nasal bone. Motor vehicle accident and assault are the most common causes. More than half of mandibular fractures are complex (communicating to the skin surface or the oral cavity) and bilateral (related to somewhat "bony ring" structures). 40% to 50% of fractures are unifocal. 15% of fractures are associated with other facial fractures.

Body, symphysis, angle (often secondary to direct trauma), and mandibular condyles (often secondary to transmitted force) are commonly fractured locations. Forces created by elevators of the mandible (pterygomasseteric sling) and the depressors (geniohyoid, mylohyoid and digastric muscles) commonly result in displacement and/or rotation of the fracture fragments.

CT scan with multiplanar reformats and 3-D volume–rendered imaging is the investigation of choice for fracture assessment. Comminuted fractures often have triangular fragment along the inferior margin of the mandible (basal triangle), which tend to show lingual displacement (butterfly fracture or lingual fragments).

Imaging assessment of this fracture is necessary as this fragment cannot be easily visualized surgically. The fracture line that crosses mandibular canal (which extends from the lingula to the mental foramen, which is at the level of the second premolar), particularly when there is more than 5-mm displacement, is associated with a high risk of inferior alveolar nerve injury.

Flail mandible refers to fractured free anterior mandibular segment (seen with bilateral angle fractures, bilateral body fractures, and parasymphyseal and bicondylar fractures), which often shows posterior and inferior displacement with loss of support to the tongue. These factors together with adjacent soft tissue injury/hemorrhage may contribute to airway compromise. Attention should be paid to the relationship of fracture to the tooth.

Management is often surgical correction—occlusal reduction (mandibulomaxillary fixation), direct internal fixation, and less commonly external fixation (with complex comminuted fractures). Postsurgical imaging is often done to evaluate for adequate reduction.

Fusion should normally occur by 8 weeks. Nonunion and osteomyelitis are the common complications. Hardware failure (fracture, bending, loosening, migration) should be assessed.

References: Buch K, Mottalib A, Nadgir RN, et al. Unifocal versus multifocal mandibular fractures and injury location. *Emerg Radiol* 2016;23(2):161–167. doi:10.1007/s10140-015-1375-9

Dreizin D, Nam AJ, Tirada N, et al. Multidetector CT of mandibular fractures, reductions, and complications: a clinically relevant primer for the radiologist. *Radiographics* 2016;36(5):1539–1564. doi:10.1148/rg.2016150218

12 Answer C. Cephalohematoma. Typical appearance limited by suture lines. Signal characteristics are that of late subacute blood and not that of CSF (option A) or venous structure (option D). This is an extracranial finding and not in epidural intracranial location (option B).

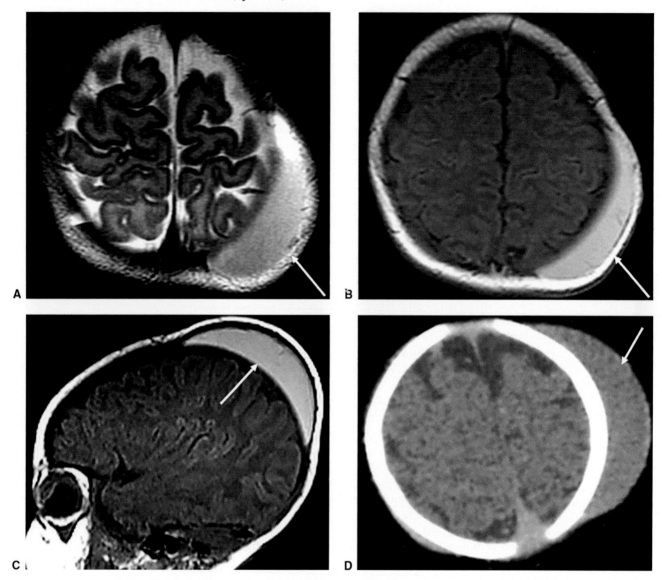

Imaging Findings: Scalp collection showing typical density/signal characteristics of subacute blood. The hematoma is well circumscribed and is limited by suture lines.

Discussion: Scalp is a multilayered soft tissue covering of the calvarial vault. The layers can be defined by the word itself:

    S—skin
    C—connective tissue (dense)
    A—aponeurotic layer (includes the galea aponeurotica)
    L—loose connective tissue
    P—pericranium

With scalp lacerations, attention needs to be paid for foreign bodies. Foreign bodies can have variable density on CT (e.g., metallic foreign bodies and glass appear hyperdense; wood pieces are hypodense).

Scalp hematomas are generally of no clinical significance, the exception being newborns and young infants. There are two types of scalp hematomas: cephalohematomas and subgaleal hematomas.

Cephalohematomas are subperiosteal hematomas that lie along the calvarial surface and elevate the periosteum. These are limited by the sutures and usually of no clinical significance. They occur in about 1% of newborns and are more common following instrumented delivery. CT scan shows somewhat lentiform hematoma that overlies the calvarium and limited by sutures. Parietal and occipital regions are the common locations. Most of cephalohematomas completely resolve within a few weeks. Rarely, chronic cephalohematoma may show peripheral calcification and present as firm palpable mass.

Subgaleal hematomas are subgaleal blood collections and a common finding with trauma in all ages. Bleeding into the subgaleal space can be very extensive as these are not anatomically limited by suture lines. The hematomas tend to spread diffusely over the entire calvarium. In newborns, these can cause hypovolemia and hypotension.

References: Drake RL, Vogl W, Mitchell AWM, et al. *Gray's anatomy for students: [online access + interactive extras; studentconsult.com].* Philadelphia, PA: Elsevier/Churchill Livingstone, 2005.

Naidich TP, ed. *Imaging of the brain.* Expert Radiology Series. Philadelphia, PA: Saunders/Elsevier, 2013.

Osborn AG. *Osborn's brain: imaging, pathology, and anatomy,* 1st ed. Salt Lake City, UT: Amirsys Pub, 2013.

13a **Answer B.** Left squamosal sutural diastases. Comparison to the normal side (image 2) clearly shows diastases of the left squamosal suture. At this age, the suture should have fused; therefore, synostosis is the incorrect choice. There is no leptomeningeal cyst.

13b **Answer A.** High risk of venous thrombosis. These are sutural fractures and can result in a higher risk of dural venous sinus thrombosis. The leptomeningeal cyst formation is seen in children. There is no specific direct association of subarachnoid hemorrhage and intracranial hypotension.

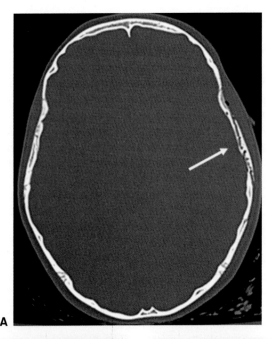

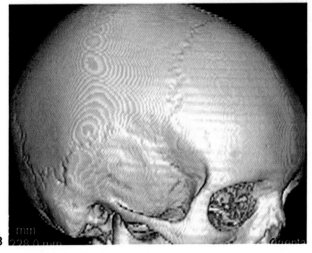

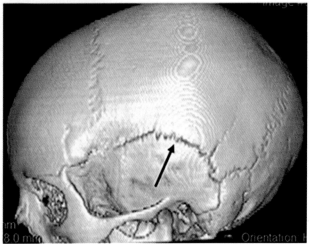

Imaging Findings: Diastasis of left squamosal suture. Fracture line is also involving inferior parietal bone. Three dimensional volume–rendered images aid in visualization.

Discussion: Calvarial fracture-sutural diastasis. Skull fracture is a common finding following trauma. The diagnosis of the fracture by itself is generally not clinically more important than the intracranial damage. However, it is an important indicator for associated intracranial injury.

Skull fractures can be simple or comminuted, closed to open. From imaging perspective, skull fractures can be described as linear fractures, depressed fractures, elevated fractures, and diastatic fractures.

Linear fractures are caused by a relatively low-intensity blunt trauma delivered over a wide area of the skull. They generally do not require specific treatment. Linear fractures crossing the vascular grooves for the middle meningeal artery or dural venous sinuses carry a higher association with epidural hematomas.

Depressed fractures are commonly caused by high-energy force to a small portion of the skull, like injury with baseball bat, hammer, etc. They often require surgical correction, especially when the displacement is more than the thickness of the skull.

Diastatic fractures are fractures that widen a suture or synchondrosis. They generally result from extension of a linear fracture into the suture or synchondrosis. In adults, sutural widening of more than 2 to 3 mm and asymmetric widening compared to the contralateral side are the indicators for sutural diastasis. With sutural fracture/diastasis, epidural hematoma can cross the suture line.

If fracture overlies the venous sinus, there is higher risk of venous thrombosis. There is a high risk of infection if there is an open fracture or the fracture involves the posterior frontal sinuses or mastoid air cells. Temporal and cribriform plate fractures predispose to CSF leak.

Growing skull fracture (also known as posttraumatic leptomeningeal cyst) occurs exclusively during childhood. It results when the dura is torn and retracts, exposing the bony margins of the fracture to the pulsation of arachnoid and subarachnoid CSF. Protrusion of CSF space into the fracture disrupts normal bony healing and CSF pulsation results in continued fracture widening.

CT scan is the modality of choice for diagnosis of skull fractures. Nondisplaced fractures can be missed on thick axial slices of the CT, especially if the fracture is in the plane of the imaging. Routine review of thin sections and 3-D volume-rendered images will help in easier detection. In sutural diastasis, 3-D volume-rendered images are specifically useful. Volume-rendered images are also helpful in better understanding of spatial relationships of fracture fragments and for surgical planning.

Cranial sutures (more so in pediatric age group because of accessory sutures) can be confused for fractures. Lack of overlying soft tissue swelling is a clue. Fractures show sharp lucencies with nonsclerotic edges, as opposed to sclerotic and wavy margins of sutures. Accessory sutures are more common in parietal and occipital bones. When a fracture extends to a major suture, there could be widening of the fracture line as it approaches the suture, and also, there could be associated diastasis of the suture. An accessory suture will usually not produce this appearance. Fractures can cross suture lines and extend from one major suture to the other, whereas accessory sutures join and merge with the suture. Accessory sutures are often bilateral and fairly symmetric.

References: Dundamadappa SK, Thangasamy S, Resteghini N, et al. Skull fractures in pediatric patients on computerized tomogram: comparison between routing bone window images and 3D volume-rendered images. *Emerg Radiol* 2015;22(4):367–372.

Naidich TP, ed. *Imaging of the brain*. Expert Radiology Series. Philadelphia, PA: Saunders/Elsevier, 2013.

14 **Answer B.** Posttraumatic subdural hygromas. Given history of recent trauma, this most likely is posttraumatic subdural hygroma. This is not a chronic hematoma, as no collection was evident in a scan done 3 days ago. Lack of complexity argue against empyema.

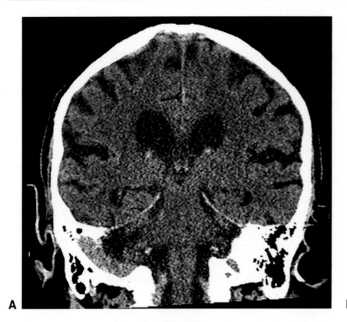

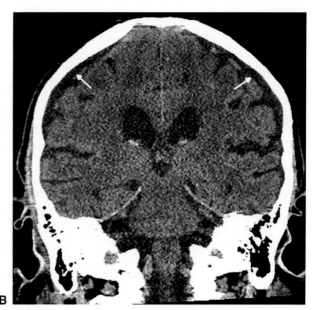

A

B

Imaging Findings: Scan done a few days following trauma shows new subdural collections over bilateral cerebral convexities showing density similar to CSF. No significant associated mass effect. No frank hemorrhage within these collections.

Discussion: Traumatic subdural hygroma. Subdural hygroma refers to collection of CSF or CSF-like fluid in the subdural space. They have similar signal characteristics to CSF and may have a higher-protein content.

Traumatic acute subdural hygroma (SHG) is not an uncommon finding, occurring in 5% to 20% of patients with closed head injury. They are generally delayed in their appearance starting a day to several days following the episode of trauma. The exact pathogenesis is uncertain. The most commonly accepted theory is a break in the arachnoid membrane, "flap-valve" mechanism of this tear, and collection of CSF in the subdural space. The other theories include leakage of fluid from damaged blood vessels and defect in CSF absorption. This is reported to be more common in extremes of age group, felt to be related to preexisting prominent CSF spaces. But this is commonly in adults, because of higher occurrence of trauma in this age group.

Majority of SHGs are small and asymptomatic. Rarely, they can grow to be a larger collection and can cause mass effect. They are collections of CSF with generally modified composition. Initially, they are thin CSF-like subdural collections and can be bilateral or unilateral, more common in frontal regions, and without any associated mass effect. Some authors refer to these early collections as small subdural effusions. They can increase in size over next several days and then progressively get absorbed over next 3 months. Membranes can develop within these collections after a couple of weeks. Fragile neovasculature in these membranes and also in the arachnoid can rupture and bleed into the collection resulting in increased density of the collection and also frank hemorrhage. Up to 33% of SHG evolve into subdural hematomas. Conversion into subdural hematoma is the most notable complication.

On imaging, these collections show typical features of subdural location and "near" CSF density/signal characteristics. In cases of hemorrhage, they can show increased CT density and conversion into frank subdural hematoma.

References: Herold TJS, Taylor S, Abbrescia K, et al. Post-traumatic subdural hygroma: case report. *J Emerg Med* 2004;27(4):361–366. doi:10.1016/j.jemermed.2004.03.018

Zanini MA, de Lima Resende LA, de Souza Faleiros AT, et al. Traumatic subdural hygromas: proposed pathogenesis based classification. *J Trauma* 2008;64(3):705–713. doi:10.1097/TA.0b013e3180485cfc

15a **Answer A.** Epidural hematoma. The location is typical for venous epidural hematoma. Epidural hematoma from middle meningeal artery injury is more posterior and lateral and typically underlies squamous temporal bone. This patient did not have lesion in this location on recent prior to suggest a meningioma. This lenticular morphology favors epidural over subdural location.

15b **Answer C.** Conservative management because of typically a benign course. Benign course is typical. Expansion and surgical evacuation are rare occurrences. For any type of epidural hematoma, a CTA or short interval follow-up are not appropriate choices.

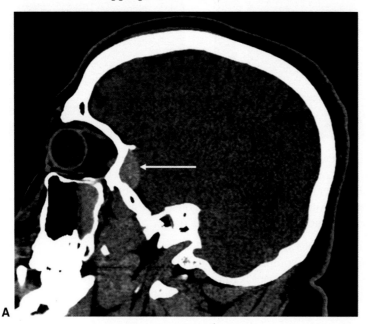
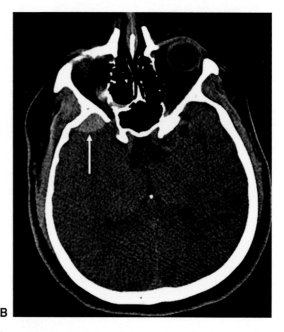

A   B

Imaging Findings: Small lentiform extra-axial hematoma overlying right temporal pole. The location is typical for a venous epidural hematoma.

Discussion: Venous epidural hematoma. Epidural hematomas are caused by high-energy direct-impact results in deformation of the skull, stripping of the dura from the endosteal margin, and arterial/venous disruption.

In the supratentorial compartment, 90% of epidural hematomas are arterial in origin and an associated fracture is seen in more than 90% of cases. Majority result from disruption of middle meningeal artery and hence the typical location beneath the squamous temporal bone.

About 10% of supratentorial epidural hematomas are venous in origin caused by fractures that cross the venous sinus such as at the skull base and in anterior temporal region. Venous epidural hematomas are more common in infratentorial compartment because of the abundance of dural veins and venous sinuses. In contrast to arterial epidural hematoma, venous epidural hematomas can cross suture lines and also dural reflections can straddle supra- and infratentorial compartments.

The anterior temporal epidural hematomas are thought to result from injury to sphenoparietal sinus or its major territories. On imaging, these are not seen biconvex CT hyperdense extra-axial collection of blood adjacent to the anterior temporal tip without significant mass effect or herniation. These are typically smaller and do not pose a risk of rapid expansion. They tend to have an indolent clinical course and may be managed conservatively.

Reference: Gean AD, Fischbein NJ, Purcell DD, et al. Benign anterior temporal epidural hematoma: indolent lesion with a characteristic CT imaging appearance after blunt head trauma. *Radiology* 2010;257(1):212–218.

16 **Answer A.** Craniocervical disassociation. Craniocervical dissociation (CCD) with disruption of atlantoaxial and atlanto-occipital articulation. The discontinuity seen in the clivus is the normal unossified sphenooccipital synchondrosis. No bony fractures are seen.

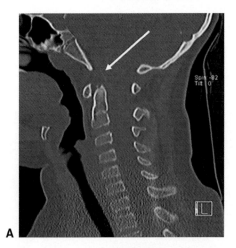 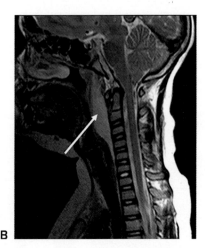 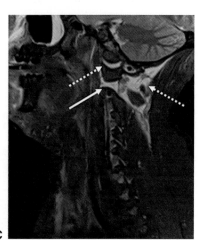

A   B   C

Imaging Findings: Sagittal CT cervical spine again shows increased basion dens interval (BDI) (A). Sagittal midline T2 obtained several hours after the initial CT shows an interval large prevertebral hematoma (B). Sagittal STIR images shows widening and fluid in atlanto-occipital and atlantoaxial joints consistent with capsular injury (C). Note prominent adjacent soft tissue edema (C).

Discussion: Craniocervical dissociation (CCD) is the disruption of the craniocervical junction and its ligamentous complex, due usually to hyperextension or hyperflexion–distraction injuries. Children are at higher risk for atlanto-occipital injury because of large head size, hypoplastic occipital condyles, and ligament laxity.

Injuries can be unilateral and bilateral and usually occur at occiput–C1, C1–C2, or both. The injury has a predominant ligamentous component.

Abnormal findings include basion dens interval (BDI) > 12 mm on radiographs (10 mm on CT) and basion posterior axial line interval (BAI) > 12 mm on radiographs (unreliable on CT).

Distraction of atlanto-occipital and atlantoaxial articulations and soft tissue/ligamentous injury is seen. These injuries are characterized by disruption of the articular capsules, alar ligaments, transverse ligament, tectorial membrane, and sometimes a type 1 dens fracture.

CCD is often a fatal or devastating injury. Survival rates are better for children. Early diagnosis, cervical spine stabilization, and cardiorespiratory support are imperative for improved survival.

References: Riascos R, Bonfante E, Cotes C, et al. Imaging of atlanto-occipital and atlantoaxial traumatic injuries: what the radiologist needs to know. *Radiographics* 2015;35(7):2121–2134.

Rojas CA, Bertozzi JC, Martinez CR, et al. Reassessment of the craniocervical junction: normal values on CT. *AJNR Am J Neuroradiol* 2007;28(9):1819–1823.

Warner J, Shanmuganathan K, Mirvis SE, et al. Magnetic resonance imaging of ligamentous injury of the cervical spine. *Emerg Radiol* 1996;3:9–15.

Brain Infections

LEE FINKELSTONE • ERNST GARCON • GAURAV JINDAL • GUL MOONIS

QUESTIONS

1 A previously healthy 30-year-old presents with seizures and recent travel history.

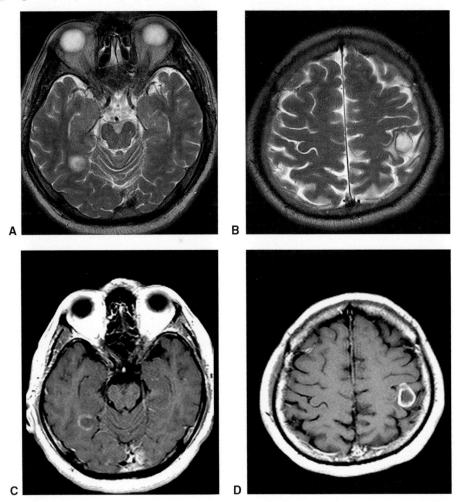

1a What is the most likely diagnosis?

A. Toxoplasmosis
B. Neurocysticercosis
C. Metastatic disease
D. Tumefactive multiple sclerosis

1b In regard to neurocysticercosis, edema surrounding the cystic lesions is greatest in which stage of the disease?

A. Vesicular

B. Colloidal vesicular

C. Granular nodular

D. Nodular calcified

2 A 50-year-old presents with fever, headaches, and new-onset seizures. Brain MRI with gadolinium was done, and selected images are submitted for review.

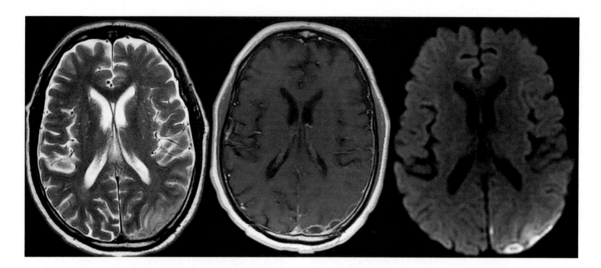

2a The abnormal MRI findings are:

A. Parenchymal

B. Intraventricular

C. Extra-axial

D. Parenchymal and extra-axial

2b What is the most likely diagnosis?

A. Herpes encephalitis

B. Cerebral abscess

C. Subdural empyema

D. Gangliocytoma

3 A 63-year-old status post bone marrow transplant (BMT) for plasmacytoma of the skull base complains of new headaches. Selected images from MRI are presented below.

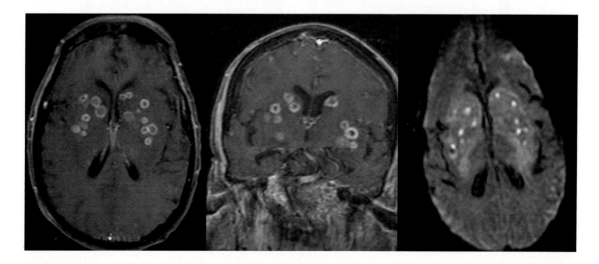

3a What is the best explanation for the imaging findings taking into account the patient's clinical history and presentation?

    A. Ischemic lacunar infarcts
    B. Hemorrhagic infarcts
    C. Hematogenous metastases
    D. Multiple small abscesses

3b What is the most likely diagnosis?

    A. CNS cryptococcal infection
    B. Herpes encephalitis
    C. Acute stroke
    D. Multiple sclerosis

4 A 30-year-old with HIV not compliant with HAART therapy presents with confusion and ataxia.

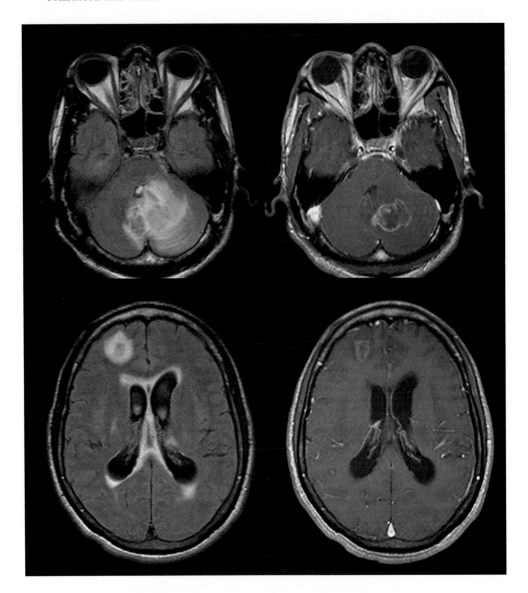

4a What is the most likely diagnosis?

    A. Metastatic disease

    B. Toxoplasmosis

    C. Lymphoma

    D. Active demyelinating disease

4b In regard to imaging findings on thallium 201 SPECT in toxoplasmosis and lymphoma, which statement is correct?

    A. Toxoplasmosis and lymphoma are both hypometabolic.

    B. Toxoplasmosis is hypometabolic and lymphoma is hypermetabolic.

    C. Toxoplasmosis is hypermetabolic and lymphoma is hypometabolic.

    D. Toxoplasmosis and lymphoma are both hypermetabolic.

5 A 4-year-old presents with fever, failure to thrive, and altered mental status.

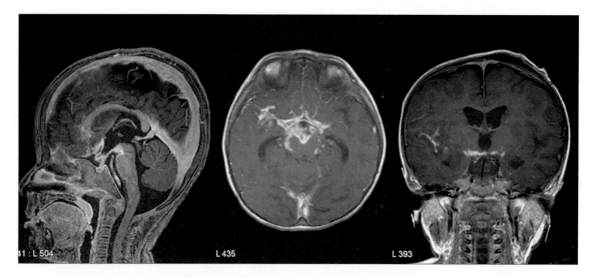

5a What best describes the imaging findings?

    A. Basilar pachymeningeal enhancement with hydrocephalus

    B. Basilar pachymeningeal enhancement without hydrocephalus

    C. Basilar leptomeningeal enhancement with hydrocephalus

    D. Basilar leptomeningeal enhancement without hydrocephalus

A chest x-ray was obtained.

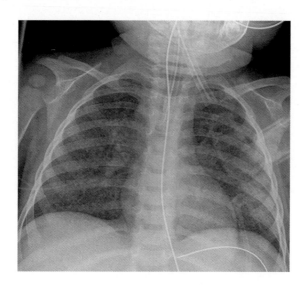

5b   Given the chest x-ray, what is the most likely diagnosis for the brain imaging findings?

   A. Neurosarcoid
   B. TB meningitis
   C. CNS lymphoma
   D. Subarachnoid hemorrhage

6   A 23-year-old male with a history of intravenous drug use presents with septic shock. An MRI of the brain is performed.

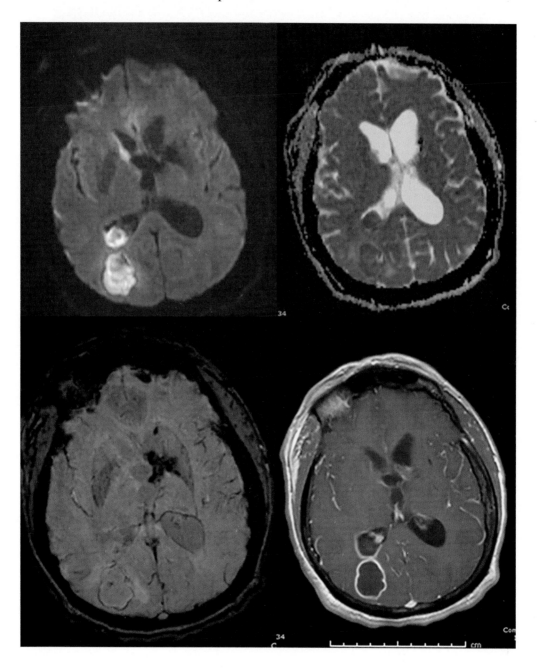

6a What is the most likely diagnosis?

    A. Acute right PCA/MCA watershed infarct

    B. Acute intracranial hemorrhage with intraventricular extension

    C. Right parietal lobe abscess with intraventricular extension

    D. Glioblastoma multiforme with intraventricular spread

7 A 35-year-old presents with headaches and seizures.

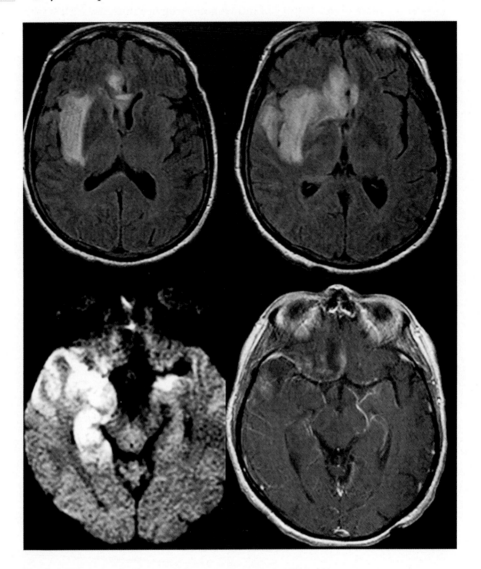

7a What is the most likely diagnosis?

    A. Anaplastic astroctyoma

    B. Acute infarction

    C. Paraneoplastic limbic encephalitis

    D. HSV encephalitis

7b The next best step to confirm the diagnosis is:

    A. CT scan of the brain

    B. Paraneoplastic antibody workup

    C. PCR (polymerase chain reaction) of CSF

    D. MRA of the circle of Willis

8 A 60-year-old man presents with progressive memory problems and abnormal movements.

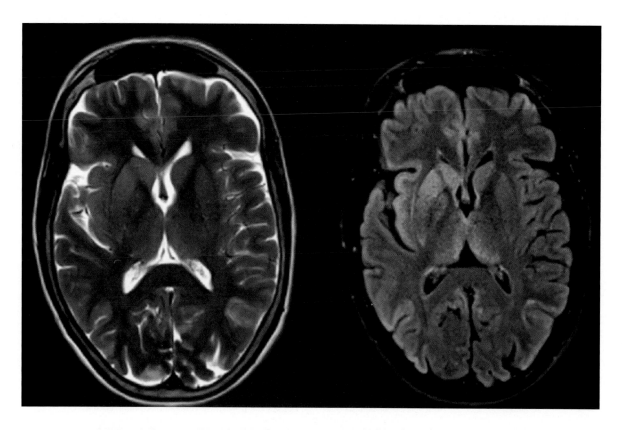

8a What is the most likely diagnosis?

A. Creutzfeldt-Jakob disease (CJD)
B. Hypoxic ischemic injury
C. Leigh syndrome
D. Wernicke encephalopathy

8b Which imaging sequence is most sensitive for diagnosing CJD?

A. T2
B. FLAIR
C. DWI
D. Postcontrast T1

ANSWERS AND EXPLANATIONS

1a **Answer B.** Neurocysticercosis. In a young patient with travel history, seizures, and multiple peripherally enhancing cystic lesions, neurocysticercosis is the most likely diagnosis. Also, there is a suggestion of enhancing nodules at the posterior aspect of the lesions, likely representing the scolex.

1b **Answer B.** Colloidal vesicular. There are four stages of neurocysticercosis: vesicular, colloidal vesicular, granular nodular, and nodular calcified. Surrounding edema is greatest in the colloidal vesicular phase.

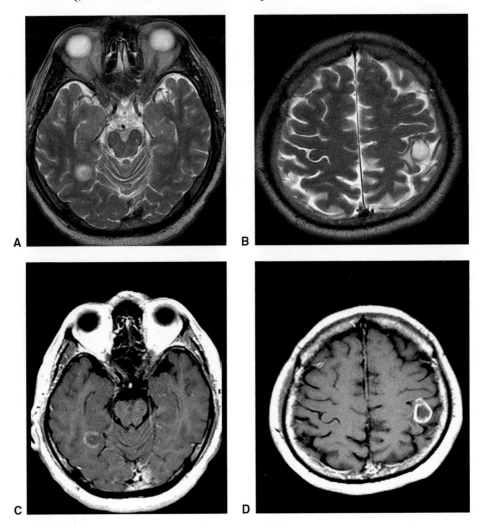

Imaging Findings: Figures A and B show T2 hyperintense cystic lesions in the medial right temporal lobe and left parietal lobe at the convexity, although the hyperintense signal is not as bright as CSF and is heterogeneous. Figures C and D show peripheral ring-like enhancement of the cystic lesions.

Discussion: Neurocysticercosis is caused by a parasitic infection from the pork tapeworm *Taenia solium*. It is the most common parasitic disease of the central nervous system worldwide, and travel and globalization have caused the disease to now spread beyond endemic regions. Patients most commonly present with seizures. Treatment depends on viability of the lesions, number of lesions, and extent of surrounding edema but is often with albendazole and steroids. Surgical intervention may be needed if hydrocephalus has developed.

Lesions can be parenchymal, intraventricular, or within the subarachnoid spaces. When parenchymal, the cysts are most commonly located at the gray-white matter junction. When intraventricular, the cysts are often solitary with predilection for the fourth ventricle. When subarachnoid, cysts tend to occur at the cortical sulci. When in the basilar cisterns, cysts may be racemose or "grape-like."

There are four stages of the disease with distinct imaging findings. In the vesicular stage, the cyst is thin walled and has signal characteristics similar to CSF without contrast enhancement or edema. An eccentric, discrete scolex can be seen. In the colloidal vesicular phase, the larva begins to degenerate creating an inflammatory response and resultant surrounding edema. The hyperintense cyst at this stage will demonstrate ring-like peripheral enhancement. In the granular nodular stage, the cyst decreases in size and the cyst wall retracts, surrounding edema decreases, and nodular or ring-like enhancement persists. Finally in the nodular calcified stage, the cyst is shrunken and calcified with hypointensity on T2 and gradient echo sequences.

References: Kiumura-Hayama ET, et al. Neurocysticercosis: radiologic-pathologic correlation. *Radiographics* 2010;30(6):1705–1720.

Lucato LT, et al. The role of conventional MR imaging sequences in the evaluation of neurocysticercosis: impact on characterization of the scolex and lesion burden. *AJNR Am J Neuroradiol* 2007;28:1501–1504.

Zhao JL, et al. Imaging spectrum of neurocysticercosis. *Radiol Infect Dis* 2015;1(2):94–102.

2a **Answer D.** Parenchymal and extra-axial. The prioritization of differential diagnosis considerations in the evaluation of a neuroimaging study depends on the anatomic location of the findings, whether intra-axial/parenchymal, extra-axial, or both. The images provided clearly identify parenchymal and extra-axial signal abnormalities and enhancement (option D).

2b **Answer C.** Subdural empyema. The extra-axial loculated enhancing collection with associated restricted diffusion and adjacent parenchymal edema favors a subdural empyema with cerebritis.

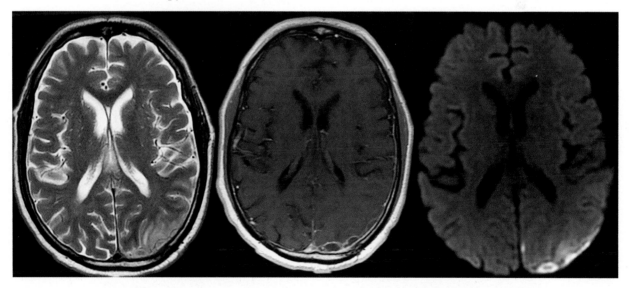

Imaging Findings: Axial T2-weighted image demonstrates gyral crowding in the left parietal lobe with prolonged T2 signal in the involved subcortical white matter consistent with vasogenic edema/cerebritis. Please note the preservation of the normal cortical thickness. Axial postgadolinium T1-weighted image demonstrates a small loculated extra-axial collection with a rim of enhancement in the left parietal region. The crescentic shape of the collection suggests a subdural location. In addition, there is diffuse smooth thickening and enhancement of the adjacent left frontoparietal pachymeninges. Diffusion-weighted image shows restricted diffusion in the extra-axial collection consistent with an empyema.

Discussion: Subdural empyema (SDE) is an uncommon infected extra-axial fluid collection located in the subdural space. SDE usually occurs as a complication of acute sinusitis, mastoiditis, meningitis, or trauma and can result in severe complications such as cortical vein thrombosis, venous infarcts, cerebritis, or abscess.

The clinical presentation depends on the etiology and anatomic location of the SDE. The patient is usually very sick with seizures, headaches, focal neurologic deficits, or altered sensorium.

The imaging evaluation may start with a noncontrast head CT that will demonstrate diffuse or focal brain swelling. If the clinical suspicion of SDE is high, a contrast-enhanced CT or MRI is preferred. The postcontrast images demonstrate enhancement of the wall of a crescentic-shaped extra-axial collection. SDE crosses the calvarial sutures like any other types of subdural collection. On MRI, the diffusion-weighted images (DWI) will establish the infected nature of the fluid.

The treatment is surgical evacuation and appropriate antibiotic therapy.

Differential Diagnosis: The main differential diagnosis is an epidural empyema that is meniscal in shape. Other extra-axial fluid collections containing blood products or cerebrospinal fluid should also be considered. Subdural lymphoma may occasionally be a diagnostic challenge on imaging (restricted diffusion), but clinical findings are very different from an acutely infected patient.

Reference: Wong AM, Zimmerman RA, Simon EM, et al. Diffusion-weighted MR imaging of subdural empyemas in children. *AJNR Am J Neuroradiol* 2004;25(6):1016–1021.

3a   **Answer D.**   Multiple small abscesses. The best explanation is multiple small abscesses in an immunocompromised patient.

3b   **Answer A.**   CNS cryptococcal infection. The most likely diagnosis in an immunocompromised patient with enhancing cystic lesions and restricted diffusion at the base of the brain is CNS cryptococcal infection (option A).

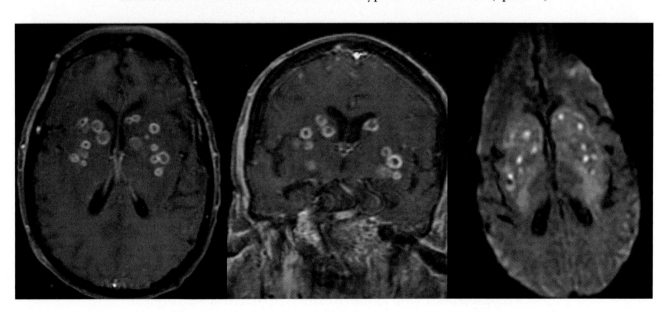

Imaging Findings: Axial DWI of the brain shows punctate foci of hyperintense signal in the bilateral basal ganglia that may represent restricted diffusion or T2 shine through. After correlation with dark ADC map signal (not shown) that confirmed true restricted diffusion, the postgadolinium images in axial and coronal planes demonstrate multiple ring-enhancing lesions in the basal ganglia that are consistent with parenchymal cryptococcoma.

Discussion: CNS cryptococcosis is a fungal infection of the brain caused by *Cryptococcus neoformans*. It is predominately seen in immune-suppressed patient with AIDS or cancer or after bone marrow transplant.

The histology of CNS involvement is primarily meningeal, less frequently parenchymal with typical distribution in the basal ganglia and midbrain, resulting in the three most common imaging patterns of meningitis, cryptococcoma, or gelatinous pseudocysts.

Clinically, the patient may present with signs and symptoms of meningitis or meningoencephalitis including headaches, seizures, blurry vision, or altered mental status.

CT scan is nonspecific and may demonstrate hydrocephalus or localized brain swelling. This case illustrates the typical MRI appearance of parenchymal cryptococcomas with accumulation of a mucinous exudate in the dilated perivascular spaces of the basal ganglia. DWI and postgadolinium images are sufficient to suggest the diagnosis and start appropriate therapy.

The treatment is amphotericin B or fluconazole with a 20% mortality rate in AIDS patients despite antifungal treatment. A fatal outcome will occur without prompt diagnosis and treatment.

Differential Diagnosis: The differential diagnoses include other CNS infections like toxoplasmosis and tuberculosis, which also occur in immunocompromised patients. A lumbar puncture with CSF analysis, culture, and sensitivity may confirm the diagnosis for targeted antibiotic therapy. Other diagnostic considerations will include primary or secondary CNS lymphoma.

Reference: Charlier C, Dromer F, Lévêque C, et al. Cryptococcal neuroradiological lesions correlate with severity during cryptococcal meningoencephalitis in HIV-positive patients in the HAART era. *PLoS One* 2008;3(4):e1950.

4a **Answer B.** Toxoplasmosis. Given that there are multiple lesions with distribution including the basal ganglia, corticomedullary junction, and cerebellum, the diagnosis favors toxoplasmosis over lymphoma. Metastatic disease can have a similar imaging appearance, but given the provided history of a young patient with HIV, toxoplasmosis is the most likely diagnosis.

4b **Answer B.** Toxoplasmosis is hypometabolic and lymphoma is hypermetabolic. Similarly, lymphoma is hypermetabolic on 18F-FDG PET and demonstrates increased relative cerebral blood flow on MR perfusion. An easy way to remember this is that lymphoma is an active tumor, so no matter how you image it, it should be "hot!"

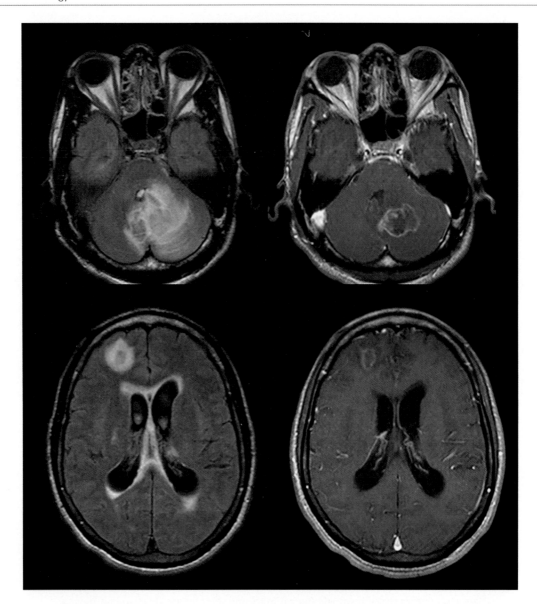

Imaging Findings: Axial FLAIR and postgadolinium images through the posterior fossa show a large rim-enhancing left cerebellar lesion with surrounding vasogenic edema and resultant mass effect on the fourth ventricle. The lesion is centrally mildly T2 hyperintense with hypointense rim. Higher axial scans demonstrate an additional right frontal rim-enhancing lesion. The multiplicity of the ring-enhancing lesions in an HIV patient favors toxoplasmosis as the leading diagnosis.

Discussion: Toxoplasmosis is an opportunistic infection caused by the parasite *Toxoplasma gondii*. It is the most common opportunistic CNS infection in AIDS patients, often when the CD4 count is <200. Toxoplasmosis is often spread by eating poorly cooked meat exposed to infected cat feces and can be transferred from mother to fetus leading to congenital toxoplasmosis. Patients with CNS toxoplasmosis can present with fever, malaise, headaches, and seizures. Treatment for toxoplasmosis is pyrimethamine and sulfadiazine.

On imaging, toxoplasmosis and lymphoma can look very similar in AIDS patients. Toxoplasmosis tends to reveal multiple ring-enhancing lesions in the basal ganglia and corticomedullary junction. Lymphoma is usually a single, solid-enhancing periventricular lesion in immunocompetent patients but is more often multifocal and irregularly enhancing or rim enhancing in AIDS patients. Both can restrict diffusion; however, it has been shown that toxoplasmosis demonstrates greater restriction on average when compared to lymphoma.

Given the overlap of imaging findings, advanced MR imaging and nuclear medicine are both helpful tools. On MR perfusion, lymphoma has increased perfusion and toxoplasmosis has decreased perfusion. On MR spectroscopy, both can have lipid–lactate peaks, but lymphoma tends to have significantly increased Cho/Cr ratio. On thallium 201 SPECT and 18F-FDG PET, lymphoma is hypermetabolic and toxoplasmosis is hypometabolic.

References: Camacho D, et al. Differentiation of toxoplasmosis and lymphoma in AIDS patients by using apparent diffusion coefficients. *AJNR Am J Neuroradiol* 2003;24:633–637.

Haldorsen IS, et al. Central nervous system lymphoma: characteristic findings on traditional and advanced imaging. *AJNR Am J Neuroradiol* 2011;32:984–992.

Ruiz A, et al. Use of thallium-201 brain SPECT to differentiate cerebral lymphoma from toxoplasma encephalitis in AIDS patients. *AJNR Am J Neuroradiol* 1994;15:1885–1894.

5a **Answer C.** Basilar leptomeningeal enhancement with hydrocephalus. Pachymeningeal enhancement refers to **dura**-arachnoid enhancement adjacent to the inner table of the skull, in the falx, and in the tentorium. On the other hand, leptomeningeal enhancement refers to **pia**-arachnoid enhancement, which follows the pial surface of the brain in the subarachnoid spaces of the sulci and cisterns. As a result of the basilar leptomeningeal meningitis, hydrocephalus has developed with dilated temporal horns for the patient's age.

5b **Answer B.** TB meningitis. Given the diffuse miliary nodules on the chest x-ray in a sick child with fever, the most likely diagnosis for the brain imaging findings is TB meningitis.

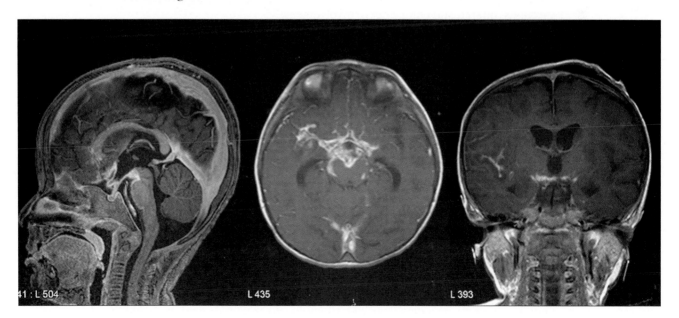

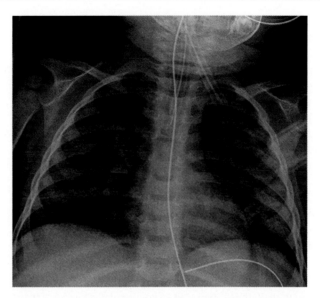

Imaging Findings: Sagittal, axial, and coronal postgadolinium images demonstrate robust basilar leptomeningeal enhancement along the surface of the midbrain, within the suprasellar cistern, and extending to the right sylvian fissure. The chest x-ray demonstrates an intubated child with innumerable bilateral miliary nodules. Although both basilar leptomeningeal enhancement and miliary nodules can have their own differential considerations, when the two findings are seen together, TB meningitis is the most likely diagnosis.

Discussion: TB meningitis is caused by infection by the acid-fast bacillus *Mycobacterium tuberculosis*. TB within the CNS involvement is most frequently secondary to hematogenous spread of disease, most often from pulmonary source. The most common manifestation of CNS TB is meningitis and is most frequently seen in children. The radiologist should have a high index of suspicion for diagnosing the complications from the meningitis including hydrocephalus, vasculitis, infarct, and cranial nerve involvement.

The other main imaging manifestation of CNS TB is intraparenchymal involvement with a tuberculoma, which can be solitary or multiple. Parenchymal tuberculomas can be isolated or be seen along with meningitis. When the two are seen together, it is highly suggestive of TB. Tuberculomas typically demonstrate heterogeneous hypointensity on MR with ring-like peripheral enhancement. CNS miliary TB can also be seen in severely immunocompromised patients.

The most common osseous manifestation of TB is within the vertebral spinal column, Pott disease with the most common location at L1. Typically, more than one vertebral body is affected with the spread of infection occurring along the anterior or posterior longitudinal ligaments, although single-level involvement can occur.

Differential Diagnosis: Neurosarcoid, other infectious etiologies including fungal disease, and leptomeningeal carcinomatosis can all have basilar leptomeningeal enhancement. Clinical correlation with the patient's presentation, lab work, and imaging outside of the CNS is often necessary to make the correct diagnosis. Given the high morbidity and mortality of TB meningitis, rapid diagnosis and treatment are vitally important. Mycobacteria tend to grow slowly in culture, and thus, imagers may be the first to suggest the diagnosis. Treatment is with multidrug therapy including isoniazid, rifampin, pyrazinamide, and often additional medications.

References: Engin G, et al. Imaging of extrapulmonary tuberculosis. *Radiographics* 2000;20: 471–488.

Smirniotopoulos JG, et al. Patterns of contrast enhancement in the brain and meninges. *Radiographics* 2007;27:525–551.

6a **Answer C.** Right parietal lobe abscess with intraventricular extension. These MRI findings are diagnostic of a cerebral abscess.

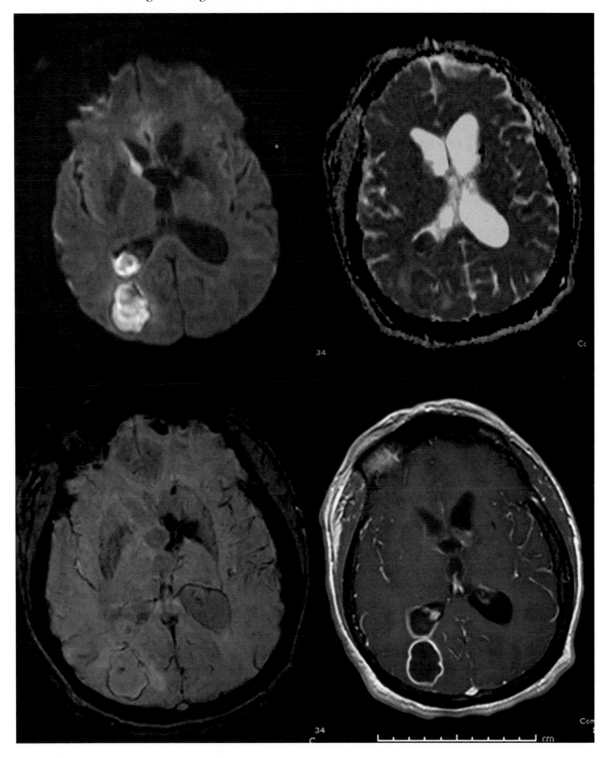

Imaging Findings: Axial DWI, ADC, SWI, and postcontrast T1-weighted images are shown. There is a rim-enhancing lesion in the right parietal lobe, which extends into the atrium of right lateral ventricle. Thin ependymal enhancement along the ventricular surface is also seen. There is slow diffusion in the center of the lesion and abnormal susceptibility in the enhancing capsule. These findings are diagnostic of a cerebral abscess.

Discussion: A ring-enhancing intra-axial lesion with central slow diffusion is most suggestive of a brain abscess. Brain abscesses may arise from the spread of infection from contiguous sinus disease/otomastoiditis, from hematogenous spread of infection, or as a complication of neurosurgical procedure. Imaging findings reflect the host immune response in an attempt to contain the infection. Four stages of abscess evolution are described, which include:

Early cerebritis: Ill-defined vasogenic edema with minimal or no enhancement
Late cerebritis: Central slow diffusion with ill-defined rim enhancement
Early capsule stage: More well-defined rim-enhancing capsule
Late capsule: Thicker rim enhancement, decreasing vasogenic edema

The medial wall of the abscess cavity may be thinner than lateral wall owing to differential blood supply, which predisposes to intraventricular rupture and satellite abscess formation. The abscess rim often shows low signal on T2-weighted and SWI images. On MR spectroscopy, there is a decrease in *N*-acetylaspartate (NAA), choline, and creatine, and elevated cytosolic amino acids and succinate.

Differential Diagnosis: A high-grade necrotic neoplasm would be expected to demonstrate decreased diffusion in the periphery within the viable tumor.

An acute infarct shows slow diffusion, but intraventricular extension or rim enhancement is not expected at this stage. Acute intracranial hemorrhage would demonstrate markedly abnormal susceptibility. Other ring-enhancing lesions such as tumefactive demyelination and radiation necrosis usually do not demonstrate diffusion abnormalities.

Reference: Mishra AM, Gupta RK, Jaggi RS, et al. Role of diffusion-weighted imaging and in vivo proton magnetic resonance spectroscopy in the differential diagnosis of ring-enhancing intracranial cystic mass lesions. *J Comput Assist Tomogr* 2004;28(4):540–507.

7a **Answer D.** HSV encephalitis. The imaging findings are most compatible with HSV encephalitis.

7b **Answer C.** PCR (polymerase chain reaction) of CSF. The next step to confirm the diagnosis of HSV encephalitis is a lumbar puncture to obtain CSF for HSV PCR (option C).

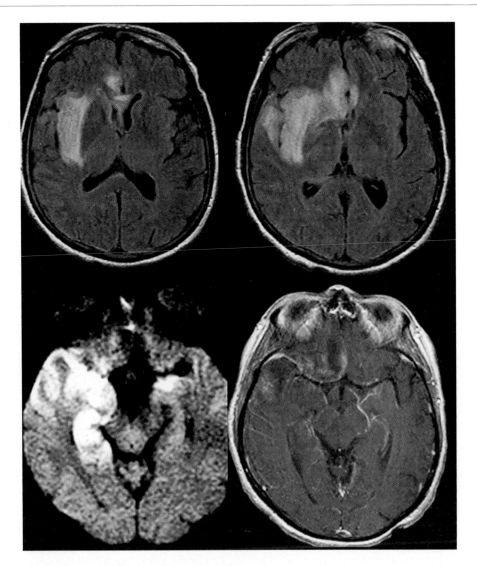

Imaging Findings: Axial FLAIR-weighted images of the brain demonstrate hyperintense signal in the right insular cortex, anterior right temporal cortex, right greater than left inferior frontal, and mesial temporal cortices. There is associated gyral swelling with effacement of the right MCA cistern and sylvian fissure. Axial diffusion-weighted images show restricted diffusion in the right insular cortex, medial right frontal cortex, and right greater than left anterior temporal cortices. The postgadolinium T1-weighted image shows a subtle leptomeningeal enhancement in the right greater than left frontotemporal regions.

Discussion: HSV encephalitis is a viral infection caused by the herpes simplex virus (HSV). The inhaled virus may remain dormant in the trigeminal ganglion for a long time and is reactivated by changes in the host's immune status to invade the brain, typically the insular cortex, anterior temporal and inferior frontal cortices. The clinical presentation is nonspecific with fever, headaches, seizures, and alteration of consciousness.

   Imaging plays an important role to suggest the diagnosis and start appropriate therapy. CT scan of the head will show asymmetric brain swelling that can be confused for an acute MCA distribution infarct. MRI of the brain with gadolinium is the imaging modality of choice and will show a cortical pattern of restricted diffusion sparing the basal ganglia. The lesions are diffuse, bilateral, asymmetric and iso- to hypointense in signal on T1WI and hyperintense in signal on FLAIR/T2WI with petechial blood products on T2* or GRE sequences. Leptomeningeal, gyral, or heterogeneous patchy enhancement is present in the late phase of the disease process. The identification of the virus in the CSF by PCR technique will confirm the diagnosis. Intravenous acyclovir is the treatment of choice.

Differential Diagnosis: The main differential diagnostic consideration on imaging is an acute MCA distribution infarct that involves the basal ganglia in addition to the insula and frontotemporal cortices and limbic encephalitis that involves the insular cortex less commonly.

Reference: Burke JW, et al. Contrast-enhanced magnetization transfer saturation imaging improves MR detection of herpes simplex encephalitis. *AJNR Am J Neuroradiol* 1996;17(4):773–776.

8a **Answer A.** Creutzfeldt-Jakob disease (CJD). The distribution of signal abnormality within the bilateral thalami suggests CJD. The associated basal ganglia and right insula cortical hyperintensity in a patient with progressing dementia and abnormal movements (myoclonic jerks) makes CJD the most likely diagnosis.

8b **Answer C.** DWI. Diffusion-weighted imaging has been shown to be the most sensitive imaging sequence in diagnosing CJD. DWI abnormality may be the only imaging finding early in the disease before T2/FLAIR signal abnormality develops.

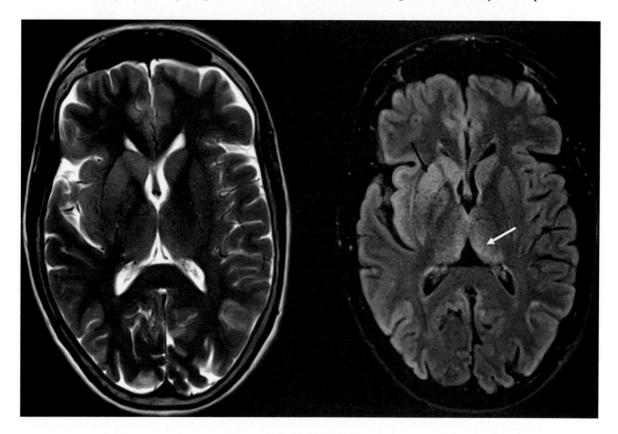

Imaging Findings: Bilateral symmetric hyperintense T2 and DWI signal is seen within the thalami, specifically within the pulvinar and dorsomedial thalamic nuclei—"hockey stick sign" (white arrow). There is also T2 and DWI hyperintense signal within the caudate heads and basal ganglia, right greater than left (black arrow). Right insula hyperintensity and more subtle posterior right temporal cortical hyperintensity are also present. These findings with the appropriate clinical history favor CJD as the most likely diagnosis.

Discussion: Creutzfeldt-Jakob disease (CJD) is a fatal disease caused by prion accumulation in the brain. Patient's present with rapidly progressing dementia and myoclonic jerks with varying pyramidal and extrapyramidal symptoms. Later in the disease, akinetic mutism develops, and patient's die usually within a year of onset of symptoms.

The disease can be sporadic, inherited, or acquired. Sporadic CJD accounts for approximately 85% to 90% of cases, familial CJD approximately 10% to 15% of cases, and acquired approximately 1% of cases including from cornea and dura transplantation. There is also variant CJD predominantly found in Western Europe that is similar to bovine spongiform encephalopathy and likely transmitted from cattle to human. CSF analysis can aid in the diagnosis with detection of protein 14-3-3 along with other markers. The classic EEG finding is of periodic synchronous discharges.

On imaging, CJD classically demonstrates bilateral basal ganglia T2 and DWI hyperintense signal with the caudate and putamen affected more commonly than the globus pallidus. Cortical distribution is often asymmetric. The thalami are affected either with pulvinar involvement or with both pulvinar and dorsomedial thalamic nuclei involvement. T1-weighted imaging tends to be normal and without enhancement, which can help differentiate from other differential considerations. White matter is often spared. Cerebral atrophy is not a prominent finding in CJD in comparison to other dementias.

Differential Diagnosis: The basal ganglia and thalami imaging findings of CJD each by themselves can have broad differential considerations, but when seen together with cortical involvement and appropriate clinical history, the diagnosis can be favored. Hypoxic ischemic injury can have similar basal ganglia findings, but the "hockey stick" thalamic involvement is not classic. Leigh syndrome affects the basal ganglia, but this is a pediatric disease usually presenting by 2 years of age. Wernicke encephalopathy can have medial thalamic involvement, but the basal ganglia is typically spared.

References: Kallenberg K, et al. Creutzfeldt-Jakob disease: comparative analysis of MR imaging sequences. *AJNR Am J Neuroradiol* 2006;27:1459–1462.

Tschampa HJ, et al. Thalamic involvement in sporadic Creutzfeldt-Jakob disease: a diffusion weighted MR imaging study. *AJNR Am J Neuroradiol* 2003;24:908–915.

Ukisu R, et al. Diffusion-weighted MR imaging of early-stage Creutzfeldt-Jakob disease: typical and atypical manifestations. *Radiographics* 2006;26:S191–S204.

6 Inherited and Neurodegenerative Abnormalities

ANDREA PORETTI • LEE FINKELSTONE • GUL MOONIS

QUESTIONS

1 A 40-year-old immunocompetent otherwise healthy male presents with recurrent migraine and progressive cognitive decline. An MRI was performed; key images are provided below.

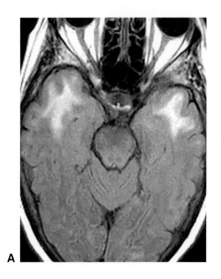
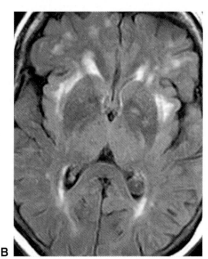
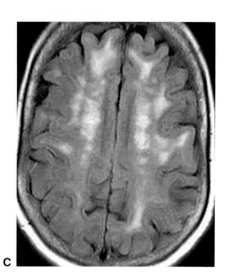

A   B   C

1a What is the most likely diagnosis?

A. Alzheimer disease
B. Creutzfeldt-Jakob disease
C. CADASIL
D. Progressive multifocal leukoencephalopathy

1b What is the mechanism for developing CADASIL?

A. Etiology is unknown and felt to be idiopathic.
B. Inherited mutation on chromosome 17
C. Sporadic mutation in the p53 gene
D. Inherited mutation in the NOTCH3 gene

2 A 55-year-old male with a palatal tremor presented for further evaluation to a neurologist. Key images from an MRI are provided below.

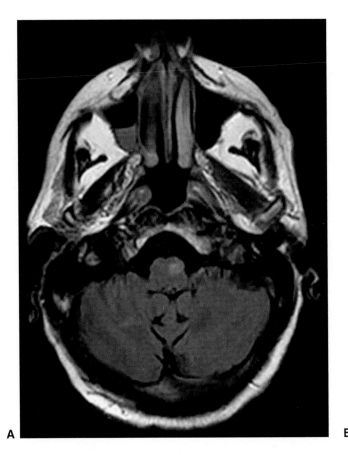
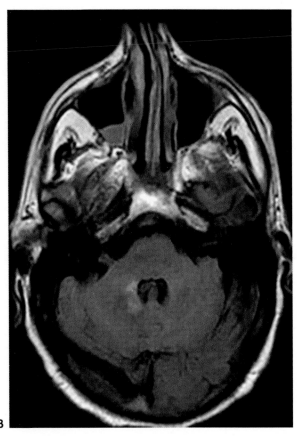

A   B

2a The location of pathology in the medulla (above) is bordered on either side by these structures.

A. Retroolivary sulcus and preolivary medullary sulcus
B. Fascicles of hypoglossal nerve and vagal, glossopharyngeal, and accessory nerves
C. Inferior cerebellar peduncle and lateral fossa of the medulla
D. Pyramid and fascicles of hypoglossal nerve

2b What is the most likely diagnosis?

A. Neoplasm
B. Demyelination
C. Hypertrophic olivary degeneration
D. Medullary infarction

3 An 8-year-old boy presents with hearing loss, decreasing school performance, attention problems, and progressive gait abnormalities.

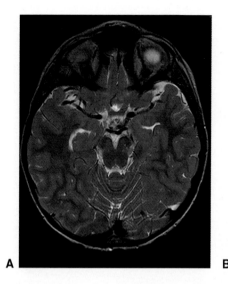 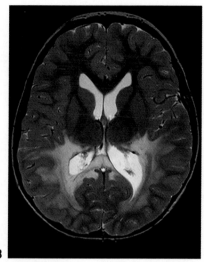 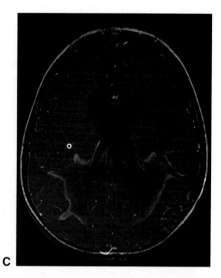

A   B   C

What is the most likely diagnosis?

A. Metachromatic leukodystrophy
B. X-linked adrenoleukodystrophy
C. Canavan disease
D. MELAS
E. Alexander disease

4 A 17-year-old teenager presents with a 4-year history of worsening psychiatric and cognitive issues and acute-onset hallucinations.

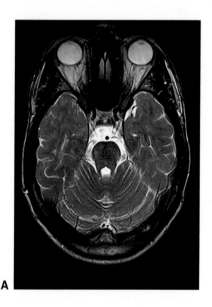 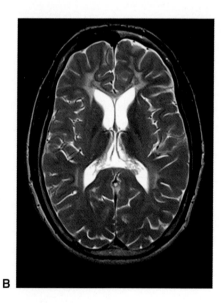 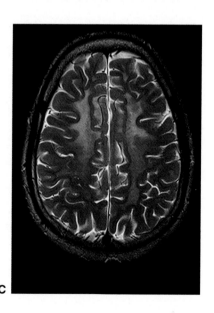

A   B   C

What is the most likely diagnosis?

A. Metachromatic leukodystrophy
B. X-linked adrenoleukodystrophy
C. Canavan disease
D. MELAS
E. Alexander disease

5 A 9-year-old boy with acute onset of headache, vomiting, impaired visual acuity, and focal seizure.

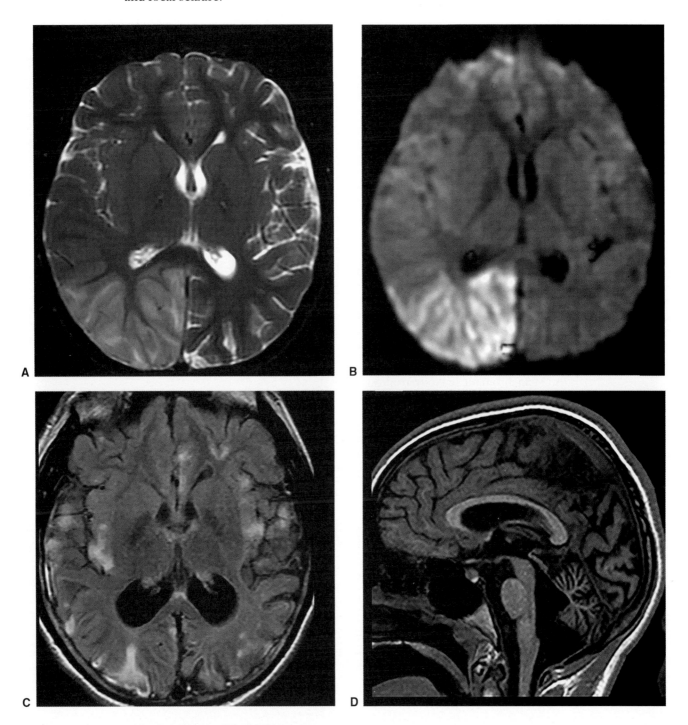

What is the most likely diagnosis?

A. Metachromatic leukodystrophy
B. X-linked adrenoleukodystrophy
C. Canavan disease
D. MELAS
E. Alexander disease

6   A 6-month-old child with hypotonia, poor head control, loss of milestones, and macrocephaly.

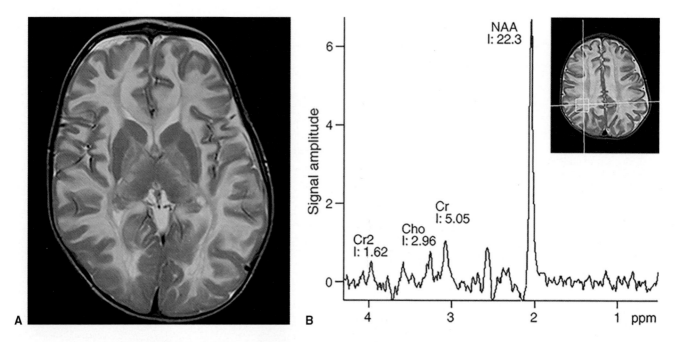

What is the most likely diagnosis?

A. Metachromatic leukodystrophy
B. X-linked adrenoleukodystrophy
C. Canavan disease
D. MELAS
E. Alexander disease

7   A 15-year-old girl presents with coarse tremors and dysarthric speech. Images are presented from an MRI scan.

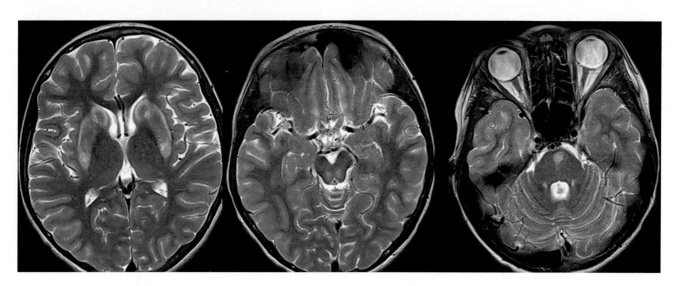

7a   The most likely diagnosis based on imaging findings is:

A. Hypoxia
B. Carbon monoxide poisoning
C. Renal failure
D. Wilson disease

7b Besides the liver, which organ system involvement is characteristic of Wilson disease?

A. Heart
B. Spleen
C. Eye
D. Kidney

8 A 10-year-old girl with progressive loss of developmental milestones, macrocephaly, and swallowing disorder; unremarkable until the age of 5 years.

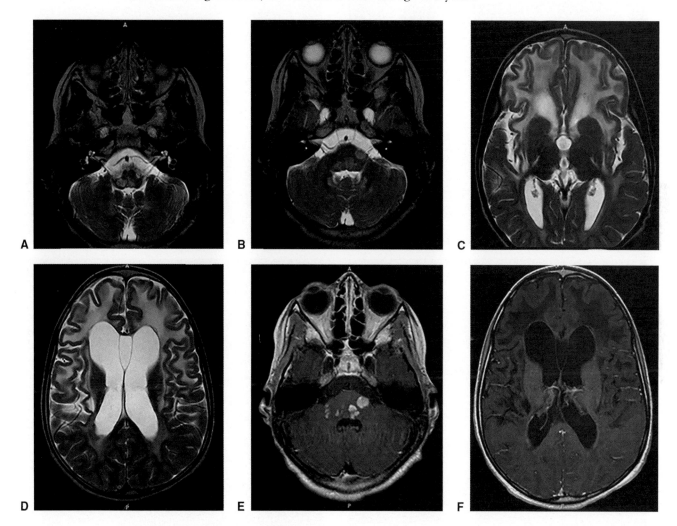

What is the most likely diagnosis?

A. Metachromatic leukodystrophy
B. X-linked adrenoleukodystrophy
C. Canavan disease
D. MELAS
E. Alexander disease

9   A 6-year-old presents with vision problems and skin discolorations.

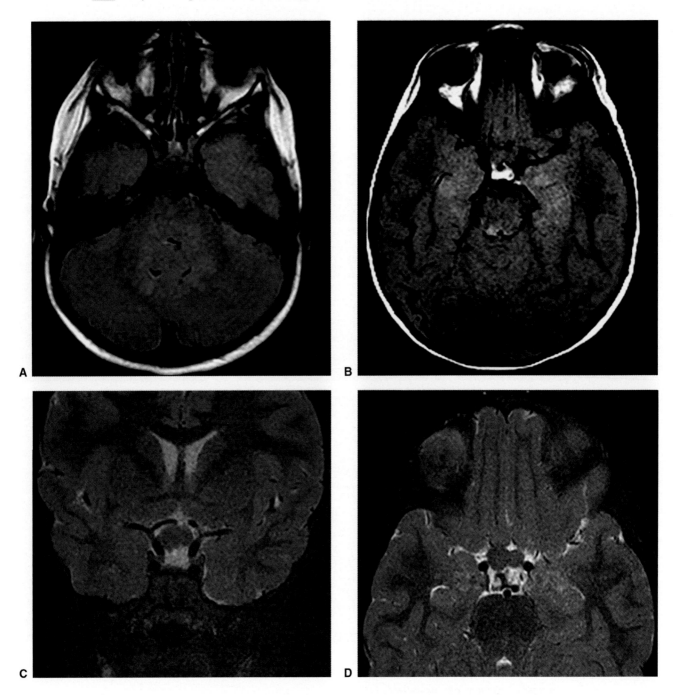

9a   What is the most likely diagnosis?

   A. PHACES syndrome
   B. NF1
   C. NF2
   D. Metastatic disease

9b In regard to optic pathway glioma prognosis, which statement is correct?

   A. NF1-related optic pathway glioma has the best prognosis.
   B. Childhood sporadic optic pathway glioma not associated with NF1 has the best prognosis.
   C. Adult optic pathway glioma has the best prognosis.
   D. All of the above optic pathway gliomas have the same prognosis.

10a A 6-year-old girl presents with progressive dystonia and dysphagia. An MRI was performed.

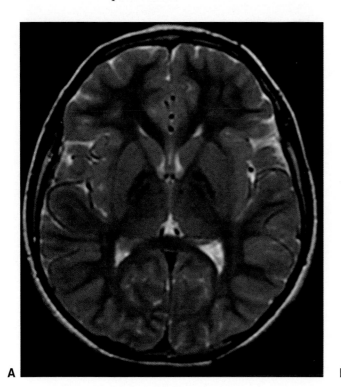 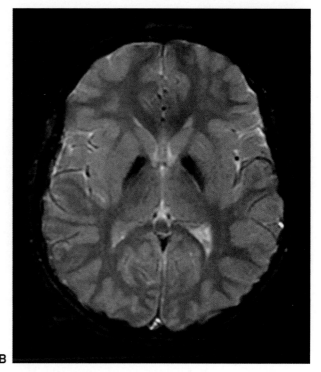

A   B

What is the most likely diagnosis based on the images?

   A. Wilson disease
   B. PKAN (pantothenate kinase–associated neurodegeneration also known as Hallervorden-Spatz syndrome)
   C. Alexander disease
   D. Canavan disease

10b Regarding Hallervorden-Spatz disease, which of the following is responsible for the hypointensity in the globus pallidus?

   A. Deposition of manganese
   B. Deposition of calcium
   C. Deposition of iron
   D. Deposition of copper

11 A 20-year-old presents with hearing loss.

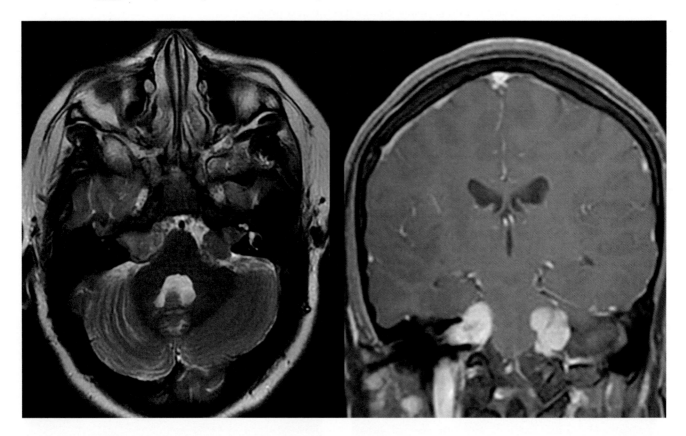

11a Which statement is correct in regard to the figure?

    A. Findings are suggestive of but not diagnostic for NF1.

    B. Findings are diagnostic for NF1.

    C. Findings are suggestive of but not diagnostic for NF2.

    D. Findings are diagnostic for NF2.

11b On what chromosome is the mutation for NF2?

    A. 3

    B. 17

    C. 22

    D. Mitochondrial mutation

12 A 15-year-old presents with seizures and skin discoloration.

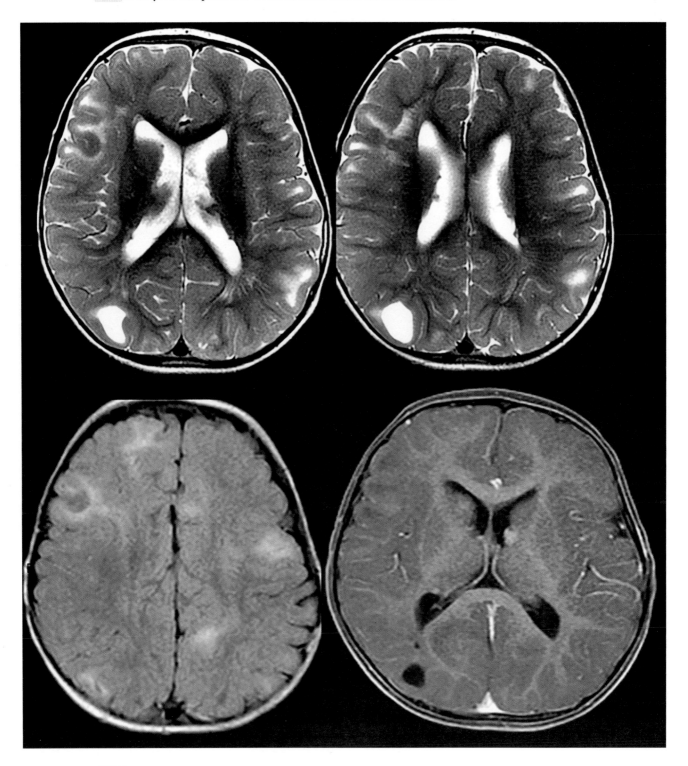

12a What is the most likely diagnosis?

A. Cortical dysplasia and gray matter heterotopia

B. Tuberous sclerosis

C. TORCH infection

D. Neurofibromatosis 1

12b In regard to diagnosing a subependymal giant cell astrocytoma (SEGA) in patients with tuberous sclerosis, what is the most important diagnostic imaging feature to look for?

A. Serially growing mass or mass >1 cm in size
B. MR imaging signal characteristics
C. Avid enhancement
D. Calcifications

13a A 65-year-old woman presents with blank face, decreased blinking, and repeated falls. What is the characteristic imaging findings based on the following images?

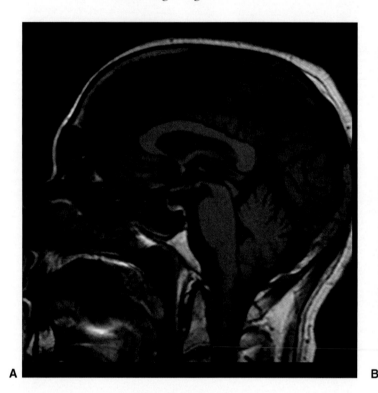
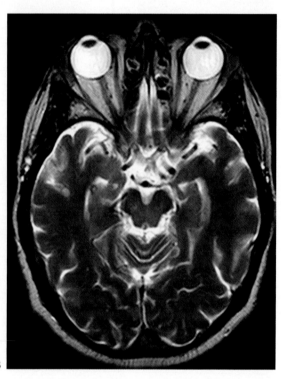

A

B

A. Hot crossed bun sign
B. Hummingbird sign
C. Panda sign
D. Lemon sign

13b Which of the following is true about the hummingbird sign?

A. Seen at the level of the medulla
B. Represents degeneration of the corticospinal tract
C. Seen in patients with progressive supranuclear palsy
D. Imaging findings are highly specific for the disease.

14 A 40-year-old presents with complex partial seizures.

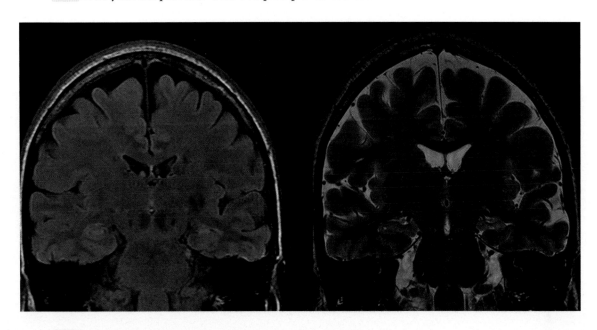

14a What is the imaging abnormality?

    A. Enlarged and hypointense right hippocampus

    B. Enlarged and hyperintense right hippocampus

    C. Atrophied and hypointense left hippocampus

    D. Atrophied and hyperintense left hippocampus

14b What is the most likely diagnosis?

    A. Mesial temporal sclerosis

    B. Focal cortical dysplasia

    C. Astrocytoma

    D. Choroidal fissure cyst

15 A 15-year-old presents with seizures and skin discoloration.

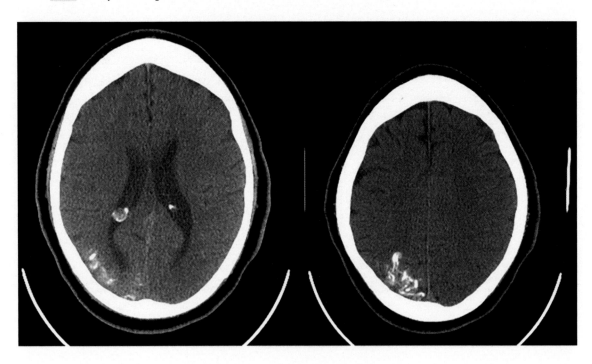

15a What is the next best imaging step?

    A. CT head with contrast

    B. CT angiogram of the head

    C. MRI of the brain with contrast

    D. Dedicated cerebral angiogram

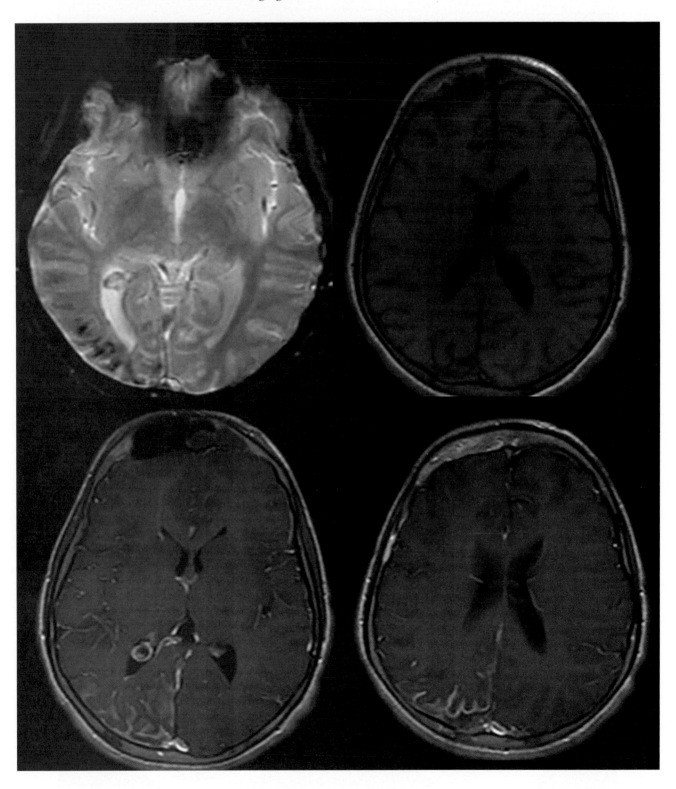

15b Based on the MRI shown what is the most likely diagnosis?

    A. Encephalotrigeminal angiomatosis
    B. Tuberous sclerosis
    C. Arteriovenous malformation
    D. Meningitis

16 A 45-year-old man presents with increasing muscle weakness and cramps. The following MR images are presented.

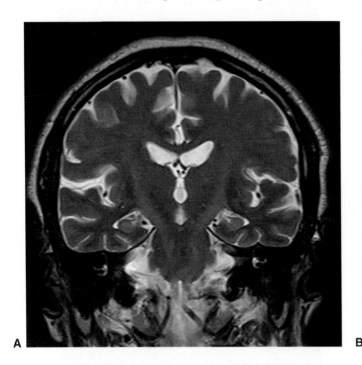
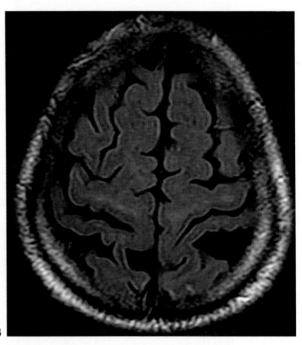

A   B

16a Which structure demonstrates abnormal signal?

    A. Spinothalamic tract
    B. Corticospinal tract
    C. Medial longitudinal fasciculus
    D. Medial lemniscus

16b Regarding amyotrophic lateral sclerosis, which of the following is true?

    A. Death occurs due to respiratory failure.
    B. Most cases are inherited.
    C. Conventional MR imaging is very sensitive in diagnosis.
    D. Corticospinal signal intensity changes correlate with clinical symptoms.

17 A 73-year-old man presents with gradually progressive cognitive decline.

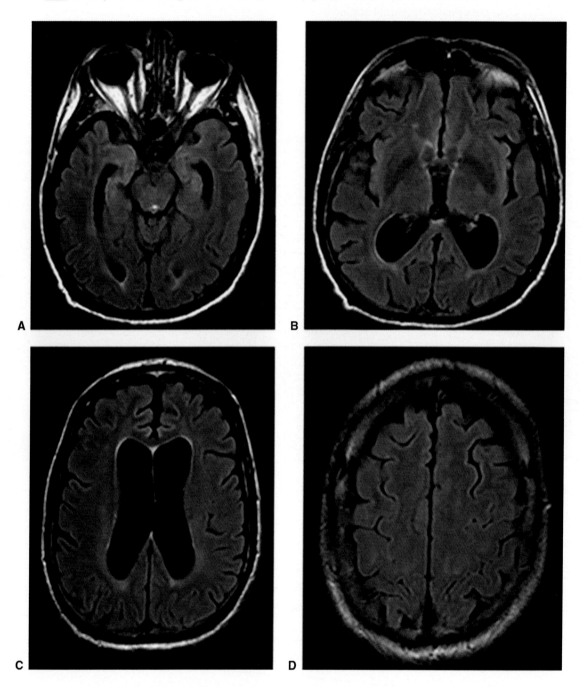

Based on the above findings, which of the following etiologies can be excluded?

A. Alzheimer dementia
B. Normal pressure hydrocephalus
C. Vascular dementia
D. Frontotemporal lobar degeneration

ANSWERS AND EXPLANATIONS

1a **Answer C.**   CADASIL. In a young patient with FLAIR abnormality most notably within the anterior temporal lobes and frontal subcortical white matter, CADASIL is the most likely diagnosis.

1b **Answer D.**   Inherited mutation in the NOTCH3 gene. CADASIL is a hereditary disease with mutation in the NOTCH3 gene. NF1 is a disease with an inherited mutation on chromosome 17, and p53 is an important tumor suppressor gene.

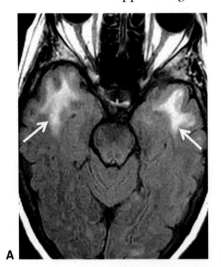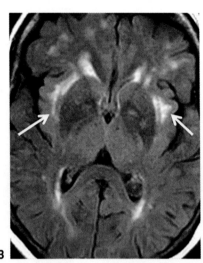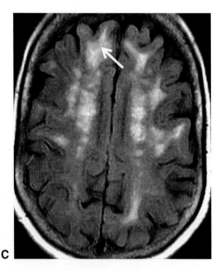

A   B   C

Imaging Findings: Multifocal hyperintense FLAIR signal abnormality is primarily within the bilateral anterior frontal lobe and temporal subcortical white matter (Figures A and C). In a young patient, this distribution of disease favors CADASIL as the diagnosis.

Discussion: CADASIL is short for cerebral autosomal dominant arteriopathy with subcortical infarcts and leukoencephalopathy. CADASIL is a hereditary disease secondary to a mutation in NOTCH3 gene on chromosome 19 leading to strokes in young to middle age adults who are otherwise healthy without stroke risk factors. CADASIL typically presents at age 30 to 50 with TIA/stroke-like symptoms, and many patients also present with migraine headaches with aura. The disease is progressive with cognitive decline and early death. Lacunar infarct burden has been shown to have an important impact on cognitive function and disability.

On imaging, CADASIL classically demonstrates relatively bilaterally symmetric FLAIR hyperintense signal abnormality within the paramedian superior frontal lobe subcortical white matter, anterior temporal lobes, and external capsules. The anterior temporal lobe involvement has been shown to be both highly specific and sensitive for aiding in the diagnosis of CADASIL. Cerebral microbleeds on gradient echo imaging are often also seen.

Differential Diagnosis: The main differential considerations for CADASIL include other vascular disorders or demyelinating disease. In atherosclerotic microvascular change, patients tend to be older and with white matter changes in the corona radiate/centrum semiovale as well as deep gray matter structures with sparing of the anterior temporal lobes. Demyelinating disease white matter hyperintensities are classically periventricular, oriented perpendicular to the ventricular system, and with corpus callosum involvement as well as the brainstem, cerebellum, and spinal cord.

References: Markus HS, et al. Diagnostic strategies in CADASIL. *Neurology* 2002;59(8):1134–1138.

Stojanov D, et al. Imaging characteristics of cerebral autosomal dominant arteriopathy with subcortical infarcts and leucoencephalopathy (CADASIL). *Bosn J Basic Med Sci* 2015;15(1):1–8.

Viswanathan A, et al. Lacunar lesions are independently associated with disability and cognitive impairment in CADASIL. *Neurology* 2007;69(2):172–179.

2a   **Answer A.**   Retroolivary sulcus and preolivary medullary sulcus. The pathology is located in inferior olivary nucleus, which is bordered by preolivary sulcus (12th nerve emerges from this sulcus) and retro-olivary sulcus (9, 10, and 11 nerve fibers are in this sulcus).

2b   **Answer C.**   Hypertrophic olivary degeneration. Location is the key for diagnosis. Search for a causative lesion in Guillain-Mollaret triangle shows signal abnormality in contralateral dentate nucleus (probably representing gliosis).

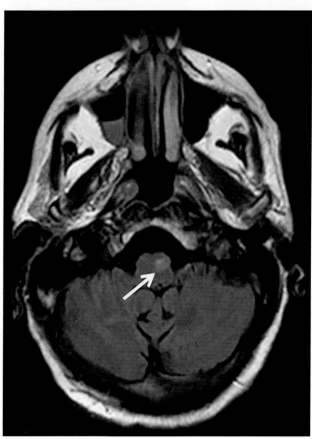
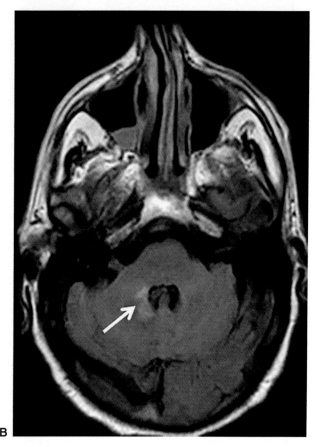

A   B

Imaging Findings: Axial FLAIR images demonstrate enlargement and increased signal within the left olive in A, with gliosis in the right dentate nucleus in B.

Discussion: Hypertrophic olivary degeneration (HOD) is caused by lesion in the triangle of Guillain and Mollaret. Patients can be asymptomatic or present with palatal tremor.

The triangle of Guillain and Mollaret (dentato-rubro-olivary pathway) contains a set of connecting tracts and is defined by the contralateral dentate nucleus (DN), ipsilateral inferior olivary nucleus (ION), and ipsilateral red nucleus (RN). The red nucleus is functionally not a part of the circuit. The efferent fibers from the DN ascend in the superior cerebellar peduncle (SCP) and after superior cerebellar peduncular decussation descend to the contralateral ION via central tegmental tract. Efferents from the ION go across the midline, travel via the inferior cerebellar peduncle cerebellar cortex, and then to the dentate nucleus, completing the triangle.

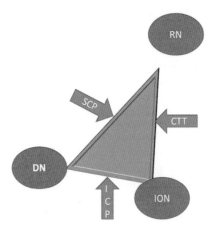

HOD is associated with lesions in afferent fibers to ION (first two limbs of the triangle). So, HOD is seen with lesions in contralateral dentate nucleus and ipsilateral brain stem. Transsynaptic degeneration is the proposed mechanism for HOD. Lesions of the olivodentate fibers can cause cerebellar atrophy. During the first month or so following the ictus, generally, there won't be any imaging changes in ION. Then, three distinct stages of HOD have been described on MRI.

1. Acute stage with increased T2 signal without hypertrophy, first 6 months after ictus
2. Both increased signal and hypertrophy of ION, 6 months to 3 to 4 years after ictus
3. Disappearance of hypertrophy with some persistence of increased signal

Reference: Goyal M, Versnick E, Tuite P, et al. Hypertrophic olivary degeneration: metaanalysis of the temporal evolution of MR findings. *Am J Neuroradiol* 2000;21(6):1073–1077.

3 **Answer B.** X-linked adrenoleukodystrophy.

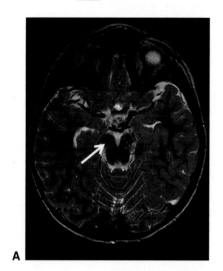 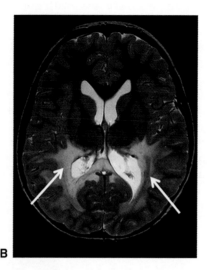 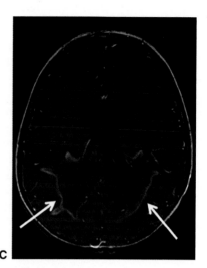

A B C

Imaging Findings: Axial T2-weighted MR image shows symmetric T2 hyperintense signal in the medial geniculate nuclei. Axial T2-weighted MR image shows symmetric T2 hyperintense signal in the parietooccipital white matter with sparing of the U-fibers. Axial contrast-enhanced T1-weighted MR image shows a rim of enhancement surrounding the parietooccipital white matter.

Discussion: X-linked adrenal leukodystrophy (ALD) is caused by a pathogenic variant within the *ABCD1* gene on chromosome Xq28 mutation. This gene codes for a peroxisomal membrane protein that plays a key role in the transport of very long chain fatty acids into the peroxisome, where they are normally metabolized. Hence, the analysis of very long chain fatty acids in plasma can be used as a diagnostic biomarker for ALD.

There are various clinical phenotypes among patients with X-linked ALD including the childhood cerebral form, adrenomyeloneuropathy (an adult form of ALD that presents with slowly progressive spastic paraparesis, impaired vibratory sense in the lower extremity, and bladder or bowel dysfunction and is characterized by a primary spinal cord involvement), and ALD with Addison disease only. The childhood cerebral variant of ALD presents at the age of 4 to 8 years with behavior problems, difficulties in school, and rapid regression of auditory discrimination, spatial orientation, speech, and writing.

The most common neuroimaging pattern in the childhood cerebral form of ALD consists of symmetric and predominantly parietooccipital white matter abnormalities that typically start in the splenium of the corpus callosum. The U-fibers and the cerebellum are relatively spared in the early onset of the disease, whereas the geniculate bodies, the lateral inferior part of the thalamus, and the posterior limb of the internal capsule may be affected early. In about 20% of the patients, the primary involvement involves the frontal white matter. After injection of contrast, a rim of enhancement may be noted surrounding the abnormal white matter. Enhancement seems to be associated with clinical worsening of the disease.

Differential Diagnosis: For the classic pattern of childhood cerebral ALD, there is almost no differential diagnosis. Alexander disease is a differential diagnosis of the ALD form with frontal predominance. Associated clinical features are key for differentiation.

References: Engelen M, et al. X-linked adrenoleukodystrophy (X-ALD): clinical presentation and guidelines for diagnosis, follow-up and management. *Orphanet J Rare Dis* 2012;7:51.

Loes DJ, et al. Analysis of MRI patterns aids prediction of progression in X-linked adrenoleukodystrophy. *Neurology* 2003;61(3):369–374.

Moser HW, et al. X-linked adrenoleukodystrophy. *Nat Clin Pract Neurol* 2007;3(3):140–151.

4 **Answer A.** Metachromatic leukodystrophy.

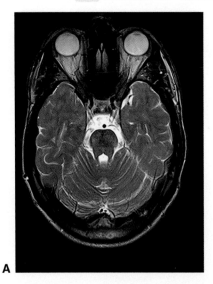
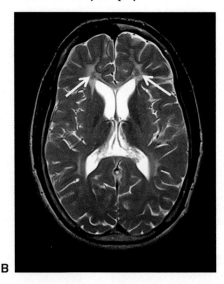
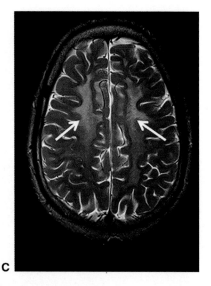

A   B   C

Imaging Findings: Axial T2-weighted MR images show a T2 hyperintense signal in the deep and periventricular white matter with sparing of the U-fibers. In addition, horizontal stripes of relatively spared white matter are noted.

Discussion: Metachromatic leukodystrophy is an autosomal recessive lysosomal disease caused by deficiency of arylsulfatase A activity leading to the accumulation of galactosylsulfatide in the white matter of the central and peripheral nervous system.

Late infantile-onset metachromatic leukodystrophy represents the most common phenotype (60% to 70%). Affected children typically present with progressive gait problems at about 14 to 16 months of age. The disease is progressive, and affected patients may lose developmental milestones and develop dysarthria, drooling, dysphagia, rigidity, and decerebrate or decorticate postures. Later, manifestations are typically characterized by behavioral abnormalities, cognitive deficits, and dementia.

MR images are nonspecific and may show areas of T2/FLAIR hyperintense signal in the deep and periventricular cerebral white matter, whereas the subcortical white matter (U-fibers) is spared until late in the course of the disease. Stripes of affected and unaffected myelin (called a "tigroid" pattern) may be seen and represent relatively spared myelin and lipid-containing glial cells in the perivascular spaces.

Differential Diagnosis: Periventricular predominance of white matter signal changes may be seen in several (hereditary and acquired) white matter diseases including Krabbe disease, Sjögren-Larsson disease, leukoencephalopathy with brainstem and spinal cord involvement and high lactate (LBSL), periventricular leukomalacia, and HIV leukoencephalopathy. The "tigroid pattern" may be seen in Krabbe disease and GM1 gangliosidoses. Hematopoietic stem cell transplant, if performed early in metachromatic leukodystrophy, can not only stabilize but even improve cerebral white matter abnormalities.

References: Eichler F, et al. Metachromatic leukodystrophy: a scoring system for brain MR imaging observations. *AJNR Am J Neuroradiol* 2009;30(10):1893–1897.

Eichler FS, et al. Metachromatic leukodystrophy: an assessment of disease burden. *J Child Neurol* 2016;31(13):1457–1463.

Groeschel S, et al. Cerebral gray and white matter changes and clinical course in metachromatic leukodystrophy. *Neurology* 2012;79(16):1662–1670.

Martin A, et al. Toward a better understanding of brain lesions during metachromatic leukodystrophy evolution. *AJNR Am J Neuroradiol* 2012;33(9):1731–1739.

5 **Answer D.** MELAS. Mitochondrial encephalomyopathy with lactic acidosis and stroke-like episodes.

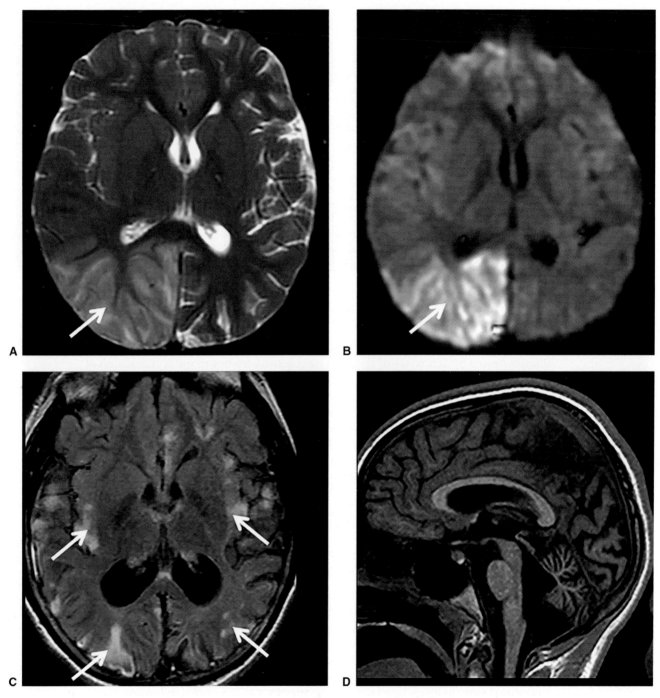

Imaging Findings: A. Axial T2-weighted MR image shows a T2 hyperintense signal in the cortical and subcortical white matter within the left occipital and posterior parietal lobes that are not restricted to a specific arterial distribution. B. Axial diffusion image shows matching-restricted diffusion. C. Follow-up axial FLAIR at 14 years of age shows multiple additional hyperintense lesions within the cortex and white matter. D. Follow-up sagittal T1-weighted MR image at 14 years of age shows cerebellar atrophy.

Discussion: Mitochondrial encephalomyopathy with lactic acidosis and stroke-like episodes (MELAS) is a maternally inherited mitochondrial disorder that is caused by point mutations within the mitochondrial DNA affecting transfer RNA genes. The A3243G mutation in the tRNAleu(uur) gene of the mitochondrial DNA is responsible for about 80% of MELAS cases.

Most patients become symptomatic before the age of 40 years. The early development is usually normal, followed by the onset of exercise intolerance, stroke-like episodes, seizures, and dementia. Almost all patients have lactic acidosis and had ragged red fibers in skeletal muscle biopsy specimens. Recurrent migraine-like headaches preceded by nausea and vomiting, hearing loss, short stature, learning difficulties, hemiparesis and hemianopia, and limb weakness are additional common features.

In the acute phase, MRI typically shows swelling and T2/FLAIR hyperintense signal and matching-restricted diffusion in the affected areas, which usually involve the parietal and occipital cortex and subcortical white matter as well as the basal ganglia. Cerebellar atrophy typically develops over time. Follow-up MR studies may show additional new lesions. The lesions are not restricted to a specific arterial distribution, and single lesions often cross vascular boundaries. [1]H-MR spectroscopy shows high lactate in affected areas of the brain.

Differential Diagnosis: Ischemic lesions from embolic or thrombotic infarction are typically not restricted to a specific arterial distribution and do not cross vascular boundaries. Urgent administration of nitric oxide precursors (e.g., arginine) in patients with MELAS ameliorates the clinical symptoms associated with stroke-like episodes.

References: El-Hattab AW, et al. MELAS syndrome: clinical manifestations, pathogenesis, and treatment options. *Mol Genet Metab* 2015;116(1–2):4–12.

Ito H, et al. Neuroimaging of stroke-like episodes in MELAS. *Brain Dev* 2011;33(4):283–288.

Tschampa HJ, et al. Neuroimaging characteristics in mitochondrial encephalopathies associated with the m.3243A>G MTTL1 mutation. *J Neurol* 2013;260(4):1071–1080.

6 **Answer C.** Canavan disease.

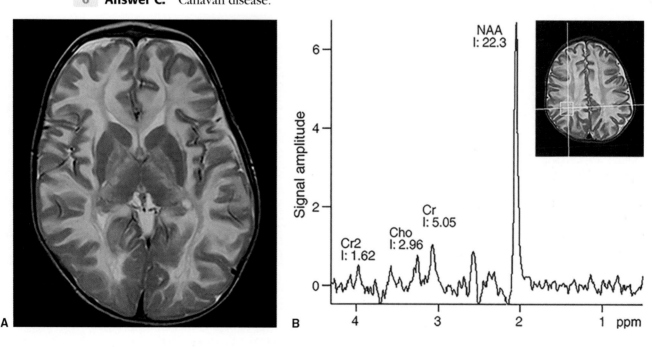

A   B

Imaging Findings: A. Axial T2-weighted MR image shows diffuse T2 hyperintense signal of the white matter, absence of any myelination in the internal capsules, and abnormal T2 hyperintense signal of the globi pallidi and thalami. B. ¹H-magnetic resonance spectroscopy shows a marked increase in *N*-acetylaspartate.

Discussion: Canavan disease or spongiform leukodystrophy is an autosomal recessive disorder caused by a deficiency of aspartoacylase. This enzyme is important for the hydrolysis of *N*-acetylaspartate (NAA).

Children with Canavan disease are typically normal for the first 1 to 2 months of life. Then, they develop hypotonia, poor head control, poor contact, seizures, macrocephaly, and loss of early milestones. In most patients, neurologic abnormalities and macrocephaly are apparent by 6 months of age. Later features of the disorder may include spasticity, opisthotonus, and decerebrate or decorticate posturing.

MR images usually reveal diffuse, symmetric T1 hypointense, and T2/FLAIR hyperintense abnormalities of the cerebral white matter without any focal predominance. The subcortical white matter is preferentially affected early in the course of the disease. The globi pallidi are nearly always affected with sparing of the adjacent putamen. Thalami are frequently involved. The dentate nuclei may also be affected. Proton spectroscopy shows increased NAA peak: this finding is strongly suggestive of Canavan disease and is already present when the rest of the MRI is still normal (neonatal age).

Differential Diagnosis: Preferential involvement of the subcortical white matter may be also seen in ʟ-2-hydroxy glutaricaciduria, Kearns-Sayre disease, propionic acidemia, and urea cycle disorders. Canavan disease occurs more frequently among patients of Ashkenazi Jewish descent.

References: Janson CG, et al. Natural history of Canavan disease revealed by proton magnetic resonance spectroscopy (1H-MRS) and diffusion-weighted MRI. *Neuropediatrics* 2006;37(4):209–221.

Kumar S, et al. Canavan disease: a white matter disorder. *Ment Retard Dev Disabil Res Rev* 2006;12(2):157–165.

Van der Knaap MS. Magnetic resonance in childhood white-matter disorders. *Dev Med Child Neurol* 2001;43:705–712.

7a **Answer D.** Wilson disease.

7b **Answer C.** Eye.

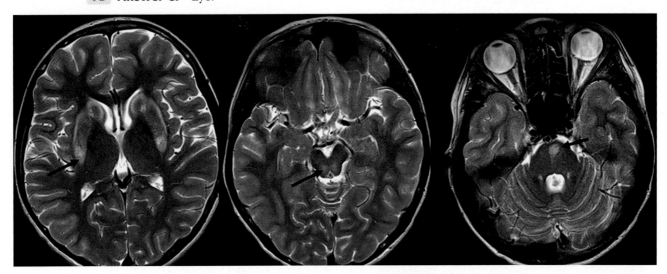

Imaging Findings: Axial T2-weighted images demonstrate increased signal in the bilateral putamen, caudate nucleus, dorsal midbrain, and anterior pons.

Discussion: Wilson disease (WD) is an inborn error of copper metabolism caused by a mutation to the copper-transporting gene *ATP7B*. The disease has an autosomal recessive mode of inheritance and is characterized by excessive copper deposition, predominantly in the liver and brain. Diagnosis of the condition depends primarily on clinical features, biochemical parameters, and the presence of the Kayser-Fleischer ring along the periphery of the cornea. Patients with hepatic WD usually present in late childhood or adolescence. The mean age of onset of "neurologic WD" is in the second to third decade. Patients commonly present with extrapyramidal, cerebellar, and cerebral-related symptoms in either a subacute or a chronic fashion. MR imaging abnormality in patients with Wilson disease can be related to hepatic dysfunction manifested by increased T1 signal intensity in the globus pallidus, putamen, and mesencephalon. Increased T2 signal in the putamen, thalami, and brainstem reflects copper deposition in brain tissue, which can result in edema, necrosis, and spongiform degeneration. The midbrain can show "face of the giant panda," and dorsal pontine abnormalities resemble the "face of a panda cub."

Signal abnormalities vary according to the stage of the disease and can be reversible with therapy in the early stages.

Differential Diagnosis: Toxic and metabolic etiologies like carbon monoxide poisoning, nitrous oxide toxicity, methanol poisoning, cyanide poisoning, metronidazole poisoning, hypoglycemia, hypoxia, CJD, Leigh disease, or viral encephalitis. Age and associated clinical findings are usually helpful in establishing a diagnosis.

References: Das SK, Ray K. Wilson's disease: an update. *Nat Clin Pract Neurol* 2006;2(9):482–493. Review. PubMed PMID: 16932613.

Singh P, Ahluwalia A, Saggar K, et al. Wilson's disease: MRI features. *J Pediatr Neurosci* 2011; 6(1):27–28. doi: 10.4103/1817-1745.84402.

8 **Answer E.** Alexander disease.

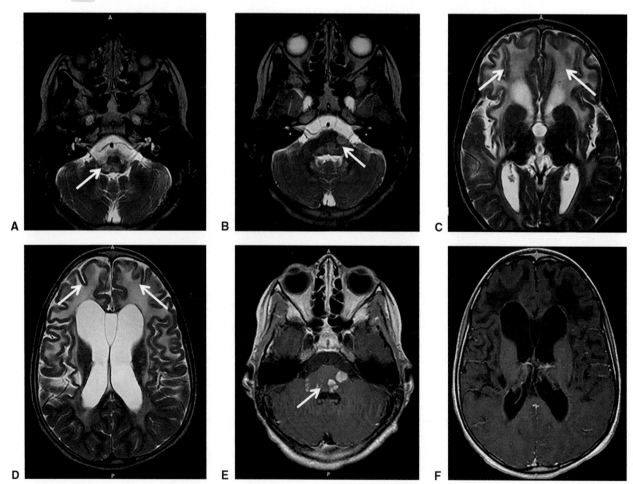

Imaging Findings: A–D. Axial T2-weighted MR images show symmetric T2 hyperintense signal of the frontal white matter and posterior limb of the internal capsule. In addition, multifocal nodular brainstem T2 hyperintense abnormalities and a T2 hypointense periventricular rim are noted. E and F. Axial contrast-enhanced T1-weighted MR images show enhancement within the periventricular regions and brainstem.

Discussion: Alexander disease is an autosomal dominant disease caused by pathogenic variants within the gene encoding the glial fibrillary acidic protein (GFAP).

Alexander disease may present with two predominant clinical phenotypes: the infantile and the juvenile or adult forms. Children with the infantile form may present with seizures, pyramidal and sometimes extrapyramidal signs, and loss of motor and cognitive milestones. Macrocephaly is an additional characteristic feature. Patients with the juvenile or adult form may present with predominant motor dysfunction, often with progressive gait disturbance or fine motor difficulties, clinically evident spasticity, and bulbar symptoms (e.g., dysphonia, dysphagia, and palatal myoclonus).

Van der Knaap et al. have described five MRI criteria by which the diagnosis of infantile Alexander disease can be made: (a) extensive cerebral white matter changes (T1 hypointensity and T2 hyperintensity) with frontal predominance, (b) a periventricular rim with hyperintense signal on T1-weighted images and hypointense signal on T2-weighted images, (c) abnormalities of the basal ganglia (particularly the caudate heads and anterior putamina) and thalami, (d) brainstem abnormalities, and (e) contrast enhancement of periventricular regions and lower brainstem. Patients with the juvenile or adult form of Alexander disease typically have regions of T1 hypointense and T2 hyperintense signal within the medulla, pons, and middle cerebellar peduncles that are intensely enhancing after intravenous injection of contrast agents.

Differential Diagnosis: The typical pattern of the infantile form of Alexander disease is quite specific and dissimilar from pattern observed in other white matter diseases. Predominant involvement of the frontal white matter may be seen in X-linked adrenoleukodystrophy. In patients with congenital muscular dystrophy because of LAMA2 pathogenic variants, extensive white matter involvement with relative sparing of the occipital white matter may be seen, but the basal ganglia and thalami are typically spared. Alexander disease should be considered in any patient with tumor-like lesion within the posterior fossa.

References: Rodriguez D, et al. Infantile Alexander disease: spectrum of GFAP mutations and genotype-phenotype correlation. *Am J Hum Genet* 2001;69:1134–1140.

Van der Knaap MS, et al. Unusual variants of Alexander's disease. *Ann Neurol* 2005;57:327–338.

Van Poppel K, et al. Alexander disease: an important mimicker of focal brainstem glioma. *Pediatr Blood Cancer* 2009;53:1355–1356.

9a **Answer B.** NF1. There are FLAIR hyperintense lesions within the pons/brachium pontis and medial temporal lobes along with a mass lesion within the right greater than left optic chiasm. In a young patient with skin discolorations, NF1 is the most likely diagnosis. PHACES is a syndrome with **P**osterior fossa malformations, **H**emangiomas, **A**rterial anomalies, **C**ardiac defects, **E**ye abnormalities, and **S**ternal (ventral) defects.

9b **Answer A.** NF1-related optic pathway glioma has the best prognosis. NF1-related optic pathway glioma has the best prognosis followed by childhood sporadic optic pathway gliomas. NF1-related optic pathway gliomas are often pilocytic astrocytomas WHO 1, whereas adult optic pathway gliomas are usually glioblastomas and have the worst prognosis.

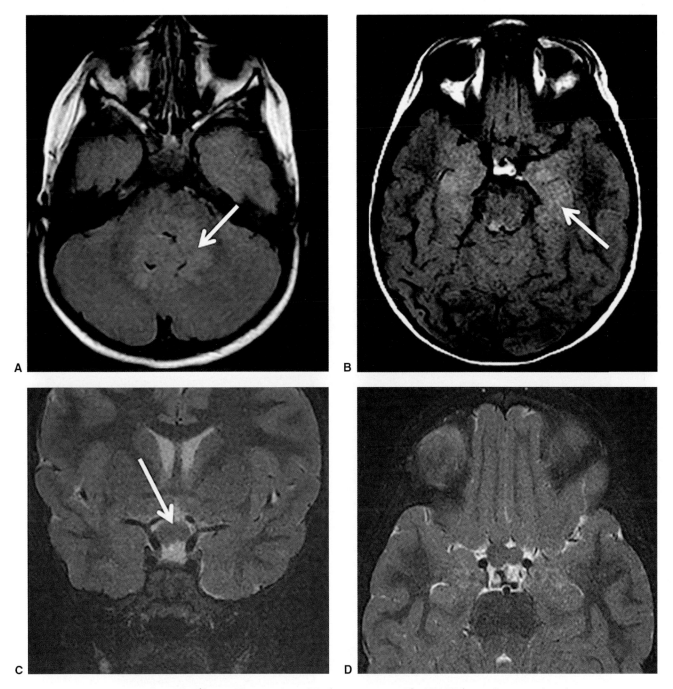

A

B

C

D

Imaging Findings: Figures A and B show nonspecific FLAIR hyperintense signal within the pons, brachium pontis, and medial temporal lobes. Figures C and D show a mass lesion centered in the right greater than left optic chiasm compatible with an optic pathway glioma. In a child with FLAIR hyperintense lesions, optic pathway glioma, and skin discolorations (café au lait spots), NF1 is the most likely diagnosis.

Discussion: Neurofibromatosis 1 is an autosomal dominant inherited disease from a mutation in the *NF1* gene located on chromosome 17. Although there is virtually 100% penetrance of the disease, the phenotypic expression can be quite variable with some expressing predominantly peripheral lesions, others with paraspinal abnormalities, and others with the intracranial findings. NF1 can be diagnosed with 2 or more of the following: 6 or more café au lait spots, 2 or more neurofibromas, or 1 plexiform neurofibroma, axillary/inguinal freckling, optic glioma, distinctive osseous lesion (sphenoid wing dysplasia, bowing of long bone with or without pseudoarthrosis), and first-degree relative with NF1.

CNS imaging characteristics of NF1 includes nonenhancing hyperintense T2/FLAIR lesions. These lesions are often found in the deep gray matter, hippocampi, brainstem, and cerebellum with little to no mass effect. They can increase in size and number as the child grows but tend to diminish in teenage years and resolve by adulthood. Optic pathway gliomas in NF1 can occur anywhere from the optic nerve through the optic radiations. Plexiform neurofibromas course along peripheral nerves and are hyperintense on T2-weighted imaging with central hypointensity—"target sign." Sphenoid wing dysplasia manifests by distortion or absence of the lateral orbital wall and often associated with an orbital plexiform neurofibroma. Rarely, NF1 patients can have a vascular dysplasia with moyamoya-like arteriopathy with vessel narrowing and collateral formation.

References: Borofsky S, et al. Neurofibromatosis: types 1 and 2. *AJNR Am J Neuroradiol* 2013;34: 2250–2251.

Czyzyk E, et al. Optic pathway gliomas in children with and without neurofibromatosis 1. *J Child Neurol* 2003;18(7):471–478.

Ferner RE, et al. Guidelines for the diagnosis and management of individuals with neurofibromatosis 1. *J Med Genet* 2007;44(2):81–88.

10a **Answer B.**   PKAN (pantothenate kinase-associated neurodegeneration also known as Hallervorden-Spatz syndrome).

10b **Answer C.**   Deposition of iron.

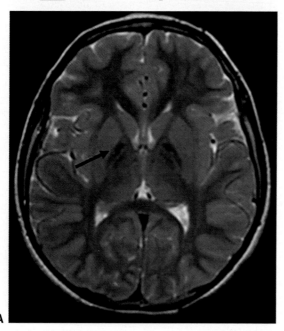 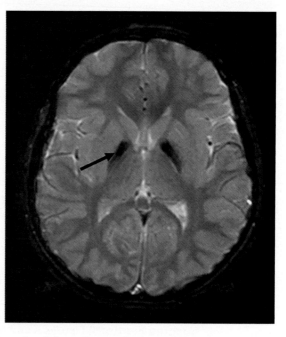

A   B

Imaging Findings: Axial T2-weighted (A) and axial gradient echo images (B) demonstrate hypointense signal in the globus pallidus with strong susceptibility effect on the GRE image.

Discussion: PKAN (pantothenate kinase–associated neurodegeneration also known as Hallervorden-Spatz syndrome) is classified as a neurodegenerative disorder with brain iron accumulation (NBIA). It involves a mutation in the PANK2 gene on chromosome 20. Most common clinical presentation occurs in the first decade of life with extrapyramidal motor disorder and intellectual deterioration. On MRI, T2-weighted images demonstrate hypointense signal in the globus pallidus with an anteromedial hyperintensity ("eye of the tiger" sign) and in the substantia nigra. Eye of the tiger appearance may precede the development of clinical symptoms. The degree of iron deposition correlates incompletely with symptoms.

Reference: Kruer MC, Boddaert N, Schneider SA, et al. Neuroimaging features of neurodegeneration with brain iron accumulation. *AJNR Am J Neuroradiol* 2012;33(3):407–414. doi: 10.3174/ajnr.A2677. Review. PubMed PMID: 21920862.

11a Answer D.   Findings are diagnostic for NF2. Neurofibromatosis 2. There are bilateral vestibular schwannomas meeting diagnostic criteria for NF2.

11b Answer C.   22. The mutation for NF2 is on chromosome 22. VHL mutation is on chromosome 3. NF1 mutation is on chromosome 17.

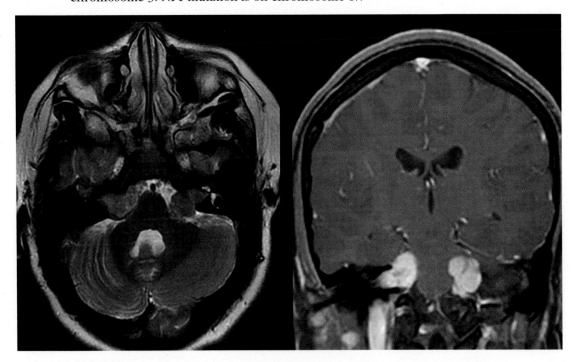

Imaging Findings: There are bilateral T2 iso to hypointense, enhancing mass lesions within the cerebellopontine angles extending into the internal auditory canal compatible with bilateral vestibular schwannomas, diagnostic of NF2.

Discussion: Neurofibromatosis type 2 is a rare autosomal dominant inherited disease from a mutation on chromosome 22 with a prevalence of approximately 1 in 60,000. The disease is really a misnomer as neurofibromas are really infrequent in the disease. Rather, the tumor manifestations of NF2 can be better remembered with the pneumonic **MISME—M**ultiple **I**nherited **S**chwannomas, **M**eningiomas, and **E**pendymomas. Thus, patients being worked up for NF2 should be screened with MRI of the brain and total spine with contrast to look for these tumors. Although the presence of a meningioma is often an isolated and incidental finding in an adult, a meningioma in a child should at least raise suspicion for NF2.

   The imaging findings of the schwannomas, meningiomas, and ependymomas in NF2 are similar to the nonsyndromic form of these tumors and are discussed in the neoplasm section.

References: Borofsky S, et al. Neurofibromatosis: types 1 and 2. *AJNR Am J Neuroradiol* 2013;34: 2250-2251.

Evans DG. Neurofibromatosis type 2 (NF2): a clinical and molecular review. *Orphanet J Rare Dis* 2009;4:4-16.

Loevner LA. *Brain imaging case review series*, 2nd ed. Mosby Elsevier, 2009:359-360.

12a Answer B.   Tuberous sclerosis. The imaging findings of multiple cortical tubers, subependymal nodules, and an enhancing mass at the level of the foramen of Monroe concerning for SEGA are classic for tuberous sclerosis.

12b **Answer A.**   Serially growing mass or mass >1 cm in size.

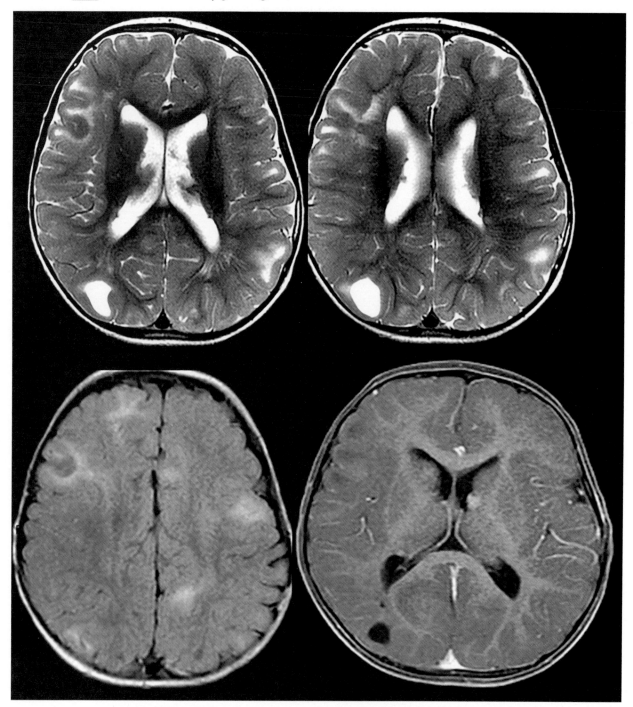

Imaging Findings: There are multifocal and bilateral T2 and FLAIR hyperintense cortical greater than subcortical lesions compatible with cortical tubers. Axial T2-weighted images show multiple bilateral small hypointense nodules lining the lateral ventricles compatible with subependymal nodules. Postgadolinium images show an enhancing mass at the level of the left foramen of Monroe suggestive of a SEGA.

Discussion: Tuberous sclerosis (TS) is an autosomal dominant inherited disease with mutations either in the TSC1 or TSC2 gene. The classic triad of seizures, mental retardation, and adenoma sebaceum is present in only a minority of patients. Thus, diagnostic criteria have been developed with both major and minor criteria with two or more major criteria meeting diagnostic criteria for TS. CNS major criteria include cortical dysplasias (including cortical tubers and radial migration lines), subependymal nodules, and SEGAs. Additional major criteria include multiple skin findings (hypomelanotic macules, angiofibromas, ungula fibromas, and shagreen patch), retinal hamartomas, cardiac rhabdomyomas, LAM, and renal AMLs.

The CNS imaging findings of cortical tubers, subependymal nodules, radial migration lines, and SEGA are classic for TS. Cortical tubers are T2/FLAIR hyperintense and are located most commonly supratentorially with greatest predilection for the frontal lobe, although infratentorial lesions can occur. Subependymal nodules tend to line the lateral ventricles, have lower T2-weighted signal intensity than cortical tubers, and often calcify. Subependymal nodules can enhance, and thus, serial imaging to look for interval growth is key to diagnosing SEGAs. SEGAs are most commonly located at the foramen of Monroe with a peak age at 8 to 18 years of age. It is important to diagnose these lesions as patients can present acutely with obstructive hydrocephalus and increased intracranial pressure if there is obstruction at the foramen of Monroe. White matter abnormalities include radial white matter bands that reflect altered migratory development of neurons and glial cells. They are thin curvilinear or straight T2 hyperintense lines extending from the ventricles to the deep surface of cortical tubers. White matter cystic spaces can also be seen and follow CSF on all imaging sequences.

Differential Diagnosis: Although cortical dysplasia and gray matter heterotopia can certainly cause seizures, gray matter heterotopia should follow gray matter on all imaging sequences and not enhance. TORCH infection, especially CMV, can have periventricular calcification, cortical dysplasia, and white matter abnormalities.

References: Northrup H, et al. Tuberous sclerosis complex diagnostic criteria update: recommendations of the 2012 International Tuberculosis Complex Consensus Conference. *Pediatr Neurol* 2013;49(4):243-254.

Roth J, et al. Subependymal giant cell astrocytoma: diagnosis, screening, and treatment. Recommendations from the International Tuberous Sclerosis Complex Consensus Conference 2012. *Pediatr Neurol* 2013;49(6):439-444.

Umeoka S, et al. Pictorial review of tuberous sclerosis in various organs. *Radiographics* 2008;28(7):e32.

13a Answer B. Hummingbird sign.

13b Answer C. Seen in patients with progressive supranuclear palsy.

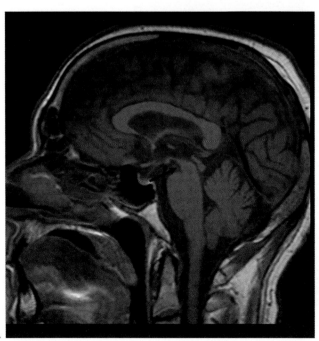

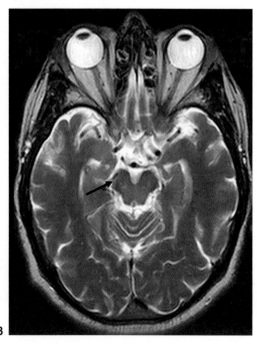

A   B

Imaging Findings: On the sagittal T1-weighted image (A), there is atrophy of the midbrain tegmentum and preserved profile of the pons compatible with the head and body of a hummingbird, the so-called hummingbird sign. On the axial T2-weighted image (B), atrophy of the midbrain tegmentum is noted.

Discussion: Progressive supranuclear palsy is a neurodegenerative disease and is classified pathologically as a tauopathy. This is a disease of unknown etiology, and there is no gender predisposition. Patients generally present in their 60s. Pathologically, the disease is characterized by neurofibrillary tangles and/or neuropil threads in the basal ganglia and brainstem. The typical patient with PSP has reduced facial expression, with marked reduction in blank frequency and overactivity of the frontalis muscle. Patients also present with poor mobility and falls, parkinsonism, visual symptoms like double or blurred vision, and bulbar symptoms like dysarthria. Cognitive and behavioral problems may also occur.

MRI is performed to exclude other diagnoses like stroke, tumor, and hydrocephalus. Findings supportive of PSP include T2 hyperintensity and atrophy of the midbrain, thinning of the substantia nigra, and atrophy of the putamen and globus pallidus.

The hummingbird or penguin sign in PSP patients is seen on a midsagittal plane as atrophy of the midbrain tegmentum and preserved profile of the pons. The decreased ratio of the area of the midbrain to the area of pons has also been shown to differentiate patients with PSP from normals and multisystem atrophy.

Hot cross bun sign seen in patients with MSA (multisystem atrophy) refers to cruciform hyperintensity through the pons on axial T2-weighted image, representing the selective loss of myelinated transverse pontocerebellar fibers and neurons in the pontine raphe with sparing of the pontine tegmentum and corticospinal tracts (see below). It has also been described in patients with parkinsonism, CJD, and spinocerebellar atrophy.

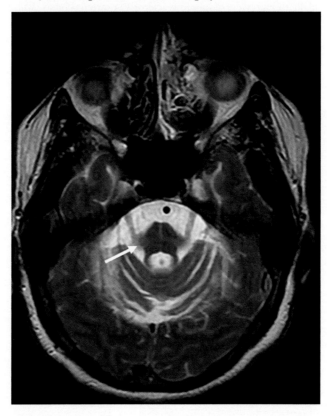

References: Kato N, Arai K, Hattori T. Study of the rostral midbrain atrophy in progressive supranuclear palsy. *J Neurol Sci* 2003;210(1-2):57-60. PubMed PMID: 12736089.

Oba H, Yagishita A, Terada H, et al. New and reliable MRI diagnosis for progressive supranuclear palsy. *Neurology* 2005;64(12):2050-2055. PubMed PMID: 15985570.

Shrivastava A. The hot cross bun sign. *Radiology* 2007;245(2):606-607. PubMed PMID: 17940314.

Warren NM, Burn DJ. Progressive supranuclear palsy. *Pract Neurol* 2007;7(1):16-23. Review. PubMed PMID: 17430861.

14a **Answer D.**   Atrophied and hyperintense left hippocampus.

14b **Answer A.**   Mesial temporal sclerosis.

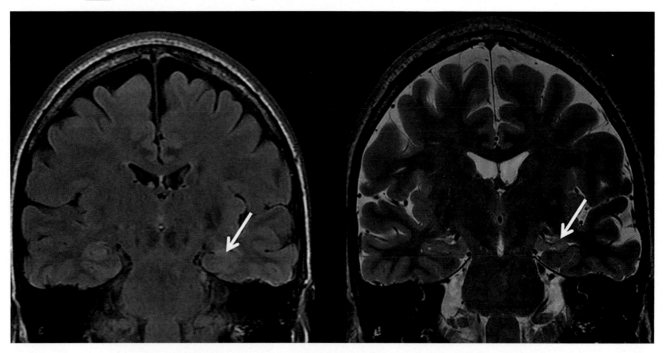

Imaging Findings: The hippocampus on the left is atrophic with loss of its normal internal architecture. There is hyperintense FLAIR signal abnormality within the left hippocampus. Imaging findings are compatible with left mesial temporal sclerosis.

Discussion: Mesial temporal sclerosis (MTS) is the most common cause of partial complex seizures in the adult population. MTS is best diagnosed with MRI with thin cut coronal T2 and coronal FLAIR imaging through the temporal lobes and hippocampi. Primary signs of MTS on imaging include hippocampal atrophy, T2/FLAIR hyperintensity, and loss of normal hippocampal internal architecture. Secondary signs of MTS include dilatation of the ipsilateral temporal horn as well as volume loss of the ipsilateral fornix and mammillary body. MTS is most often unilateral but can be bilateral approximately 20% of the time.

There is controversy in the literature in regard to whether MTS is the cause of the patient's seizures or results from the seizures themselves. There is also controversy in the literature whether febrile seizures as a child leads to MTS as an adult. Initial treatment is with antiepileptic medications. Patient's refractory to antiepileptic medication can go on to more invasive treatment options including temporal lobectomy or laser ablation.

References: Lee DH, et al. MR in temporal lobe epilepsy: analysis with pathologic confirmation. *AJNR Am J Neuroradiol* 1998;19:19–27.

Meiners LC, et al. Temporal Lobe Epilepsy: the various MR appearances of histologically proven mesial temporal sclerosis. *AJNR Am J Neuroradiol* 1994;15:1547–1555.

Shinar S. Febrile seizures and mesial temporal sclerosis. *Epilepsy Curr* 2003;3(4):115–118.

15a **Answer C.** MRI of the brain with contrast. CT shows right parietal gyral calcification suggestive of Sturge-Weber. MRI with contrast is the next best step.

15b **Answer A.** Encephalotrigeminal angiomatosis. Another name for Sturge-Weber Syndrome is encephalotrigeminal angiomatosis.

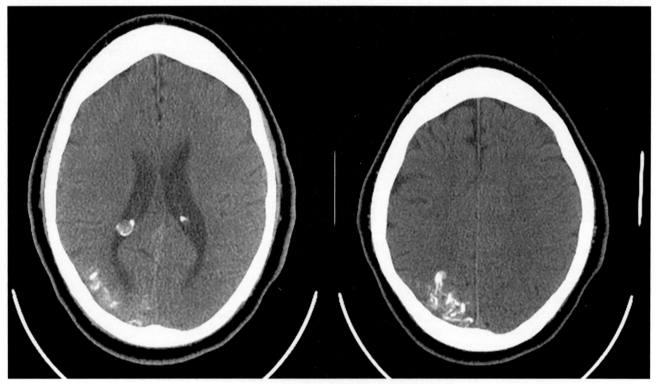

Figure 1. A noncontrast CT scan with right parietooccipital curvilinear gyral calcification as well as subcortical calcifications. There is also prominence of the right choroid in comparison to the left.

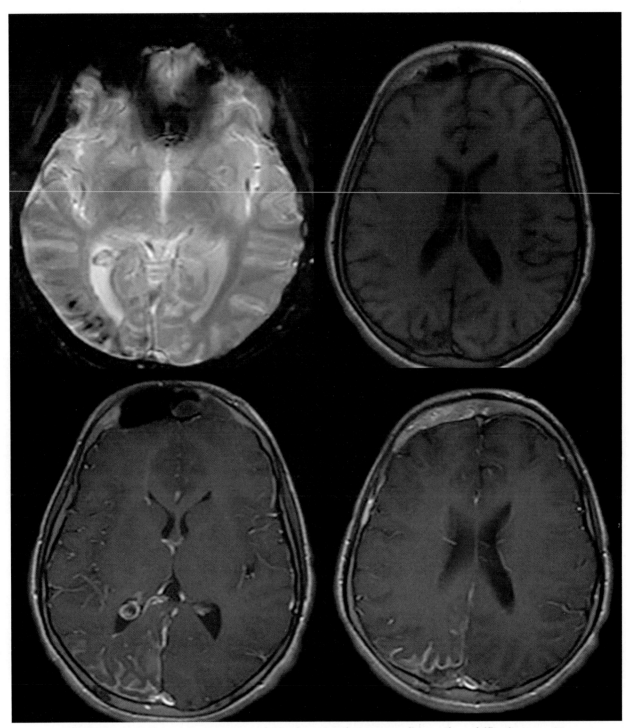

Figure 2. Gradient echo sequence shows low signal corresponding to the calcifications on CT. On the T1-weighted sequence, there is no intrinsic T1 shortening. Postgadolinium images demonstrate right-sided leptomeningeal enhancement and pial angiomatosis. The right choroid is noted to be prominent, and there is subtle volume loss of the right cerebral hemisphere in comparison to the left. Findings are compatible with Sturge-Weber Syndrome.

Discussion: Sturge-Weber Syndrome or encephalotrigeminal angiomatosis is a neurocutaneous disorder characterized by facial port-wine stain and pial angiomatosis involving one cerebral hemisphere. Sturge-Weber is a rare disease affecting approximately 1 in 50,000 to 230,000 people. Unlike the other phakomatoses, Sturge-Weber is felt not to be hereditary and rather results from a somatic mutation the GNAQ gene on chromosome 9q21.

Patients present with seizures within the first year of life, mental retardation, and glaucoma, along with the classic port-wine stain. The port-wine stain usually involves the ophthalmic division (V1) of the trigeminal nerve, unilaterally and ipsilateral to the intracranial abnormality. However, given how rare Sturge-Weber is, most patients with a port-wine stain simply have an isolated, uncomplicated finding.

Imaging findings of Sturge-Weber include gyral and subcortical calcifications, cerebral atrophy, ipsilateral choroid plexus enlargement, and leptomeningeal enhancement with pial angiomatosis all within the same cerebral hemisphere. The distribution tends to progress from posterior to anterior with the occipital and parietal lobes involved greater than the frontal and temporal lobes. Infratentorial involvement is not classic but does occur as well.

References: Adams ME, et al. A spectrum of unusual neuroimaging findings in patients with suspected Sturge-Weber syndrome. *AJNR Am J Neuroradiol* 2009;30:276–281.

Juhasz C, et al. Multimodality imaging of cortical and white matter abnormalities in Sturge-Weber syndrome. *AJNR Am J Neuroradiol* 2007;28:900–906.

Nozaki T, et al. Syndromes associated with vascular tumors and malformations: a pictorial review. *Radiographics* 2013;22:175–195.

16a Answer B. Corticospinal tract.

16b Answer A. Death occurs due to respiratory failure.

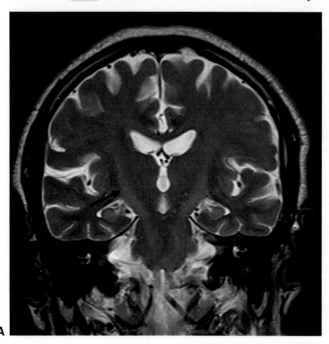 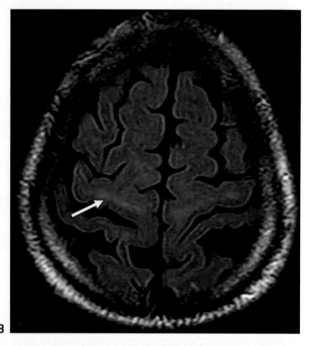

A   B

Imaging Findings: Coronal T2-weighted image (A) demonstrates increased signal in the bilateral corticospinal tracts. Axial FLAIR image (B) shows increased signal in the precentral/motor cortex.

Discussion: ALS, also known as motor neuron disease, is a neurodegenerative disorder characterized by progressive muscular paralysis secondary to degeneration of motor neurons in the primary motor cortex, brainstem, and spinal cord. Most patients with ALS have no family history and therefore have sporadic ALS. The disease is inherited in about 5% to 10% patients. The diagnosis of sporadic ALS is based on clinical signs and symptoms, and there is marked phenotypic heterogeneity. In patients who have a clinically definite disease, conventional MRI is not required. In patients who have clinically probable or possible disease, MR imaging is useful to rule out ALS mimic syndromes like multiple sclerosis, ischemia, cervical spondylotic myelopathy, and other causes of myelopathy. Death usually occurs 3 to 5 years after onset because of respiratory failure.

Conventional MR imaging in ALS patients demonstrates increased signal on T2-weighted, proton density-weighted, and FLAIR sequences in the cortical spinal tracts, a finding that is reported to be approximately 60% sensitive. This finding is not very specific and has been described in healthy subjects. Corticospinal tract signal intensity changes do not correlate with clinical scores of the disease. Additionally, a characteristic low signal intensity of the precentral cortex on T2-weighted images has been observed; again, this finding is neither very sensitive nor specific. Advanced imaging techniques including MR spectroscopy (decrease in the NAA level and NAA to creatinine ratio), diffusion tensor imaging (decrease in fractional anisotropy), and functional MRI may be helpful for prognostication.

Reference: Agosta F, Chiò A, Cosottini M, et al. The present and the future of neuroimaging in amyotrophic lateral sclerosis. *AJNR Am J Neuroradiol* 2010;31(10):1769–1777. doi: 10.3174/ajnr. A2043. Review. PubMed PMID: 20360339.

17   Answer C.   Vascular dementia.

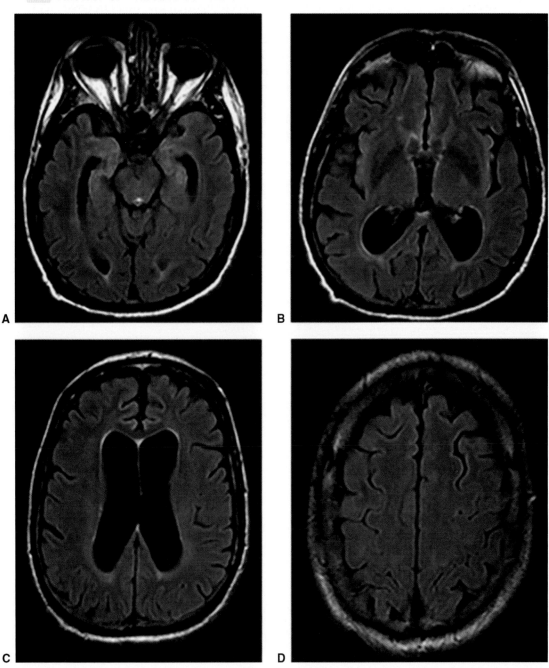

Imaging Findings: Axial FLAIR MR sequences demonstrate moderate diffuse ventriculomegaly with mild periventricular FLAIR hyperintense signal. No specific regional pattern of neurodegeneration or neocortical atrophy is obvious. No central white matter or cortical/juxtacortical signal changes. No evidence of stigmata of lacunar infarctions.

Discussion: Cognitive decline may have various etiologic underpinnings. Vascular cognitive impairment (VCI) is one of those causes. VCI is associated with FLAIR signal changes that suggest underlying small vessel disease, lacunar infarction or infarctions in strategic locations such as watershed distribution and association cortex. In this example, there are no significant white matter changes to suggest this entity, making this the least likely etiology to explain cognitive decline.

In addition, memory loss with gait difficulties and urinary incontinence may be seen with normal pressure hydrocephalus. The presence of moderate ventriculomegaly without commensurate increase in sulcal volume may be seen with normal pressure hydrocephalus. It has been reported that in infarct-free older individuals from a population-based cohort, those in the highest quartile of ratio of ventricular volume/sulcal volume were more likely to have impaired gait and cognition. Specific regional patterns of atrophy are reported with other entities such as Alzheimer dementia (medial temporal/hippocampal, parietooccipital), frontotemporal lobar degeneration (frontotemporal), and progressive supranuclear palsy (infratentorial). However, early changes from these entities may remain occult on structural imaging; therefore, despite lack of a specific pattern of neurodegeneration on these images, these other entities remain considerations in the appropriate clinical setting.

References: Harper L, et al. An algorithmic approach to structural imaging in dementia. *J Neurol Neurosurg Psychiatry* 2014;85(6):692–698.

Palm WM, et al. Ventricular dilation: association with gait and cognition. *Ann Neurol* 2009;66(4): 485–493.

7

Vascular Abnormalities

PRACHI DUBEY • ALY H. ABAYAZEED • SATHISH KUMAR DUNDAMADAPPA

QUESTIONS

1 A 41-year-old female with no prior medical history presents with new-onset seizure. Following are the key images from an MRI.

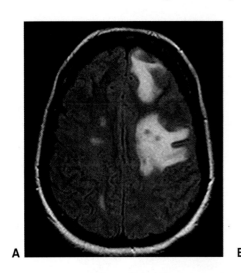
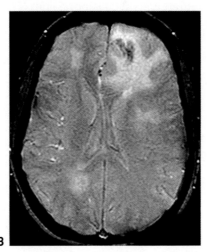
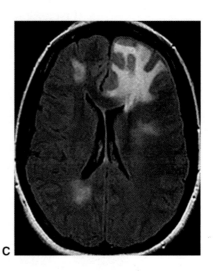

A   B   C

1a Which of the following entities is the most likely explanation for these lesions?

A. CNS vasculitis
B. Progressive multifocal leukoencephalopathy
C. Lymphoma in immunocompetent individuals
D. Multiple sclerosis

1b Which of the following tests is most useful in confirmation of the diagnosis of primary angiitis of the CNS?

A. Conventional cerebral angiography
B. MR angiography with contrast
C. High-resolution vessel wall imaging
D. Surgical biopsy

2   A 50-year-old male with neck pain and vertigo presents to the emergency department. Key images from an MRI are provided below:

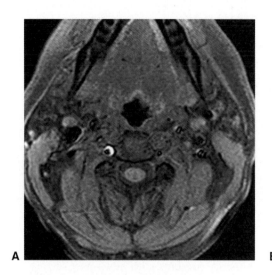

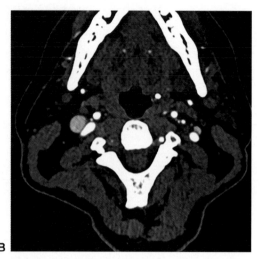

A

B

2a   What is the sequence type shown in Figure A?

A. T1w axial with contrast and blood suppression
B. T1w axial with fat saturation
C. T2w axial with fat saturation
D. T2w axial with contrast and blood suppression

2b   What is the most common imaging manifestation of the above diagnosis?

A. Arterial stenosis
B. Intimal flap
C. Intimal hematoma
D. Pseudoaneurysm

3   A 55-year-old male with sudden-onset right-sided weakness and altered mental status.

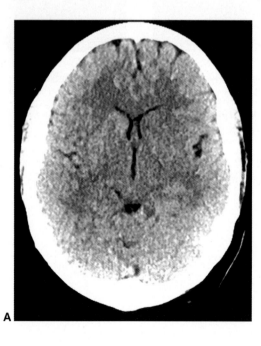

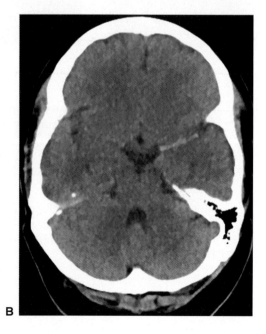

A

B

3a Given the noncontrast head CT findings, what is the next best study?

    A. Digital subtraction angiography
    B. CT angiography and CT perfusion
    C. Brain MRI and MRI perfusion
    D. No additional workup needed, only treatment

3b Below are key images from the coronal CTA, CBF, CBV, and MTT maps (in that order) from CT angiography and CT perfusion. What is the most accurate diagnosis?

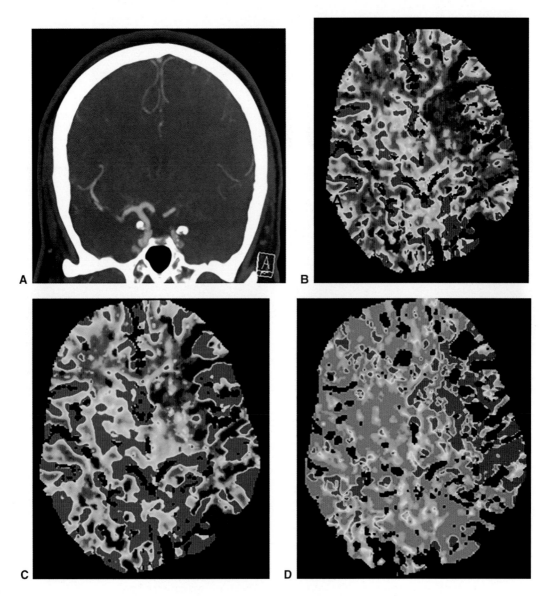

    A. Left ICA paraclinoid/terminus occlusion with LMCA ischemic penumbra
    B. Left ICA paraclinoid/terminus occlusion without an ischemic penumbra
    C. Left ICA paraclinoid/terminus occlusion with chronic LMCA infarction
    D. Left ICA paraclinoid/terminus occlusion without perfusion deficits

4   Images A, B and C were obtained during the initial presentation and Image D was obtained at 2 month follow up.

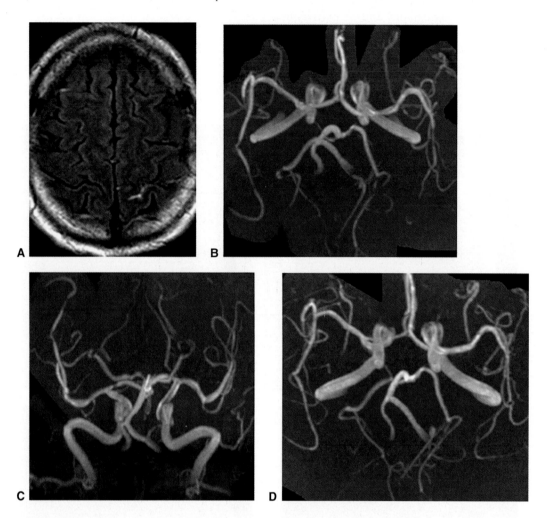

A   B

C   D

4a   Based on the above images, what is the most likely symptom in this 35-year-old otherwise healthy female?

A. Thunderclap headache
B. Positional vertigo
C. Painful visual loss
D. Gait disturbances

4b   Which of the following is the key feature in reversible cerebral vasoconstriction syndrome (RCVS)?

A. Lack of involvement of medium-/large-sized vessels
B. Complete resolution of symptoms but persistent imaging findings
C. Treatment by magnesium is crucial
D. Complete resolution of symptoms and imaging findings within 3 months

5 A 45-year-old male with conjunctival chemosis and proptosis presents for initial evaluation. Key images from a CTA head are provided below.

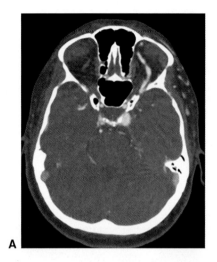

A

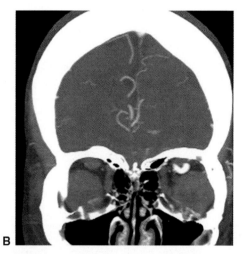

B

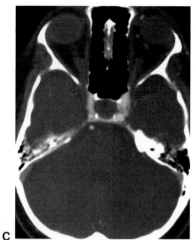

C

5a What is a common etiology for the above changes?

    A. Developmental in nature

    B. Posttraumatic etiology

    C. Postinflammatory changes

    D. Related to radiation therapy

5b What specific ocular abnormality is seen with the above diagnosis?

    A. Orbital varix

    B. Carotid cave aneurysm

    C. Engorgement of the superior ophthalmic vein

    D. Retrobulbar hemorrhage

5c What is the most likely etiology for mass-like lesion in left cavernous sinus?

    A. Lymphoma

    B. Meningioma

    C. Tolosa-Hunt syndrome

    D. Arterialized cavernous sinus

6

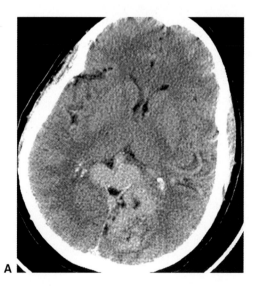

A

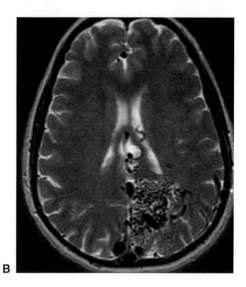

B

6a   What is the most likely diagnosis?

    A. Developmental venous anomaly (DVA)
    B. Cavernous malformation
    C. Arteriovenous malformation (AVM)
    D. Dural arteriovenous fistula (DAVF)

6b   Which of the following is one of the key differentiating features between AVM and dural arteriovenous fistula (DAVF)?

    A. Presence of intraparenchymal nidus
    B. Large-vessel arterial feeder
    C. Deep venous drainage
    D. Size

7   A 25-year-old female with recurrent transient ischemic attacks presents for an MRI/MRA. Key images are shown below.

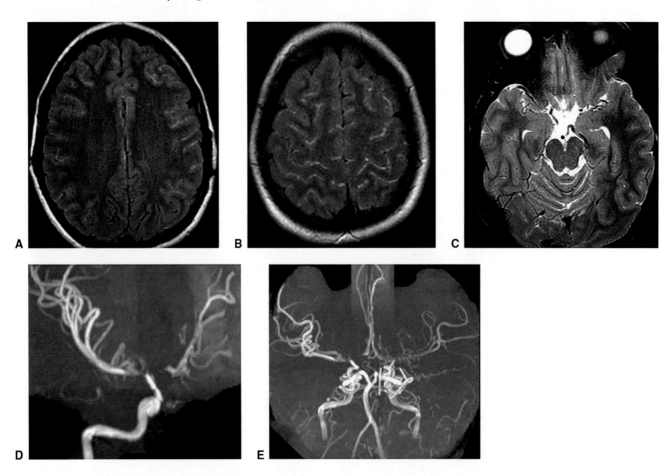

7a   Based on these images, what is the most likely explanation for the abnormality shown in Figures A and B?

    A. Abnormal oxygenation
    B. Subarachnoid hemorrhage
    C. Meningitis
    D. Pial vascular engorgement

7b Which of the following is an accepted management strategy for this condition?

    A. Vascular stenting

    B. Endovascular aneurysm coil embolization

    C. ECA (superficial temporal artery branch) to MCA anastomoses

    D. Intravenous antibiotics

8 A 35-year-old female with severe headache presents to the ER for further assessment. Key images from a CT and MRI are provided below.

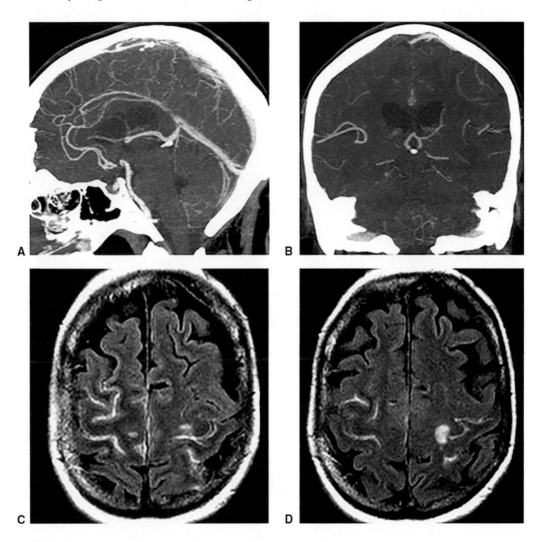

8a What is a possible relevant clinical history in this patient?

    A. High-dose aspirin use

    B. Oral contraceptive use

    C. Cocaine abuse

    D. Uncontrolled hypertension

8b Which of the following venous structures is part of deep venous drainage?

    A. Vein of Trolard

    B. Vein of Labbé

    C. Sylvian vein

    D. Internal cerebral vein

9   A 70-year-old female with acute-onset altered mental status and abnormal head CT shown below. Remaining of the workup was unrevealing including CTA head and neck, MRI, and catheter cerebral angiogram.

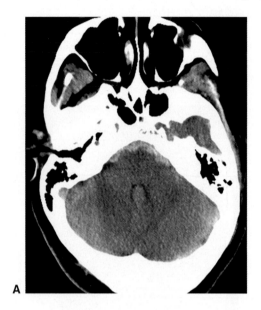
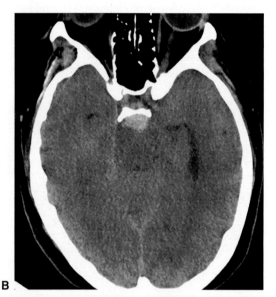

What is the most likely diagnosis?

A. Basilar meningeal exudates
B. Prepontine mass
C. Aneurysmal subarachnoid hemorrhage
D. Benign perimesencephalic hemorrhage

10   A 50-year-old female smoker and hypertensive with acute-onset severe headache presents to the ER. Key images from noncontrast head CT and cerebral angiogram are shown below.

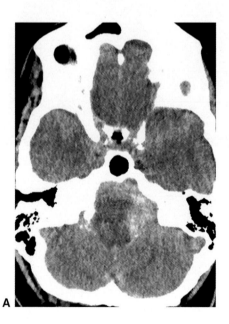
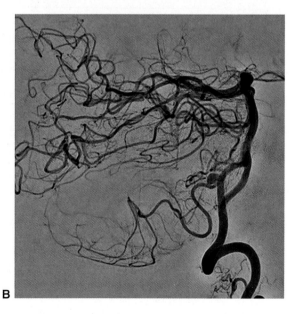

10a What is an anticipated risk that contributes to significant mortality and morbidity with the above condition?

A. Cerebral vasospasm

B. Large-vessel thrombosis

C. Associated dissection

D. Hydrocephalus

Patient had subsequent deterioration of clinical status. Following key images from a CT angiogram are shown.

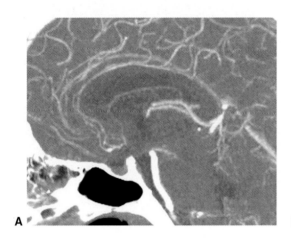
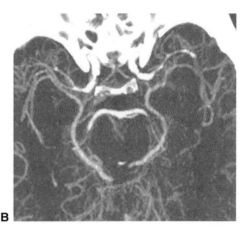

10b What is the most likely diagnosis?

A. Cerebral vasospasm

B. LMCA dissection

C. Basilar stenosis

D. Basilar thrombosis

11 A 56-year-old male presents to the ER with disorientation and ataxia. Key images from MRI and CTA are provided below.

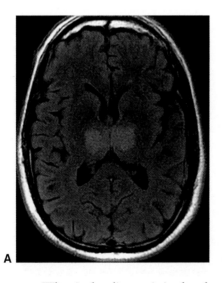
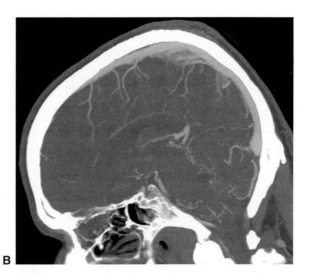

What is the diagnosis in the above case?

A. Artery of Percheron infarct

B. Deep venous sinus thrombosis

C. Creutzfeldt-Jakob disease

D. Bithalamic glioma

12 A 60-year-old diabetic female with sudden-onset headache, blurry vision, and facial numbness, and paresthesias was sent for an MRI. Key images are shown below.

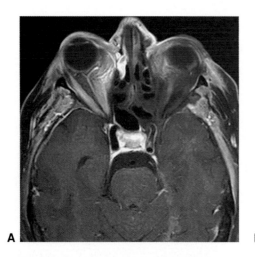

A

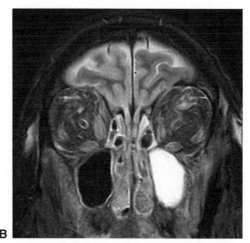

B

12a Which is the most likely diagnosis?

    A. Orbital pseudotumor
    B. Tolosa-Hunt syndrome
    C. Cavernous sinus thrombosis
    D. Carotid–cavernous fistula

12b What the additional abnormality shown on these images predisposes to this diagnosis?

    A. Skull base trauma
    B. Paranasal sinus infection
    C. Maxillary sinus mucocele
    D. Cavernous carotid dissection

13 A 45-year-old male with abnormal head CT. An MRI was performed for better assessment, as shown below.

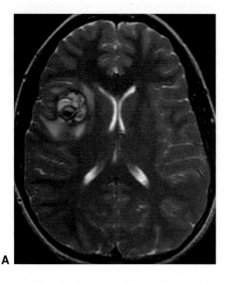

A

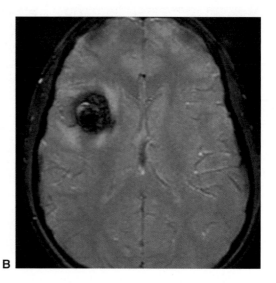

B

What is the most likely diagnosis?

    A. Cavernoma
    B. Developmental venous anomaly
    C. Arteriovenous malformation
    D. Oligodendroglioma

14 A 30-year-old female presented for evaluation of pulsatile tinnitus. On otoscopic evaluation, a retrotympanic mass with reddish hue was seen behind the tympanic membrane. A CT was performed for further assessment.

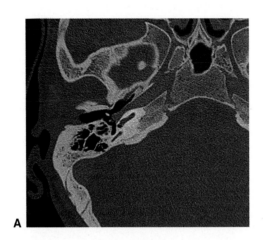

A

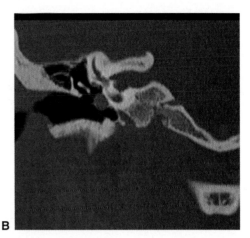

B

14a What is the diagnosis?

    A. Glomus tympanicum

    B. Aberrant internal carotid artery

    C. Congenital cholesteatoma

    D. Jugular bulb dehiscence

14b The above entity is often associated with which of the following secondary findings?

    A. Absence of cervical ICA and enlargement of inferior tympanic canaliculus

    B. Absence of the sigmoid plate of the jugular foramen

    C. Middle ear ossicular erosion or displacement

    D. Dehiscence of the tegmen tympani

15 A 75-year-old patient was found down and brought to the ER. First a CT and then MRI was performed.

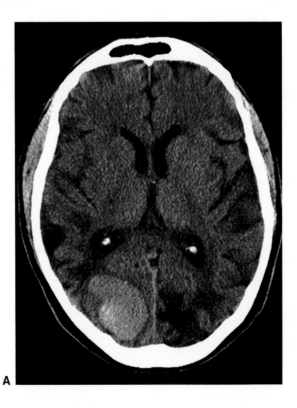

A

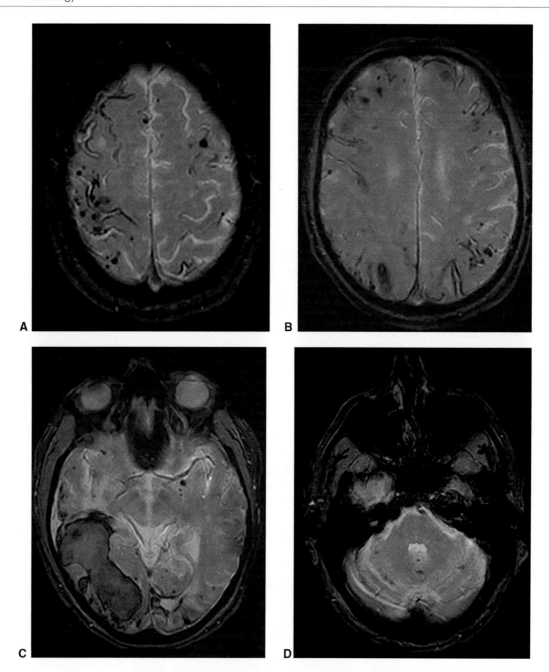

A

B

C

D

15a What is the investigation of choice for diagnosing this condition?

A. CT scan
B. Catheter angiogram
C. MR imaging with susceptibility-weighted sequence
D. Amyloid nuclear scan

15b What is true about this condition?

A. Most commonly an inherited condition with autosomal transmission. Other family members need to be screened.
B. This is a rare condition in elderly population.
C. Repeated trauma with second impact syndrome
D. Commonly involves small- and medium-sized vessels in peripheral aspect of the brain.

ANSWERS AND EXPLANATIONS

1a **Answer A.** CNS vasculitis. Presence of peripheral cortical/subcortical signal changes with presence of hemosiderin staining in the left frontal lobe, is most compatible with CNS vasculitis. The cortical extension is atypical with PML. Lymphoma can be multifocal and hemorrhagic in immunocompromised but very unlikely morphology in immunocompetent patients. Rare variant of tumefactive demyelination or ADEM can have this appearance; fulminant forms may hemorrhage but will not be a likely or usual consideration.

1b **Answer D.** Surgical biopsy. The peripheral small-vessel involvement lowers the yield of diagnostic imaging in confirming the diagnosis. Often, these studies are normal despite path-proven primary CNS angiitis changes seen on cortical and meningeal biopsy.

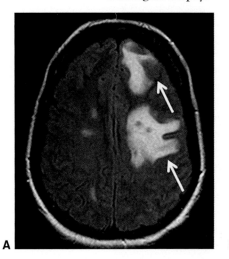 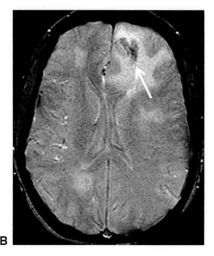 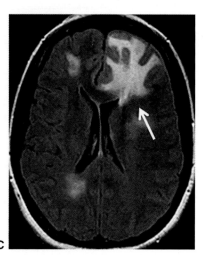

A   B   C

Imaging Findings: Axial FLAIR (A and C) showing scattered cortical/subcortical white matter lesions with left frontal lobe focus showing small hemosiderin staining (B).

Discussion: Vasculitis is a broad term, which includes multiple diseases with a common feature of inflammation of the vessel wall involving arteries, veins, or both. It is responsible for about 5% of strokes in young patients.

Vasculitis involving the nervous system is classified into primary angiitis of the central nervous system (PACNS) and secondary vasculitis. Secondary vasculitis can be primary systemic vasculitis with CNS involvement or secondary vascular involvement with a systemic disease. Vasculitis-like picture can also be seen with recreation drug use and as long-term sequel of radiation.

Vasculitis is also subclassified based on the size of the smallest involved vessel as large-vessel vasculitis (defined as vessel larger than 2 mm in size, vessels including and proximal to M1/A1/P1), medium-vessel vasculitis (vessel size of 0.5 mm), and small-vessel vasculitis (vessel size of 0.2 to 0.3 mm, leptomeningeal and cortical vessels).

Common systemic vascular diseases involving CNS are giant cell arteritis (large vessel), Takayasu disease (large vessel), Wegener granulomatosis (small vessel), polyarteritis nodosa (medium vessel), and Churg-Strauss syndrome (small vessel). Sjögren syndrome, mixed connective tissue disorders, SLE, and neuro-Behçet's are some of the systemic diseases with secondary vascular involvement.

PACNS aka primary CNS vasculitis is by definition confined to central or peripheral nervous system. This is rare disorder with peak incidence in 4th to 6th decades of life and commonly affecting small vessels and occasionally medium-sized vessels. Veins are affected less often. Histopathologically, there is focal or segmental inflammatory infiltrate accompanied by vessel wall necrosis with or without perivascular granuloma, myelin loss, and axonal degeneration. The disease is heterogeneous with varied and often nonspecific clinical presentation. Imaging is also nonspecific and reflects sequela of vessel abnormality (intervening areas of stenosis and dilation, "beaded appearance"), ischemia following luminal compromise, and hemorrhage following vessel wall disruption.

Imaging evaluation of the vasculitis should begin with MRI, evaluating the parenchymal effects. This should be followed by vascular imaging and if necessary biopsy.

The most common imaging abnormality in PACNS is bilateral, multiple, supratentorial white matter T2 hyperintensities. Basal ganglia and cortex can also be involved. Multiple infarcts in different vascular territories can be seen. Contrast enhancement of the lesions, meninges, and perivascular spaces can be seen. Mass-like lesions are seen in about 15% of cases. Parenchymal and subarachnoid hemorrhages often small and petechial can be present, best depicted by SWI images. DWI restriction can be seen in newer lesions in the background of older lesions.

Noninvasive vascular imaging is often negative in PACNS as small vessels are below the resolution of CTA/MRA. Catheter angiogram can be negative unless there is involvement of the medium-sized vessels. Meningeal or brain biopsy is the mainstay for diagnosis in small-vessel vasculitis. Given the heterogeneity of the disease, even biopsy can be false negative.

References: Birnbaum J, Hellmann DB. Primary angiitis of the central nervous system. *Arch Neurol* 2009;66(6):704–709. doi:10.1001/archneurol.2009.76

Garg A. Vascular brain pathologies. *Neuroimaging Clin N Am* 2011;21(4):897–926. doi:10.1016/j. nic.2011.07.007

Hähnel S, ed. *Inflammatory diseases of the brain*, 2nd ed. 2013 ed. New York, NY: Springer, 2013.

Law M, Som PM, Naidich TP. *Problem solving in neuroradiology: expert consult—online and print*, 1st ed. Philadelphia, PA: Saunders, 2011.

Naidich TP, ed. *Imaging of the brain*. Expert Radiology Series. Philadelphia, PA: Saunders/Elsevier, 2013.

2a **Answer B.** T1w axial with fat saturation. The axial image shows T1 weighting (note low signal from CSF in cervical canal and intermediate signal from mucosal surface). There is also suppressed signal from subcutaneous fat. There is no contrast or blood suppression.

2b   **Answer A.**   Arterial stenosis. The diagnosis here is vertebral artery dissection. Often on imaging, it manifests as an abrupt change in vessel caliber or tapering stenosis not accounted by atherosclerotic disease.

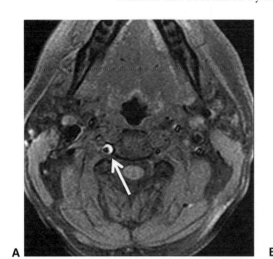

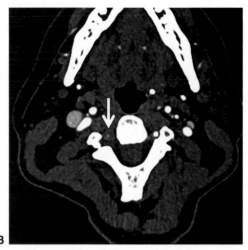

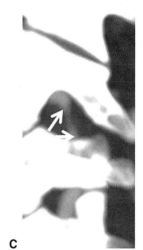

A   B   C

Imaging Findings: There is a crescenteric focus of T1 hyperintensity seen in the V2 segment of the right vertebral artery on axial T1 fat saturation without contrast (A). This corresponds to mural thickening and string-like luminal narrowing at this level on CTA (B). Note focal dilation just distal to the string-like narrowing seen on coronal CTA MIP (C).

Discussion: Vertebral artery dissection (VAD) is an important diagnostic consideration in patients with neck or head pain and vertigo/dizziness. It may also result in an ischemic stroke and should be carefully evaluated in the posterior circulation acute ischemic strokes. The causes include spontaneous, traumatic, iatrogenic neck manipulation, or having predispositions such as fibromuscular disease and collagen vascular disorders.

Clinically, these patients can present with neck pain and dizziness or vertigo. Additional neurologic deficits may be present if complication by a posterior circulation infarction or subarachnoid hemorrhage.

On imaging, CTA and MRA can be both used for noninvasive diagnosis. A T1 or T2 fat saturation sequence can be used to assess for intramural hematoma. Commonly, however, the VAD demonstrates vascular stenosis with vessel wall thickening, string sign, because of marked luminal narrowing or abrupt changes in vessel caliber. There may be vessel wall irregularity that can be better seen with high-resolution vessel wall imaging or conventional cerebral angiography, the latter considered the gold standard for VAD diagnosis.

Vertebral artery dissection itself can have a steno-occlusive or aneurysmal morphology. The aneurysmal pattern can have a focal or fusiform dilation proximal or distal to the stenotic segment. This has been most frequently found in the V4 segment and may be associated with subarachnoid hemorrhage. When the dissection progresses through the media into the subadventitial layer, it results in eccentric outer wall dilation, leading to a dissecting pseudoaneurysm. Management largely depends upon clinical symptoms, location, and morphology of the dissection. Anticoagulation can be used in patients with extradural dissection. However, it is contraindicated in patients who have hemorrhagic infarction or subarachnoid hemorrhage. Endovascular coil or surgical embolization of dissecting aneurysms can be performed.

References: Gottesman RF, Sharma P, Robinson KA, et al. Imaging characteristics of symptomatic vertebral artery dissection: a systematic review. *Neurologist* 2012;18(5):255-260.

Shin JH, Suh DC, Choi CG, et al. Vertebral artery dissection: spectrum of imaging findings with emphasis on angiography and correlation with clinical presentation. *Radiographics* 2000;20(6):1687-1696.

3a **Answer B.** CT angiography and CT perfusion. There is hypoattenuation in the left basal ganglia region with loss of definition of left caudate and putamen (Fig. A). There is also a hyperdense vessel in the LMCA region, concerning for a thrombus (Fig. B). This is compatible with acute stroke and B is therefore the next step in workup.

3b **Answer A.** Left ICA paraclinoid/terminus occlusion with LMCA ischemic penumbra. The MTT and CBF maps show ischemic region in the LMCA distribution and low CBV in the basal ganglia region, suggesting a small core infarct with a mismatch perfusion defect compatible with an ischemic penumbra.

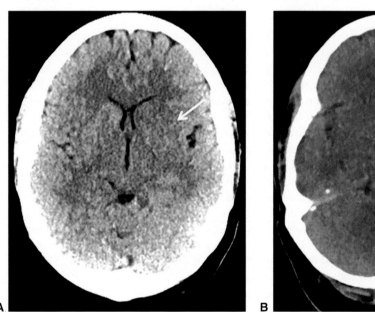

A   B

Figure 1

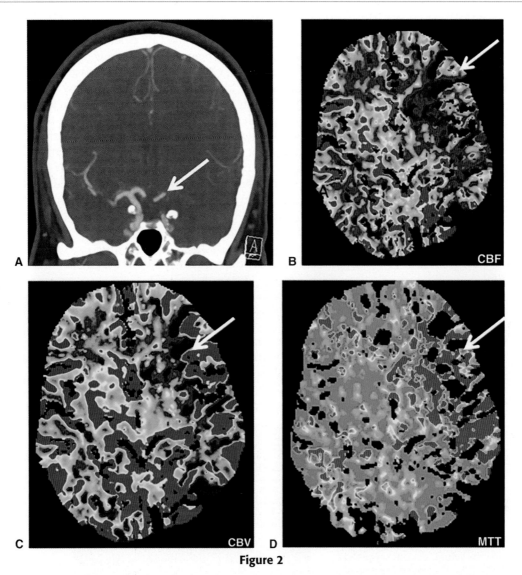

Figure 2

Imaging Findings: Figure 1. Axial noncontrast head CT demonstrates hyperdense left MCA sign because of intraluminal thrombus and cytotoxic edema/infarction in the left caudate and lentiform with loss of the normal gray–white matter differentiation.

Figure 2. Coronal MIP at the level of the carotid terminus from the CTA showing occlusion of the left carotid terminus and the left MCA. CBF, CBV, and MTT maps from the CT perfusion demonstrate a small area of core infarction (reduced CBV, which matches with severely reduced CBF, coded as dark blue on CBF map) in the left caudate and lentiform nuclei and large area of tissue at risk/penumbra (mismatched CBV/MTT) in the left frontal and parietal lobes in the vascular territory of the left MCA, which denotes patent distal pial collaterals supplying the ischemic tissue and potentially salvageable tissue.

Discussion: In cases of acute stroke, a noncontrast head CT is the first study performed to exclude intracranial hemorrhage and look for signs of intracranial ischemia. IV tPA is administered if the patient is within the therapeutic window for medical treatment and there is no intracranial hemorrhage. IA tPA can be administered in anterior circulation strokes up to 6 h from the time of onset.

It is the common practice to obtain CTA with or without CT perfusion studies in the setting of acute stroke to evaluate for possible intervention if the patient is within the therapeutic window (0 to 8 h in the anterior circulation). CTA will evaluate the site and extent of the vascular pathology (in situ thrombus, emboli, or dissection) and will show the status of the vessels proximal and distal to the site of occlusion and the status of collateral blood vessels. Core infarction (site of irreversible loss of function) will show matched CBF and CBV defects. Areas of tissue at risk (site of potentially salvageable neurons or penumbra) will show decreased CBF in mL/100 g brain tissue/min, maintained CBV in mL/100 g brain tissue (open collaterals), and prolonged MTT in seconds (it takes longer for blood to flow around the collateral vessels). Of note 4D CTA or dynamic CT angiography has been shown recently to be superior to spCTA (single-phase CTA) in evaluating the degree of vascular occlusion in ischemic lesions, tandem vascular lesions, the status of the delayed collateral circulation, and the spot sign in case of intracranial hemorrhage, a sign that is associated with increased risk of hematoma expansion. DWI-MRI is very sensitive towards accurate detection of infarct core. However due to MRI availability related limitations, CT remains the mainstay for work-up in many institutions.

References: Allen LM, Hasso AN, Handwerker J, et al. Sequence-specific MR imaging findings that are useful in dating ischemic stroke. *Radiographics* 2012;32(5):1285–1297.

Kortman HGJ, Smit EJ, Oei MTH, et al. 4D-CTA in neurovascular disease: a review. *AJNR Am J Neuroradiol* 2015;36:1026–1033; originally published online on October 29, 2014, doi:10.3174/ajnr.A4162

Lui TW, Tang ER, Allmendinger AM, et al. Evaluation of CT perfusion in the setting of cerebral ischemia: patterns and pitfalls. *AJNR Am J Neuroradiol* 2010;31:1552–1563; originally published online on February 25, 2010, doi:10.3174/ajnr.A2026

4a **Answer A.** Thunderclap headache. A classical symptom associated with RCVS. Note that this symptom is also seen with aneurysm rupture making it a challenging diagnosis based on clinical picture alone.

4b **Answer D.** Complete resolution of symptoms and imaging findings within 3 months.

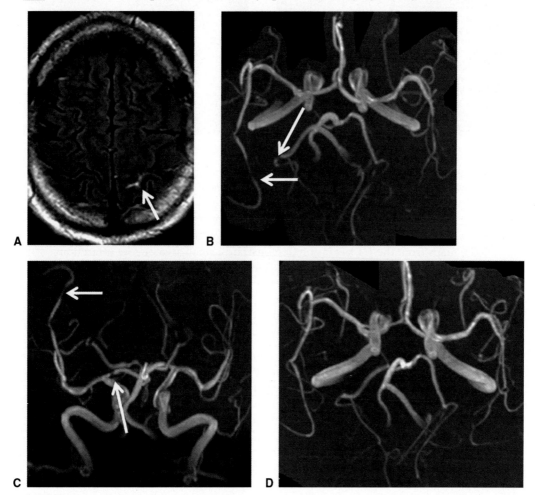

Imaging Findings: There is focal left superior parietal sulcal nonsuppression of CSF on FLAIR suggesting trace subarachnoid hemorrhage (A). There are areas of focal segmental narrowing seen on MRA indicated by arrows (B and C) with involvement of right ACA A1 segment (C). These findings in the current clinical setting and age group are most likely to represent RCVS. Two-month follow-up image from MRA in the same patient shows complete resolution of previously seen findings (D).

Discussion: Reversible cerebral vasoconstriction syndrome (RCVS) refers to a group of disorders characterized by severe headache (often thunderclap type and recurrent in first week or two of the disease) with or without other neurologic symptoms and focal and segmental noninflammatory constrictions in multiple intracranial arteries that resolve spontaneously within 1 to 3 months. It has uniphasic course without new symptoms after 1 month of onset. "Thunderclap headache" refers to acute-onset extreme headache that reaches severity in less than a minute.

A wide range of age group can be involved, the peak at about 40 years of age, with female preponderance. Less than half of the cases are spontaneous. In nearly 60% of cases, precipitating factor is present, the most common being postpartum state and exposure to several recreational drugs (cannabis, cocaine, ecstasy, LSD, amphetamine derivatives) as well medications (nasal decongestants, SSRIs, etc.) many of which are vasoactive. Binge alcohol consumption is also reported trigger. Neck arterial dissection and carotid endarterectomy are also known triggers.

Exact pathophysiology of the disease is not known. This is believed to result from transient disturbance in maintenance of vascular tone and sympathetic overreactivity. Association with reversible leukoencephalopathy (PRES) and brain edema suggests the possibility of endothelial dysfunction as a contributory factor. The disturbance is hypothesized to start with smaller arteries and then progress to medium- and large-sized arteries over the next couple of weeks. Hence, RCVS is a dynamic process and clinicoradiologic features depend on the time course of the disease. PRES on the other hand has a propensity for medium- and small-sized vessels.

Given the dynamic nature of the disease, in early stages, imaging can be negative and "headache" can be the only symptom. A short-term repeat imaging is recommended. If there is associated neck pain, neck vascular imaging is suggested to look for dissection. Transcranial Doppler can be useful in monitoring cerebral vasoconstriction. Biopsy is not recommended for RCVS as this is a noninflammatory process and should only be done if there is a strong suspicion for true vasculitis. The prognosis of the disease is determined by the presence and extent of stroke; however, usually, this disease has a self-limiting benign course and responds to calcium channel blockers in the acute phase.

Differential diagnoses:

Aneurysmal SAH: Distribution of hemorrhage is often typical and generally more central. Vasospasm is generally limited to the areas of hemorrhage and the extent somewhat proportionate to the amount of hemorrhage. In RCVS, the stenoses are widespread and disproportionate to the small peripheral SAH. Unlike, SAH, headache of RCVS is short lived.

CNS vasculitis: Small peripheral hemorrhages can also be seen with vasculitis. In vasculitis, the onset of symptoms is more gradual. MRI generally shows presence of white matter lesions as well as infarcts at the time of presentation. Headaches are frequent with vasculitis but generally not thunderclap type.

References: Ducros A. Reversible cerebral vasoconstriction syndrome. *Lancet Neurol* 2012;11(10):906–917.

Ducros A, Boukobza M, Porcher R, et al. The clinical and radiological spectrum of reversible cerebral vasoconstriction syndrome. A prospective series of 67 patients. *Brain* 2007;130(12):3091–3101.

5a **Answer B.** Posttraumatic etiology. A carotid cavernous fistula (CC fistula) is seen with aneurysmal dilation of the left supraclinoid ICA, engorged left cavernous ICA, and left superior ophthalmic vein. Trauma is a common etiologic factor leading to this condition.

5b **Answer C.** Engorgement of the superior ophthalmic vein.

5c **Answer D.** Arterialized cavernous sinus. A distended arterially enhancing left cavernous sinus is seen in the setting of a dilated left superior ophthalmic vein compatible with a CC fistula.

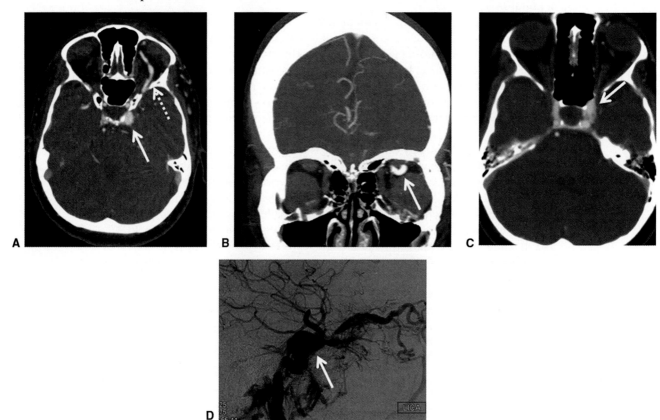

Imaging Findings: Enlarged and arterialized superior ophthalmic vein and vascular engorgement of left cavernous sinus seen on CTA source images (A to C). Catheter angiogram confirms CCF with venous congestion in orbit and in pterygoid venous plexus/masticator space (D).

Discussion: Carotid-cavernous fistula (CC fistula) is abnormal communication between the ICA and cavernous sinus shunting the carotid arterial blood into the cavernous venous system.

Carotid–cavernous sinus fistula (CCF) can be classified based on etiology (traumatic or spontaneous), rate of flow (high vs. low), or the angiographic architecture (direct, resulting from an ICA tear or indirect, which are due to meningeal branches from ICA and/or ECA shunting via a dural AV fistula).

The most commonly used calcification is by Barrow et al.:

1. Direct (type A fistula): Direct communication between internal carotid artery and cavernous sinus, usually high-flow fistula, commonly resulting from trauma. A smaller percentage (20%) can be spontaneous, resulting from rupture of either aneurysm or weakened ICA vessel wall.
2. Indirect CCF (types, B, C, and D): Dual arteriovenous fistulas, fed by meningeal branches of ICA (type B), external carotid artery (type C), or both (type D, the most common type of indirect CCF). These are more commonly low-flow fistulas, sequel of venous thrombosis.

Trauma to skull base is a common etiology for CCF. It can also be seen with ICA aneurysm rupture into the cavernous sinus. The indirect CCFs may result from revascularization of a prior cavernous sinus thrombosis. Clinically, these patients have ocular symptoms such as proptosis, conjunctival injection, chemosis, diplopia, or visual loss.

Imaging features on CTA or MRA include engorgement and arterial enhancement of the ipsilateral cavernous sinus and engorgement of the superior ophthalmic vein; bilateral cavernous sinus enlargement can also be seen due to intercavernous communications. T2-weighted MR images show abnormal flow voids within the cavernous sinus; abnormal hyperintense signal can be seen on time-of-flight MRA within the cavernous sinus.

Findings related to venous congestion are commonly seen in the orbits and include enlarged superior ophthalmic veins, enlargement of extraocular muscles, proptosis, and orbital edema. Intracranial venous congestion can present as engorged leptomeningeal and cortical veins and white matter T2 hyperintensity. One to two percent of patients can present with intracranial hemorrhage.

Conventional cerebral angiogram is the gold standard in identifying the exact site of communication, presence of dural feeders, and rate of flow.

Management depends on the type of fistula and symptoms. The direct CCF are typically high flow and have high risk for intracranial hemorrhage requiring timely intervention. Endovascular treatment with balloon, coil, or stent embolization can be performed. If needed, surgical ligation, cavernous sinus packing, or stereotactic radiosurgery can be considered. Conservative treatment is generally undertaken for indirect CCF, especially when the clinical symptoms are mild. Twenty to fifty percent of indirect CCFs heal spontaneously.

References: Gemmete JJ, Ansari SA, Gandhi D. Endovascular treatment of carotid cavernous fistulas. *Neuroimaging Clin N Am* 2009;19(2):241–255. doi:10.1016/j.nic.2009.01.006

Jindal G, Miller T, Raghavan P, et al. Imaging evaluation and treatment of vascular lesions at the skull base. *Radiol Clin North Am* 2017;55(1):151–166.

Lee JY, Jung C, Ihn YK, et al. Multidetector CT angiography in the diagnosis and classification of carotid-cavernous fistula. *Clin Radiol* 2016;71(1):e64–e71.

6a **Answer C.** Arteriovenous malformation (AVM). There is large tangle of vessels with distended vein of Galen and a proliferative nidus seen on axial T2w MR image.

6b **Answer A.** Presence of intraparenchymal nidus. This is the key feature seen with AVM but not with DAVF. Both have arterial feeders shunting into the venous system. Extent of abnormality can be variable depending on the severity of the shunt.

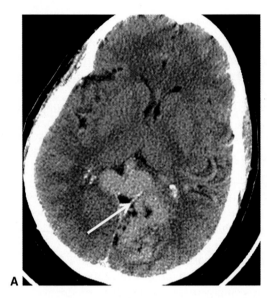
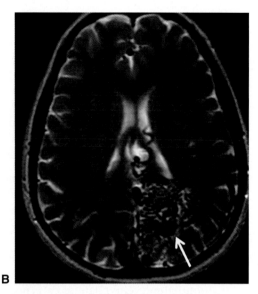

Imaging Findings: Contrast-enhanced CT shows prominent tangle of vessels in the left parieto-occipital region with a distended vein of Galen (A). There is a diffuse or proliferative intraparenchymal nidus seen on axial T2w MRI (B).

Discussion: Brain arteriovenous malformations (bAVMs) are abnormal communications between arterial feeders, specifically pial, supplying the brain tissue and venous drainage pathways. This results in shunting of arterial blood directly into the venous pathways without an intervening normal capillary network. For the diagnosis of AVMs, two characteristic features are important: first, presence of an intraparenchymal nidus and, second, presence of early venous drainage seen on dynamic imaging such as conventional catheter angiogram.

Overall, these are one of rare causes for intraparenchymal hemorrhage and stroke. However, in younger individuals, this is the most common cause of intracranial hemorrhage. It can be isolated in nature or occur in association with syndromes such as Osler-Weber-Rendu (hereditary hemorrhagic telangiectasia [HHT]) or Wyburn-Mason syndrome.

Clinically, these patients can present with seizures, headache, focal neurologic deficits, and hemorrhage. On imaging, key features are presence of a parenchymal nidus, which may be compact or be diffuse with interspersed brain tissue, presence of arterial feeders, and early venous drainage. These lesions can be further classified using the Spetzler-Martin grading system designed to predict the risk of surgery.

- Size of nidus: small <3 mm (1 point), medium 3-6 mm (2 points), and large (>6 mm) (3 points)
- Venous drainage: superficial (0 points) or deep venous system (1 point)
- Eloquence of adjacent brain: noneloquent (0 points) versus eloquent (1 point). This is determined by importance of the brain structure in terms of functional significance, such as sensorimotor cortex, visual cortex, language, thalamus/hypothalamus, brainstem, internal capsule, cerebellar peduncles, and deep cerebellar nuclei, which are all considered eloquent.

The grade is defined as sum of points in each category. Therefore, the highest possible grade is V (3+1+1). These lesions are deemed high risk with significant surgical morbidity and mortality. Management can be medical management with or without intervention such as surgery, endovascular embolization, or stereotactic radiosurgery.

References: Geibprasert S, Pongpech S, Jiarakongmun P, et al. Radiologic assessment of brain arteriovenous malformations: what clinicians need to know. *Radiographics* 2010;30(2):483–501.

Speizler RF, Martin NA. A proposed grading system for arteriovenous malformations. 1986. *J Neurosurg* 2008;108(1):186–193.

7a **Answer D.** Pial vascular engorgement. This condition is compatible with moyamoya syndrome, which is typically associated with extensive collateralization and related pial vascular engorgement. The sulcal nonsuppression of CSF shown in this case is likely resulting for vascular congestion. On contrast-enhanced MRI, this may manifest as pial enhancement, namely, the "Ivy sign."

7b **Answer C.** ECA (superficial temporal artery branch) to MCA anastomoses.

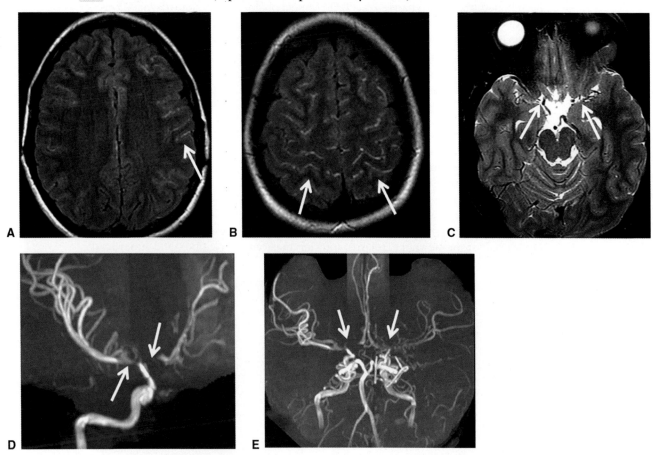

Imaging Findings: Axial FLAIR images showing sulcal nonsuppression of CSF (A and B) because of pial vascular engorgement in the setting of hypoplasia of M1-MCA bilaterally as noted on axial T2 weighted image (C) through the sylvian fissures bilaterally. 3D volume-rendered reformats from MR angiogram (D and E) confirm absent M1-MCA and A1-ACA bilaterally. These findings are consistent with moyamoya disease.

Discussion: Moyamoya disease is a progressive cerebrovascular pathology of unclear etiology. It is commonly seen in Asian population and has a female predilection. The disease has a bimodal distribution, seen in 1st and 3rd to 4th decade of life. Moyamoya-like vascular lesions can be seen with conditions such as sickle cell disease, NF1, radiation exposure, HCV infection, and cryoglobulinemia, among other numerous etiologies. In the presence of an etiologic factor, the condition is referred to as moyamoya syndrome.

Clinically, these patients can present with headaches, vertigo, transient ischemic attacks, stroke, hemorrhage, and seizures. Imaging findings include progressive nonatherosclerotic stenosis or occlusion of terminal portion of the ICA and proximal portions of ACA and MCA with extensive collateral formation, leading to the "puff of smoke" appearance on conventional angiogram. These collateral vessels are prone to both thrombotic occlusion and hemorrhage because of microaneurysm formation. FLAIR and postcontrast T1w sequences can show pial vascular congestion–related hyperintensity, namely, the "Ivy sign."

Management can range from observation in mild cases to medial management with antiplatelet medication and surgery for severe cases. Surgery involved direct and indirect anastomosis using superficial temporal artery and middle cerebral artery (direct) or through directly placing the vascularized tissue on the cortex, such as with encephaloduroarteriosynangiosis (EDAS) or encephaloduroarteriomyosynangiosis (EDAMS). Prognosis is variable ranging from slow progression with rare ischemic events to rapid neurologic deterioration with infarction and hemorrhage.

References: Tarasów E, Kułakowska A, Łukasiewicz A, et al. Moyamoya disease: diagnostic imaging. *Pol J Radiol* 2011;76(1):73–79.

Yoon HK, Shin HJ, Chang YW. "Ivy sign" in childhood moyamoya disease: depiction on FLAIR and contrast-enhanced T1-weighted MR images. *Radiology* 2002;223(2):384–389.

8a **Answer B.** Oral contraceptive use. The images show bilateral subarachnoid and small focus of parenchymal hemorrhage in superior convexities. This is seen in the setting of thrombus within the superior sagittal sinus seen on the CTA. Oral contraceptive use predisposes to sinus thrombosis.

8b **Answer D.** Internal cerebral vein. All the other veins are a part of the superficial venous drainage system. Note that the other names for these structures are superior anastomotic vein (Trolard), inferior anastomotic (Labbé), and superficial middle cerebral vein (sylvian vein).

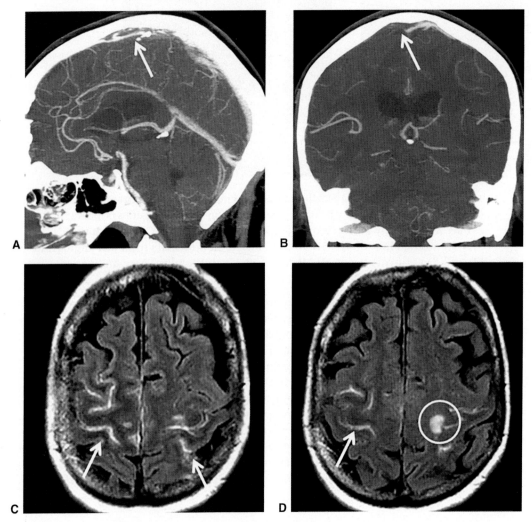

Imaging Findings: CT angiogram shows an irregular filling defect in the superior sagittal sinus (A and B), compatible with venous sinus thrombosis. Axial FLAIR images show sulcal nonsuppression of CSF with a small left posterior frontal focus of intraparenchymal hemorrhage. Both subarachnoid and intraparenchymal hemorrhagic foci can be seen with venous sinus thrombosis.

Discussion: Dural venous sinus thrombosis is a fairly uncommon disorder, typically seen in the presence of risk factors leading to hypercoagulable state, such as oral contraceptive use, underlying malignancy, protein C or S deficiency, or sinus/mastoid infections.

It is important to note that initial imaging may be a nonvascular study such as NECT or MRI without contrast, often showing findings such as parenchymal or scattered foci of subarachnoid hemorrhage with wide differential possibilities.

Venous infarctions can span multiple arterial vascular territories and present with parenchymal changes such as hemorrhage and cytotoxic and/or vasogenic edema. For this reason, presence of restricted diffusion may not be consistently seen with venous thrombosis. In addition to the parenchymal changes discussed above, NECT may show hyperdense dural venous sinus or cerebral veins. On noncontrast MRI, lack of T2 flow void through venous sinuses may also be seen. For definitive evaluation, venogram studies such as time-of-flight or contrast-enhanced MR venogram, CT venogram, or conventional angiography should be considered.

Reference: Leach JL, Fortuna RB, Jones BV, et al. Imaging of cerebral venous thrombosis: current techniques, spectrum of findings, and diagnostic pitfalls. *Radiographics* 2006;26(Suppl 1):S19–S41.

9   **Answer D.**   Benign perimesencephalic hemorrhage. There is subarachnoid hemorrhage in the basilar cisterns. In the absence of angiographic evidence of aneurysm, this is likely a benign nonaneurysmal perimesencephalic hemorrhage.

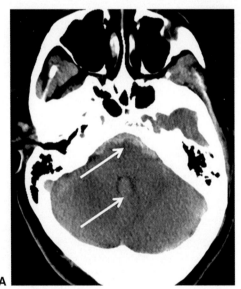 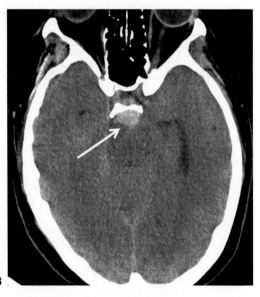

A   B

Imaging Findings: Axial noncontrast head CT shows high-density material in the prepontine and interpeduncular cistern and within the fourth ventricle compatible with subarachnoid hemorrhage with intraventricular extension.

Discussion: Benign nonaneurysmal perimesencephalic hemorrhage is a subset of subarachnoid hemorrhage seen with a negative angiogram and without other underlying etiologies such as trauma. The pathogenesis is unclear and a venous etiology is speculated. Some studies have shown an association with higher incidence of primitive venous drainage, thereby suggesting that these may be venous in nature. The diagnosis can be challenging given vasospasm and thrombus in the aneurysm sac may cause them to remain occult early on. This is particularly seen with basilar artery aneurysms; therefore, in some cases, a repeat angiogram may be needed to confirm nonaneurysmal etiology. This is particularly true for nonperimesencephalic distributions. Overall, these patients typically have significantly improved outcomes compared to the aneurysmal etiology with good functional recovery.

Reference: Boswell S, Thorell W, Gogela S, et al. Angiogram-negative subarachnoid hemorrhage: outcomes data and review of the literature. *J Stroke Cerebrovasc Dis* 2013;22(6):750–757.

10a **Answer A.** Cerebral vasospasm. There is subarachnoid hemorrhage from a ruptured vertebral artery aneurysm. One of the risks in patients with diffuse subarachnoid hemorrhage that complicates the management course is vasospasm leading to significant mortality and morbidity.

10b **Answer A.** Cerebral vasospasm. There is evidence of profound vasospasm seen in the LMCA and ACA vessels shown on CTA.

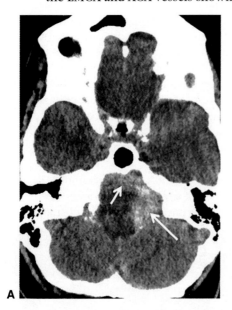
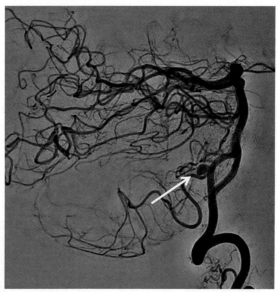

Figure 1

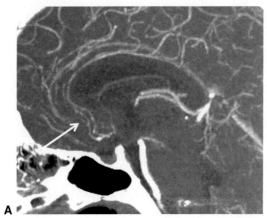
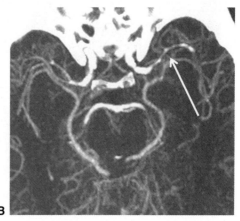

Figure 2

Imaging Findings: Figure 1. Subarachnoid hemorrhage in the basilar cisterns (A). Note a clot is noted in the left cerebellopontine angle, often indicating the site of aneurysm as noted in this case on image B, showing a left post-PICA V4 vertebral artery aneurysm.

Figure 2. There is prominent narrowing and irregularity in bilateral ACA (A) and left MCA (B), compatible with vasospasm.

Discussion: Cerebral vasospasm (cVSP) postaneurysmal subarachnoid hemorrhage (aSAH), leading to delayed cerebral ischemia (DCI), is a significant factor influencing mortality and morbidity. About one-third of the patients can die from cVSP or have significant disability. In the first 2 weeks following aSAH, patients can develop vasospasm, many times only seen as an angiographic finding; however, some of these patients can have profound neurologic deficits suggesting symptomatic cVSP.

CT Fisher or modified Fisher scale was developed to predict the risk of DCI or symptomatic cVSP. Modified Fisher scale published stroke 2001 (*completely filling ≥1 cistern or fissure):

Grade 0: No SAH or IVH
Grade 1: Minimal/thin SAH but no IVH in both lateral ventricles
Grade 2: Minimal/thin SAH with IVH in both lateral ventricles
Grade 3: Thick SAH* (cisternal clot) but no IVH in both lateral ventricles
Grade 4: Thick SAH* (cisternal clot) with IVH in both lateral ventricles

In patients with clinical features of DCI, transcranial Doppler ultrasound, CT/MR perfusion and angiography can be used for confirming diagnosis. There is evidence of hypoperfusion with corresponding significant narrowing, irregularity, and attenuation of vasculature as shown in the current case. Management is complex and multipronged, relying on volume and sodium management, calcium channel antagonist, NSAIDS, and occasionally endovascular intervention.

References: Boulouis G, Labeyrie MA, Raymond J, et al. Treatment of cerebral vasospasm following aneurysmal subarachnoid haemorrhage: a systematic review and meta-analysis. *Eur Radiol* 2016.

Claassen J, Bernardini GL, Kreiter K, et al. Effect of cisternal and ventricular blood on risk of delayed cerebral ischemia after subarachnoid hemorrhage: the Fisher scale revisited. *Stroke* 2001;32(9):2012–2020.

Janardhan V, Biondi A, Riina HA, et al. Vasospasm in aneurysmal subarachnoid hemorrhage: diagnosis, prevention, and management. *Neuroimaging Clin N Am* 2006;16(3):483–496.

11 **Answer B.** Deep venous sinus thrombosis. There is bithalamic signal abnormality seen in the setting of complete occlusion of the straight sinus and vein of Galen.

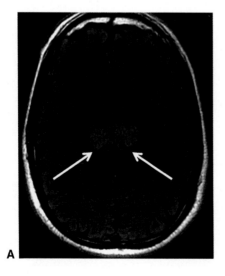
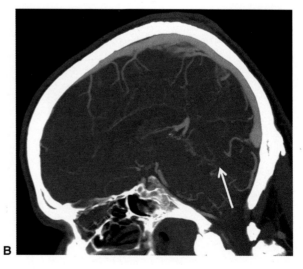

A   B

Imaging Findings: Axial FLAIR shows abnormal signal in both thalamus and complete thrombosis of the straight sinus and vein of Galen compatible with thalamic venous infarction.

Discussion: Bilateral thalamic lesions can have a wide differential diagnosis ranging from vascular, neoplastic, to infectious or metabolic etiologies (as below). Clinical features and other ancillary findings are important for understanding the etiology.

- Arterial infarction: Typically, because of a variant anatomy arising from occlusion within a solitary artery to Percheron from P1-PCA supplying the paramedian thalami and rostral midbrain bilaterally. Top of basilar syndrome may also result in bithalamic involvement but is associated with additional areas of involvement including superior cerebellum and bilateral PCA distribution.
- Venous infarction: As in this case, because of thrombosis within the straight sinus and vein of Galen. Other deep cerebral venous thrombosis involving the basal vein of Rosenthal, internal cerebral, and thalamostriate veins can also result in thalamic venous infarction.
- Creutzfeldt-Jakob disease (CJD): A rare neurodegenerative disease with rapidly progressive dementia. This condition can have bithalamic, basal ganglia, and cortical involvement.
- Wernicke encephalopathy: Vitamin B1 deficiency with involvement of medial thalami, mammillary bodies, periaqueductal gray, and dorsal medulla.
- Other metabolic abnormalities such as Fahr disease, Wilson disease, and Leigh disease. These usually also have involvement of basal ganglia. Clinical features and age group are other differentiating features.
- Neoplasms: Lymphoma and GBM can't involve bilateral thalami but appear more mass like.

Reference: Smith AB, Smirniotopoulos JG, Rushing EJ, et al. Bilateral thalamic lesions. *AJR Am J Roentgenol* 2009;192(2):W53–W62.

12a **Answer C.**   Cavernous sinus thrombosis. There is asymmetric nonopacification of the left cavernous sinus. Associated sinus inflammatory changes are also present.

12b **Answer B.**   Paranasal sinus infection. Sinonasal, orbital, and facial infections may be an underlying etiology of septic cavernous sinus thrombosis as shown in this case.

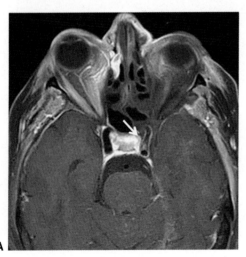 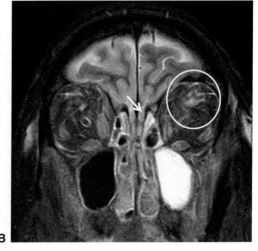

Imaging Findings: Axial contrast-enhanced postcontrast T1 fat saturation shows asymmetric nonopacification of the left cavernous sinus (A). There is evidence of sinonasal inflammatory changes suggesting a potential sinonasal etiology of the cavernous sinus thrombosis (B). Note presence of edema in the left superior orbital region, likely secondary to the cavernous sinus thrombosis.

Discussion: Cavernous sinus thrombosis as seen in this case may arise from sinus, nasal, or facial infections, commonly referred to as septic cavernous sinus thrombosis or cavernous sinus septic thrombophlebitis. Clinically, the patients can have severe headache, chemosis, proptosis, orbital or facial pain, visual symptoms, and facial numbness or paresthesias. On imaging, there is a filling defect or nonopacification within the cavernous sinus. This may be symmetric or asymmetric depending upon the extent of involvement. A dilated superior ophthalmic vein and reactive enhancement of adjacent dural or tentorial leaflets may also be present. Often, exophthalmos can also be seen on imaging. Evaluation of a source for infection in the adjacent sinonasal cavity, orbits, and face is useful. The most common reported organism is *Staphylococcus aureus*. Fungal etiology is more common in immunocompromised patients. Management depends on the etiology and relies upon antibiotics, anticoagulation, and surgical drainage of the source if needed.

References: Razek AA, Castillo M. Imaging lesions of the cavernous sinus. *AJNR Am J Neuroradiol* 2009;30(3):444–452.

Weerasinghe D, Lueck CJ. Septic cavernous sinus thrombosis: case report and review of the literature. *Neuroophthalmology* 2016;40(6):263–276.

13 **Answer A.** Cavernoma.

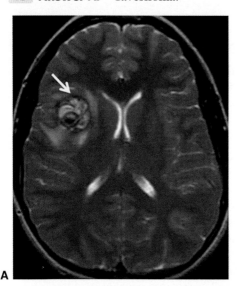
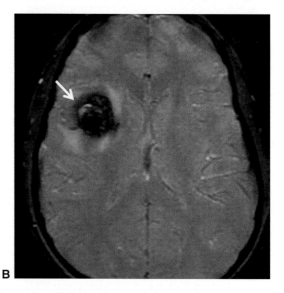

Imaging Findings: There is a right frontal well-defined rounded centrally T2 hyperintense lesion with a peripheral rim of T2 hypointensity (A) and corresponding loss of signal on gradient recall echo (B). The lesion morphology on T2w image is referred to as "popcorn" lesion with rounded foci of T2 hyperintensity and associated hemosiderin ring. There is mild surrounding vasogenic edema. Imaging features are characteristic for a cavernoma.

Discussion: Intracerebral cavernous malformations or cavernomas are distinct vascular malformations that are typically intraparenchymal, well-circumscribed, lesions containing endothelial-lined sinusoidal vascular channels. Majority of which are thrombosed. These are typically supratentorial subpial, juxtaventricular. Approximately 25% of lesions may be infratentorial, commonly cerebellar or pontine in location. These lesions may be asymptomatic and incidentally discovered or present with seizure, hemorrhage, headaches, and focal neurologic deficit. Seizures have been associated with supratentorial lesions and focal neurologic deficits with the infratentorial lesions. Annual rate of hemorrhage is variable ranging from <1% to 3%. Management includes conservative, neurosurgical excision or stereotactic radiosurgery.

References: Atlas SW. *Magnetic resonance imaging of the brain and spine*, 4th ed. Head Trauma. Vol 1. Ch 14:727–734.

Gross BA. The natural history of intracranial cavernous malformations. *Neurosurg Focus* 2011;30(6):E24.

14a Answer B. Aberrant internal carotid artery.

14b Answer A. Absence of cervical ICA and enlargement of inferior tympanic canaliculus.

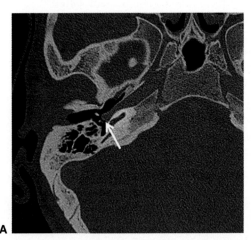 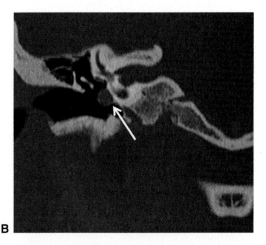

A   B

Imaging Findings: Axial contrast-enhanced CT at skull base demonstrates dehiscence of the right-sided carotid canal. The right ICA at the skull base courses laterally protruding into the middle ear cavity. The jugular bulb is intact and the tubular lesion communicates with the petrous ICA. These findings are consistent with an aberrant right internal carotid artery.

Discussion: Aberrant internal carotid artery is hypothesized to result from one of the collateral pathways typically recruited from the branches of external carotid artery in the setting of embryologic agenesis of cervical segment of the ICA. The inferior tympanic artery arising from the ascending pharyngeal artery is consequently hypertrophied and serves as a collateral pathway to supply the horizontal petrous ICA. It courses through an enlarged inferior tympanic canaliculus, passes laterally to the cochlear promontory, and anastomoses with the caroticotympanic artery (a branch of the horizontal petrous ICA) to supply the petrous ICA segment. Awareness of this entity is critical to prevent inadvertent biopsy. Typically, in the absence of injury or hemorrhage, no further intervention is indicated, even in the presence of tinnitus or conductive hearing loss. In scenarios of vascular injury, further endovascular management to control bleeding is indicated.

References: Nicolay S, et al. Aberrant internal carotid artery presenting as a retrotympanic vascular mass. *Acta Radiol Short Rep* 2014;3(10).

Sauvaget E, et al. Aberrant internal carotid artery in the temporal bone: imaging findings and management. *Arch Otolaryngol Head Neck Surg* 2006;132(1):86–91.

15a **Answer C.**   MR imaging with susceptibility-weighted sequence. This is a case of cerebral amyloid angiopathy (CAA). CT is the most frequently performed initial investigation. It helps in assessment of the hematoma size and associated mass effect. However, CT has limited utility in assessment of old hemorrhages, microhemorrhages, which are crucial in making this diagnosis.

15b **Answer D.**   Commonly involves small- and medium-sized vessels in peripheral aspect of the brain. CAA is commonly a sporadic condition and rarely an inherited disorder.

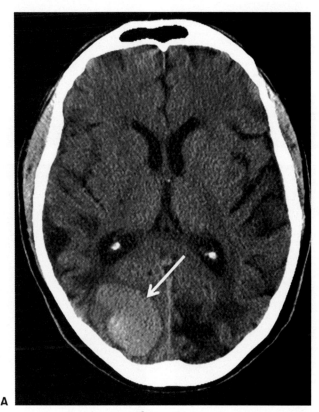

A

Figure 1

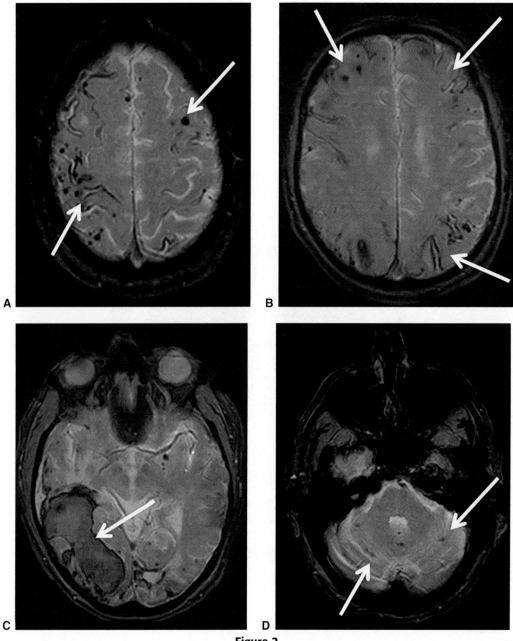

Figure 2

Imaging Findings: Figure 1. CT scan shows lobar hematoma in right occipital lobe.

Figure 2. Multiple susceptibility-weighted images are presented, which show additional scattered older hemorrhages including multiple microhemorrhages and meningeal siderosis related to old hemorrhage. Please note predominantly peripheral lobar distribution of hemorrhages with relative sparing of brainstem.

Discussion: Cerebral amyloid angiopathy (CAA) is a cerebrovascular disorder characterized by deposition of beta amyloid protein in media and adventitial layers of small- and medium-sized vessels in cortex, subcortical area, and leptomeninges. Pathologically, these vessels demonstrate fibrinoid necrosis, focal vessel wall fragmentation, and microaneurysms, which predispose patients for hemorrhage and small-vessel ischemia.

CAA is the most common of the three cerebral amyloid deposition diseases. The other 2 less common entities are beta amyloid–related angiitis (ABRA) and an amyloidoma.

CAA can be sporadic or hereditary, the former being much more common. Rarer hereditary form demonstrates autosomal dominant transmission and present in younger age group (couple of decades earlier than sporadic CAA, which is typically seen in patients past 55 years of age).

CAA is found on biopsy in about 33% of autopsy patients in 60 to 70 years age range. Many are asymptomatic. When symptomatic, typical presentation includes acute intracranial hemorrhage, TIA symptoms, or dementia.

Imaging plays a critical role in diagnosis of CAA. The commonly seen features are intracranial hemorrhages, leukoencephalopathy, and atrophy.

Macrohemorrhages: CAD-related hemorrhage shows distinct lobar cortical-subcortical location that generally spares deep white matter, basal ganglia, and brainstem. There can be associated subarachnoid and subdural hemorrhage, generally from contiguous extension of lobar hemorrhage or primary extra-axial hemorrhage secondary to diseased leptomeningeal vessels.

Microhemorrhages: Presence of multiple prior microhemorrhages in the setting of acute lobar hematoma in normotensive patient over 55 years is highly suggestive of CAA.

Leukoencephalopathy: Caused by luminal narrowing of the vessels secondary to fibrinoid necrosis. Corpus callosum and capsular white matter are generally spared. Leukoencephalopathy with sparing of subcortical fibers is the common form, which typically involves centrum semiovale. In ABRA, there can be involvement of subcortical white matter and some degree of associated mass effect.

Atrophy: Nonspecific finding, most likely the result of the microangiopathic changes and leukoencephalopathy.

Enhancement: Contrast enhancement is typically absent in CAA, unlike ABRA and amyloidoma wherein striking enhancement can be seen.

MRI is the modality of choice to evaluate for CAA. Gradient- and susceptibility-weighted images are exquisitely sensitive for peripherally located microhemorrhages. T2- and FLAIR-weighted images demonstrate leukoencephalopathy.

References: Chao CP, Kotsenas AL, Broderick DF. Cerebral amyloid angiopathy: CT and MR imaging findings. *Radiographics* 2006;26(5):1517–1531. doi:10.1148/rg.265055090

Osborn AG. *Osborn's brain: imaging, pathology, and anatomy*, 1st ed. Salt Lake City, UT: Amirsys Pub, 2013.

CNS Imaging Manifestations of Toxic, Metabolic, and Systemic Pathologies

SATHISH KUMAR DUNDAMADAPPA • ALY H. ABAYAZEED • PRACHI DUBEY

QUESTIONS

1 A 60-year-old female with acute-onset movement disorder presents for evaluation; CT and MR are performed (key images are shown below). Past medical history is significant for hypertension and type 2 DM; both are not well controlled on medication.

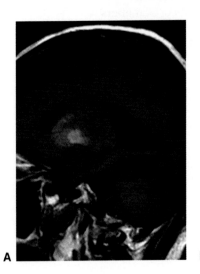
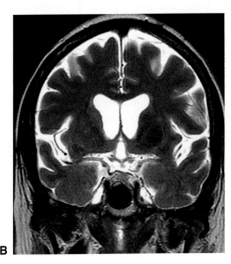
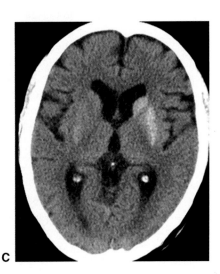

A   B   C

1a   Based on the available clinical information and the above images, what is the most likely systemic abnormality expected in this patient?

A. Elevated ammonia levels
B. Hypertensive crisis
C. Nonketotic hyperglycemia
D. Respiratory acidosis

1b   What is the usual expected clinical course after correction of the systemic abnormality?

A. Permanent residual movement dysfunction
B. Parkinsonian rigidity
C. Complete resolution of symptoms
D. Progressive neurologic deficit

2 A 45-year-old chronic alcoholic with malnutrition presents with acute alteration of mental status. Key images from MRI are shown below.

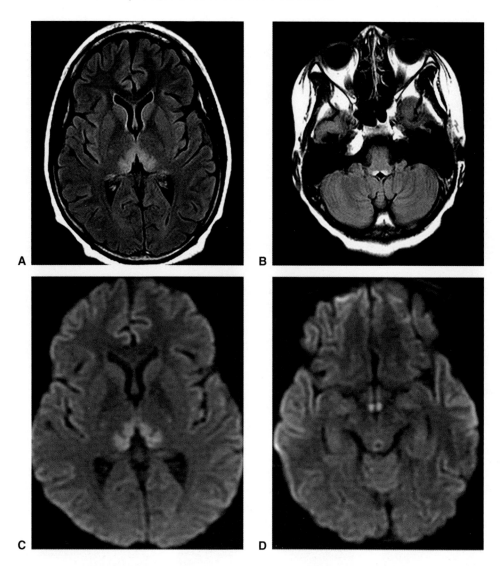

2a What is the most likely biochemical abnormality explaining these changes in the current clinical setting?

    A. Thiamine deficiency
    B. Vitamin B_{12} deficiency
    C. Hyperammonemia
    D. Hyponatremia

2b If left untreated in the chronic phase, the patient may develop which of the following conditions?

    A. Transient global amnesia
    B. Delirium tremens
    C. Korsakoff psychosis
    D. Chronic traumatic encephalopathy

3 A 25-year-old man was rescued from a residential fire with impaired consciousness and seizures. An MRI was performed; key images are shown below.

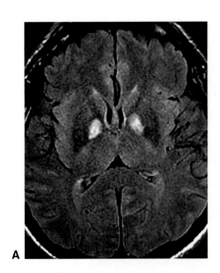
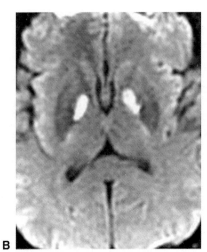
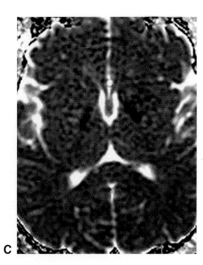

A   B   C

3a What is the characteristic structure involved with this condition?

A. Internal capsule
B. Caudate nucleus
C. Putamen
D. Globus pallidus (GP)

3b What is the most likely diagnosis?

A. Carbon monoxide poisoning
B. Nitrous oxide poisoning
C. Methanol poisoning
D. Opioid overdose

4 A middle-aged man "found down" on the side walk was brought to the ER. Initial EKG shows sinus tachycardia and nonspecific T-wave changes. A head CT was performed; key images are shown below.

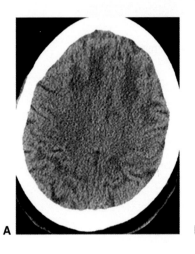
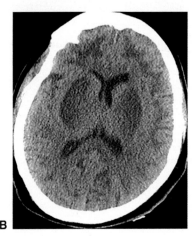
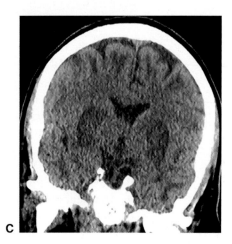

A   B   C

4a Which of the following is the most likely diagnosis?

A. Wilson Disease
B. CO monoxide poisoning
C. Postictal change
D. Methanol toxicity

4b Further investigation reveals severe metabolic acidosis. What structure is at particularly high risk for involvement with this condition?

    A. Cerebellum

    B. Thalami

    C. Hippocampus

    D. Optic nerve

5 A 60-year-old male patient presents with an abnormal MRI; key images are shown below.

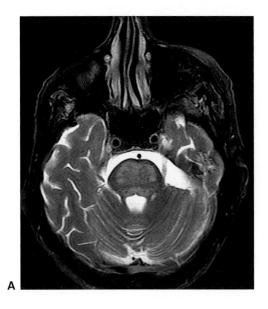 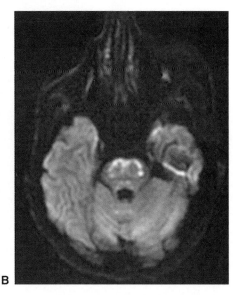

5a What is the most likely history in this patient?

    A. Recent upper respiratory tract viral infection

    B. Rapidly progressive cognitive decline

    C. Recent liver transplant

    D. Recently diagnosed small cell lung cancer

5b Following images are from a different patient with the same history. What is the most likely diagnosis?

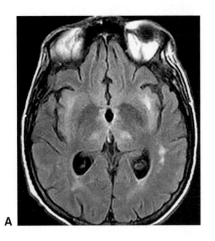 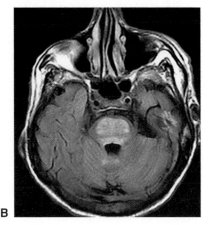 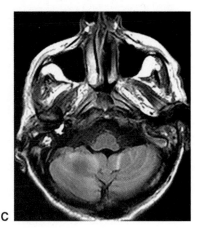

    A. Creutzfeldt-Jakob disease

    B. Osmotic demyelination

    C. Paraneoplastic limbic encephalitis

    D. Acute disseminated encephalomyelitis

6   A 67-year-old male with chronic hypertension presents with headache, visual disturbance, and seizures. Key images from an initial noncontrast head CT performed in the ER are shown below.

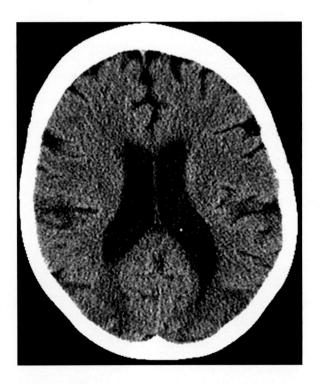

6a   What is the next best step?

    A. A contrast-enhanced CT scan
    B. CT angiogram of the head
    C. A contrast-enhanced MRI
    D. Magnetic resonance spectroscopy

6b   A contrast enhanced MRI was performed. What is the most likely diagnosis?

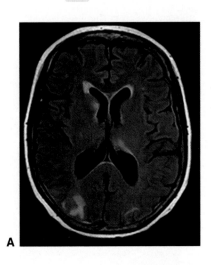
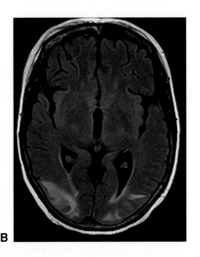
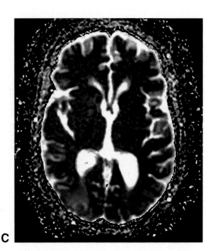

A   B   C

    A. Acute infarction in the posterior circulation
    B. Status epilepticus
    C. Posterior reversible encephalopathy syndrome (PRES)
    D. Progressive multifocal leukoencephalopathy

7 A 46-year-old female with HCV cirrhosis presents with acute-onset mental status. Key images from MRI are shown below.

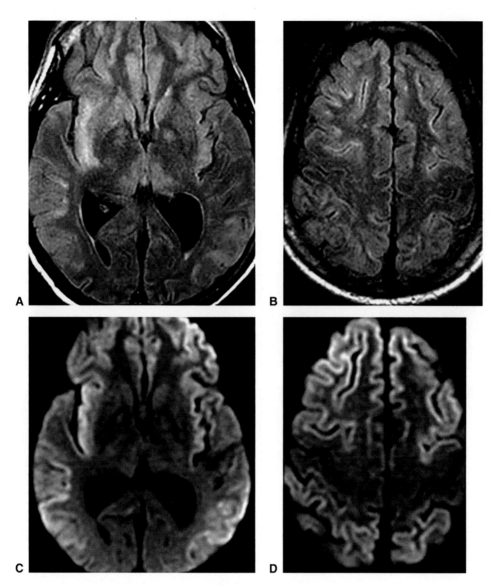

7a In view of the clinical setting, what is the most likely diagnosis?

A. Osmotic demyelination
B. Acute hyperammonemic encephalopathy
C. Limbic encephalitis
D. Watershed infarcts

7b Which of the following can be an inciting event for the above condition?

A. GI bleeding
B. Seizure
C. Exposure to CO
D. Recent cardiac arrest

8

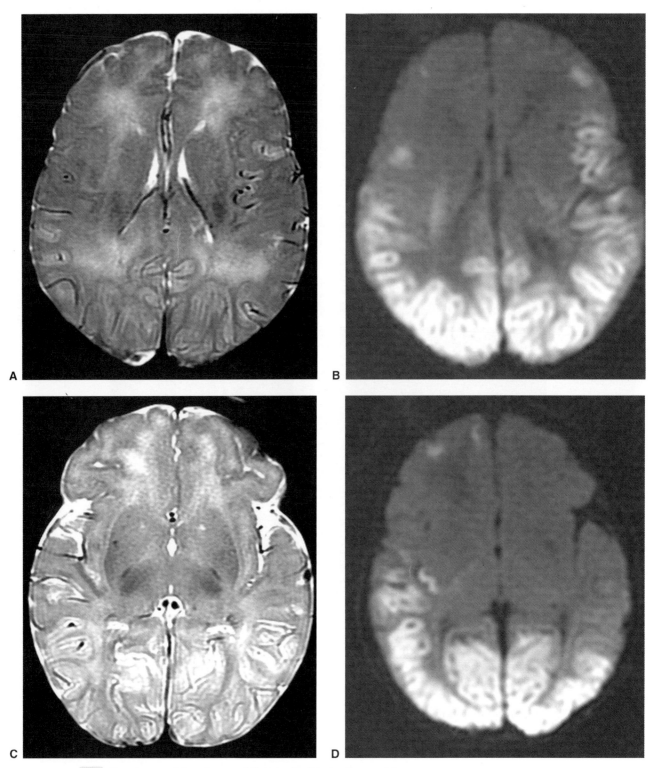

A

B

C

D

8a   Newborn with seizures. What is the likely diagnosis?

A. Mitochondrial disorder
B. Encephalitis
C. Hypoxic–ischemic injury
D. Hypoglycemic injury

8b What is true regarding this condition?

    A. Increased incidence in preterm infants, large for age infants, and infants born to diabetic mothers

    B. Shows maternal inheritance with mutations in extranuclear DNA

    C. Commonly caused by HSV-2

    D. Commonly caused by excessive maternal alcohol intake.

9 A 70-year-old male who had a cardiac arrest, s/p CPR, now presents with obtunded mental status. Key images from MRI are shown below. What is the most likely diagnosis?

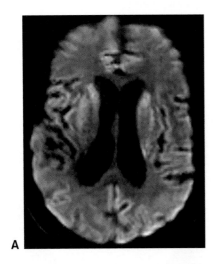 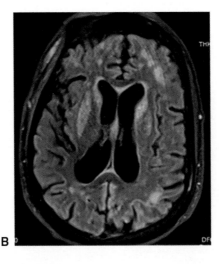 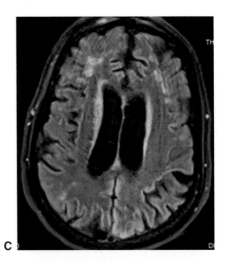

A   B   C

    A. Cardioembolic stroke

    B. Hypoxic–ischemic encephalopathy

    C. Postictal change

    D. Posterior reversible encephalopathy syndrome (PRES)

ANSWERS AND EXPLANATIONS

1a **Answer C.** Nonketotic hyperglycemia. This appearance is not typical for a hypertensive hemorrhage, attenuation is lower for hemorrhage, and morphology is not compatible with a hematoma. There are no corroborating clinical findings to support a hyperammonemic state or substrates for respiratory acidosis.

1b **Answer C.** Complete resolution of symptoms. Imaging findings and movement abnormalities resolve with treatment and correction of hyperglycemia. Rarely, imaging findings can persist for a longer time.

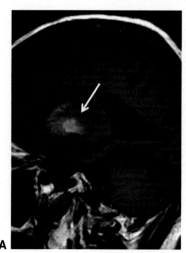
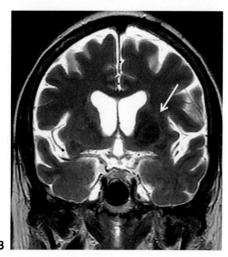
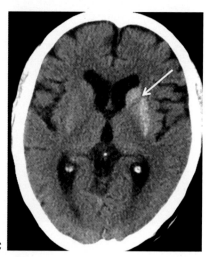

A   B   C

Imaging Findings: There is hyperintensity on T1w image (A), hypointensity on T2w image (B), and high attenuation on CT within the caudate and putamen (C), significantly more striking on the left. Findings are most likely to represent hyperglycemia-related changes in the current clinical setting.

Discussion: Nonketotic hyperglycemia with acute-onset hemiballismus–hemichorea.

Nonketotic hyperglycemia with acute-onset hemiballismus–hemichorea is usually caused by lesions in contralateral basal ganglia. Those lesions, which are caused by nonketotic hyperglycemia, are characterized by T1 hyperintensity, and are commonly seen in elderly patients with diabetes, more so in females and Asian population. The exact pathogenesis is uncertain. The proposed etiologies include altered metabolism, petechial hemorrhages, and accumulation of gemistocytic astrocytes.

Putamen is the most commonly involved region, followed by caudate nucleus. Globus pallidus and midbrain involvement can also be seen. The lesions are usually unilateral. T1 hyperintensity in the involved regions without mass effect or abnormal enhancement is the characteristic finding. T2-weighted images can be hypointense or isointense. Mild degree of blooming can be seen on susceptibility images. Mild reduction in ADC can also be seen. CT demonstrates hyperdensity. Imaging findings and movement abnormalities usually resolve with treatment and correction of hyperglycemia.

Differential diagnosis: Other cause of T1 hyperintensity in basal ganglia: the most common in being hepatic encephalopathy. Clinical history can help in differentiation.

References: Priola AM, Gned D, Veltri A, et al. Case 204: nonketotic hyperglycemia-induced hemiballism-hemichorea. *Radiology* 2014;271(1):304–308. doi: 10.1148/radiol.14120840

Rumboldt Z, Castillo M, Huang B, et al., eds. *Brain imaging with MRI and CT: an image pattern approach*. Cambridge, UK: Cambridge University Press, 2012.

2a **Answer A.** Thiamine deficiency. In the clinical setting of chronic alcoholism and malnutrition, the signal changes shown in the medial thalami, dorsal medulla, and mammillary body are typical for Wernicke encephalopathy because of thiamine deficiency. Another classic location is periaqueductal gray matter not shown in this case.

2b **Answer C.** Korsakoff psychosis. In the chronic phase, patients may develop confabulation, amnestic episodes with memory loss, and difficulty learning new information.

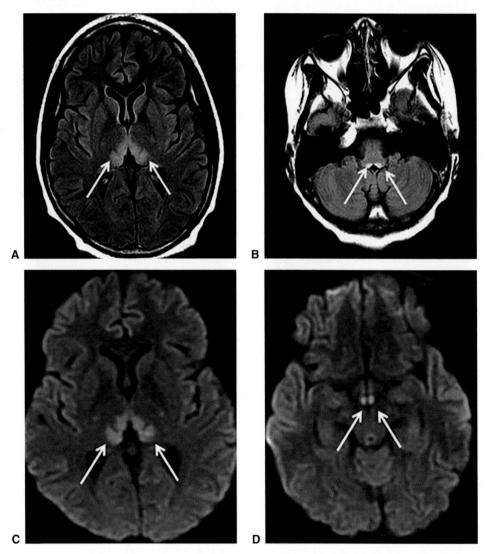

Imaging Findings: There is FLAIR hyperintense signal present in the medial thalami and dorsal medulla bilaterally (A and B). Restricted diffusion is seen in bilateral medial thalami and mammillary bodies (C and D). These findings in the current clinical setting are suggestive of Wernicke encephalopathy, because of thiamine deficiency. Note that low signal on ADC map must be assessed to confirm restricted diffusion (images not shown here).

Discussion: Wernicke encephalopathy.

Wernicke encephalopathy (WE) is an acute neurologic disorder caused by thiamine deficiency. There is about 17% mortality, and the prognosis depends on the timing of thiamine supplementation. The classic clinical triad of "ocular dysfunction, altered consciousness, and ataxia" is only seen in a minority of patients, and neuroimaging plays a critical role in diagnosis.

Deficiency of thiamine is commonly seen in alcoholics (related to dietary deficiency, and not to alcohol per se) and in other disorders associated with malnutrition or decreased absorption (malignancy, GI surgeries, etc.).

Imaging reflects intracellular as well as extracellular edema (cytotoxic and vasogenic edema) and break in blood–brain barrier. Typically, the abnormality is bilaterally symmetrical and the sites involved are periaqueductal gray matter, medial thalami, periventricular region of the third ventricle, tectal plate, and mammillary bodies. Basal ganglia involvement is more common in children.

CT has limited sensitivity for WE and shows hypodensity in involved areas. Long TR MR images (T2/FLAIR) are most sensitive and show hyperintensity in the involved areas. Diffusion restriction (reversible cytotoxic edema) can be seen in acute stages. Some of these regions (typically the mammillary bodies) can show contrast enhancement.

Differential diagnoses:

- Artery of percheron infarction: Different clinical presentation. Medial thalamic and mesencephalic involvement seen. The other sites that can be involved with WE are spared.
- Deep vein thrombosis: Swelling is more pronounced. Hemorrhage is more common. Deep vein thrombosis can be demonstrated on venogram and with lesser sensitivity in routine imaging.
- Osmotic demyelination syndrome: More prominent pontine involvement. Basal ganglia and external capsule are often affected. Can coexist with WE.
- Acute disseminated encephalomyelitis (ADEM): Multifocal involvement in white and gray matter.
- Variant Creutzfeldt-Jakob disease: Abnormality in thalamic pulvinar, basal ganglia, and cortex. Persistent and more striking diffusion restriction.
- Thalamic involvement in hypoxic–ischemic encephalopathy: Clinical picture other sites of involvement that are typical for diffuse ischemic injury including the cortical ribbon and hippocampi.
- Metronidazole toxicity: Sites of involvement in the posterior fossa are similar to WE, particularly cerebellar dentate involvement.

References: Ha ND, Weon YC, Jang JC, et al. Spectrum of MR imaging findings in Wernicke encephalopathy: are atypical areas of involvement only present in nonalcoholic patients? *AJNR Am J Neuroradiol* 2012;33(7):1398–1402. doi: 10.3174/ajnr.A2979

Rumboldt Z, Castillo M, Huang B, et al., eds. *Brain imaging with MRI and CT: an image pattern approach.* Cambridge, UK: Cambridge University Press, 2012.

Zuccoli G, Pipitone N. Neuroimaging findings in acute Wernicke's encephalopathy: review of the literature. *AJR Am J Roentgenol* 2009;192(2):501–508. doi: 10.2214/AJR.07.3959

Zuccoli G, Santa Cruz D, Bertolini M, et al. MR imaging findings in 56 patients with Wernicke encephalopathy: nonalcoholics may differ from alcoholics. *AJNR Am J Neuroradiol* 2009;30(1):171–176. doi: 10.3174/ajnr.A1280

3a **Answer D.**   Globus pallidus (GP). This the most characteristic structure involved with CO poisoning. The clinical history of exposure to fumes in the fire makes this the most likely consideration.

3b **Answer A.**   Carbon monoxide poisoning. As explained above, it is the most likely reason for this appearance in the current clinical setting. Nitrous oxide poisoning typically results in neurotoxicity because of vitamin B_{12} inhibition; the pattern of abnormalities is very similar to vitamin B_{12} deficiency, such as the presence of dorsal column involvement in the spinal cord. Methanol tends to favor putaminal involvement, and opioid overdose can lead to a pattern similar to hypoxic–ischemic encephalopathy.

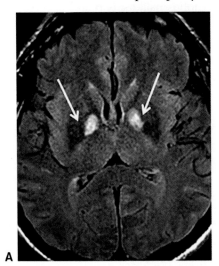 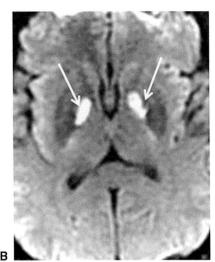 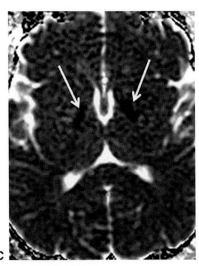

A   B   C

Imaging Findings: There is FLAIR hyperintensity in the region of globus pallidus (A) and corresponding restricted diffusion seen on DWI (B) and ADC map (C).

Discussion: Carbon Monoxide Poisoning.

Carbon monoxide (CO) is the most common lethal poison worldwide, either suicidal or accidental inhalation. Mechanism of injury is both hypoxic and cellular toxicity.

Its affinity to hemoglobin is about 250 times that of oxygen. Formation of carboxyhemoglobin reduces oxygen-carrying capacity of the blood, causing tissue hypoxia. Cardiotoxicity can result in ischemia, contributing to hypoxic–ischemic damage.

The globus pallidus is the most common and characteristic site of involvement.

Acute and intense poisoning can also result in involvement of other basal ganglia structures, thalami, cortex, hippocampi, brainstem, and cerebellum. In this situation, the pattern can be similar to diffuse ischemic injury from other causes.

In subacute stage, typically 2 to 3 weeks following the insult, up to a third of patients develop leukoencephalopathy related to myelin break down. Bilateral nearly symmetrical lesions are present commonly involving centrum semiovale and periventricular white matter. If the injury is severe, subcortical and posterior fossa white matter can also be involved.

In acute stages, the involved regions are hypodense on CT, hypointense on T1, and hyperintense on T2 and show restricted diffusion. Hemorrhagic products, if present, can result on heterogeneous appearance and some T1 shortening. Acute/ subacute stage can show inhomogeneous or peripheral mild contrast enhancement. White matter injury shows up as diffuse T2 hyperintensity and exhibits mild diffusion restriction in early stages. In late stages, atrophy ensues if there is severe enough injury, as a sequel of neuronal necrosis and apoptosis.

Differential considerations:

- Cyanide poisoning: Can look identical. Hemorrhagic necrosis of putamen is more commonly seen with cyanide and methanol poisoning.
- Diffuse hypoxic–ischemic injury: Preferential globus pallidal involvement is unlikely.
- Methanol intoxication: Characteristic putaminal necrosis. Globus pallidus is typically spared. White matter involvement may be seen with methanol.
- Mitochondrial disorders, Leigh disease: Younger age group. Putaminal and brain-stem involvement is more common.

References: Kinoshita T, Sugihara S, Matsusue E, et al. Pallidoreticular damage in acute carbon monoxide poisoning: diffusion-weighted MR imaging findings. *AJNR Am J Neuroradiol* 2005;26(7):1845–1848.

Lo CP, Chen SY, Lee KW, et al. Brain injury after acute carbon monoxide poisoning: early and late complications. *AJR Am J Roentgenol* 2007;189(4):W205–W211. doi: 10.2214/AJR.07.2425

Rumboldt Z, Castillo M, Huang B, et al, eds. *Brain imaging with MRI and CT: an image pattern approach*, 1st ed. Cambridge, UK: Cambridge University Press, 2012.

4a **Answer D.** Methanol toxicity. Of the available options, the prominent putaminal and white matter involvement is most commonly seen with methanol toxicity.

4b **Answer D.** Optic nerve.

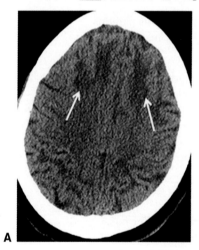 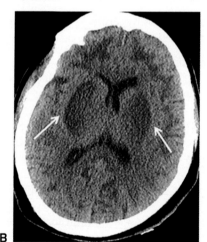 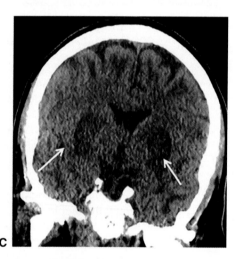

A   B   C

Imaging Findings: There is bilateral putaminal hypodensity and hypoattenuation in frontal subcortical and deep white matter on CT.

Discussion: Methanol is found in antifreeze solutions, varnishes, and paint fuel and also in bootlegged alcohol. Poisoning can result from intentional or accidental ingestion. Its metabolites formic acid/formate ion are responsible for toxicity by mitochondrial enzyme inhibition and resultant tissue hypoxia and also by causing metabolic acidosis.

Bilateral putaminal necrosis is the typical imaging presentation. Nonhemorrhagic lesions show CT hypodensity, T2 hyperintensity, T1 hypointensity, and diffusion restriction. Associated hemorrhage is quite common. Optic nerve involvement is common and may show up on dedicated imaging as T2 hyperintensity. The less common sites of involvement are globus pallidus, brainstem, subcortical white matter, and rarely peripheral lesions without central involvement. Peripheral mild contrast enhancement can be seen in acute/subacute stages.

The exact reason for putaminal predilection is not known. The proposed theories include high metabolic rate, venous drainage pattern, and high regional accumulation of methanol.

Differential Diagnosis:

- Diffuse ischemic injury: Generally bilateral, involvement of basal ganglia and cortical ribbon, T2 hyperintensity, and T1 hypointensity with diffusion restriction. History of a contributory event such as cardiac arrest, drug overdose, or drowning can be helpful.
- Cyanide poisoning: Also has characteristic putaminal involvement; however, white matter changes are more typical with methanol poisoning.
- Mitochondrial disorders: Pediatric population is more commonly affected. Movement disorder is not a common presenting symptom.
- Wilson disease: Putaminal T2 hyperintensity is also common in Wilson disease. Other common areas of involvement include caudate, globus pallidus, and ventrolateral thalamus. Rarely cortical/subcortical region, brainstem, and cerebellar vermis may also be involved.

References: Gupta N, Sonambekar AA, Daksh SK, et al. A rare presentation of methanol toxicity. *Ann Indian Acad Neurol* 2013;16(2):249–251. doi: 10.4103/0972-2327.112484

Zakharov S, Kotikova K, Vaneckova M, et al. Acute methanol poisoning: prevalence and predisposing factors of haemorrhagic and non-haemorrhagic brain lesions. *Basic Clin Pharmacol Toxicol* 2016;119(2):226–238. doi: 10.1111/bcpt.12559

5a   **Answer C.**   Recent liver transplant. The images show central pontine signal changes, typically seen with osmotic demyelination, which may occur in posttransplant setting. Recent upper respiratory tract viral infection history is typically seen with acute disseminated encephalomyelitis (ADEM). The images are not typical for Creutzfeldt-Jakob disease or paraneoplastic limbic encephalitis to suggest options B and D, respectively.

5b   **Answer B.**   Osmotic demyelination. It is to be emphasized that although central pontine involvement is typical, extrapontine and mixed central and extrapontine involvement may also be seen with osmotic demyelination, as shown in this companion case.

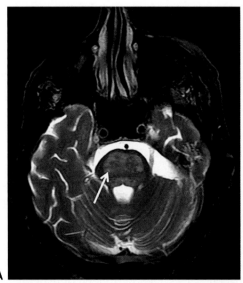 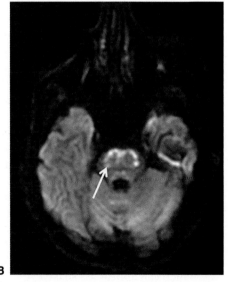

Figure 1

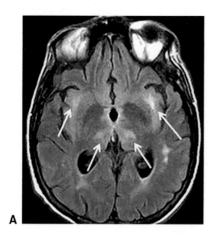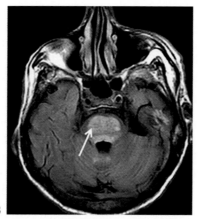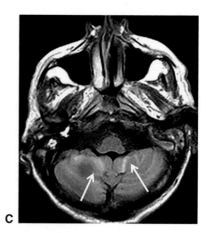

Figure 2

Imaging Findings: Figure 1. Axial T2-weighted imaging demonstrates increased signal in the pons with sparing of the periphery and corticospinal tracts (A) and associated restricted diffusion (B), consistent with central pontine myelinolysis (osmotic demyelination).

Figure 2. FLAIR hyperintensity seen in bilateral thalami, bilateral insular, and cerebellar regions, compatible with a combination of pontine and extrapontine myelinolysis.

Discussion: Osmotic demyelination.

Osmotic demyelination is a rare disorder commonly in middle-aged patients characterized by symmetrical and noninflammatory demyelination involving pons and extrapontine sites (pontine and extrapontine myelinolysis). It is thought to be caused by aggressive correction of hyper- or hyposmolar states. The classic clinical scenario is rapid correction of hyponatremia (by more than 12 mmol/L/day) in an alcoholic. Though rapid correction of hyponatremia is the classic scenario, the disease can be seen in other osmolar abnormalities and in chronic diseases. Isonatremia doesn't rule out the disease. Associated conditions include malnutrition, prolonged diuretic use, liver failure, organ transplant, and extensive burns.

Pons is the classical site of involvement.

Pontine tegmentum and corticospinal tracts are generally spared. Extrapontine involvement is fairly common, with an incidence close to that of pontine involvement, but is generally seen with pontine involvement. The sites commonly involved are cerebellum, basal ganglia, thalami, external capsule, lateral geniculate bodies, hippocampi, and cerebral gray–white junction. The periventricular and subpial sites are typically spared. Isolated extrapontine disease is seen in a minority, about 20%.

Histologic studies have shown that oligodendroglial cells are most susceptible to CPM-related osmotic stresses.

Conventional imaging findings (MR and CT) typically lag clinical manifestations, limiting the utility of imaging in early diagnosis of CPM. CT is insensitive and can show symmetrical hypodensities in the involved regions. MRI is the investigation of choice. DWI can show restriction as soon as 24 hours following clinical symptoms, the diffusion restriction resolving over 1 to 2 weeks. T2 signal abnormality develops over several days following clinical symptoms. MR imaging findings include symmetric signal intensity abnormality in the central pons on T2-weighted and FLAIR imaging. This may progress to classic hyperintense "trident-shaped" central pontine abnormality, with sparing of the ventrolateral pons and corticospinal tracts, which can appear as "snake eye." In subacute stages, mild peripheral or ill-defined enhancement can be seen in a small percentage of patients.

The clinical presentation is variable and depends on the site of involvement. "Biphasic presentation" (initial encephalopathy followed by improvement with correction of osmolyte disturbance and then sudden deterioration) is often seen. The pontine involvement is characterized by tetraplegia, bulbar and pseudobulbar palsies, altered mental status, and coma. Movement disorders can be seen with basal ganglia involvement. Historically, the disease was thought have a dismal prognosis. But recent literature points to variable prognosis, with up to 50% patient survival, many without long-term adverse effects. Extent of imaging abnormality does not predict clinical outcome. Patients who survive show residual signal abnormality or cavitation in the pons.

Differential diagnoses:

- Pontine infarction: Generally reaches anterior pontine margin and rarely symmetrical.
- Demyelination: Rarely symmetrical and typical morphology and distribution can be seen in supratentorial white matter lesions.
- Neoplasm: Generally pontine glioma is a disease of the young. Associated pontine enlargement is typical.

References: Abbott R, Silber E, Felber J, et al. Osmotic demyelination syndrome. *BMJ* 2005;331(7520):829–830.

Alleman AM. Osmotic demyelination syndrome: central pontine myelinolysis and extrapontine myelinolysis. *Semin Ultrasound CT MR* 2014;35(2):153–159. doi: 10.1053/j.sult.2013.09.009

Rumboldt Z, Castillo M, Huang B, et al., eds. *Brain imaging with MRI and CT: an image pattern approach*. Cambridge, UK: Cambridge University Press, 2012.

Ruzek KA, Campeau NG, Miller GM. Early diagnosis of central pontine myelinolysis with diffusion-weighted imaging. *AJNR Am J Neuroradiol* 2004;25(2):210–213.

Singh TD, Fugate JE, Rabinstein AA. Central pontine and extrapontine myelinolysis: a systematic review. *Eur J Neurol* 2014;21(12):1443–1450. doi: 10.1111/ene.12571

6a **Answer C.** A contrast-enhanced MRI.

6b **Answer C.** Posterior reversible encephalopathy syndrome (PRES).

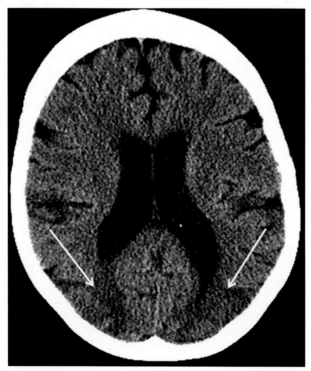

Figure 1

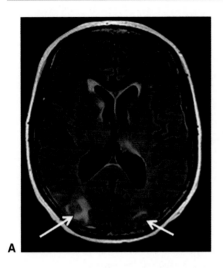
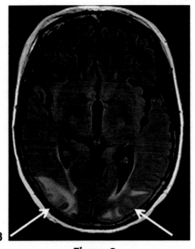
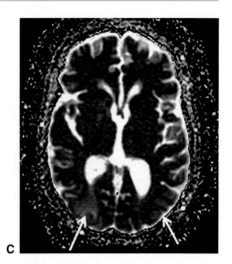

A   B   C

Figure 2

Imaging Findings: Figure 1. Noncontrast CT showing bilateral parieto-occipital symmetric subcortical and white matter hypoattenuation.

Figure 2. Bilateral parieto-occipital with involvement of the subcortical U-fibers.

Discussion: Posterior reversible encephalopathy syndrome (PRES).

Patients typically present with altered mental status, headache, focal neurologic deficits, visual disturbances, and seizures. PRES is classically associated with clinical conditions such as preeclampsia/eclampsia, cyclosporine use, and hypertension. Other less common clinical associations include infection, sepsis, shock, autoimmune disease, and other pharmacologic agents (such as tacrolimus).

The most widely accepted theory of the pathophysiology of PRES is that of hypertension, resulting in a breakdown of the blood–brain barrier causing fluid leaking across capillary membranes in the setting of disordered cerebral autoregulation. Treatment of PRES is directed toward the underlying etiology with resolution of symptoms and imaging findings in uncomplicated cases.

PRES presents as areas of predominately subcortical low attenuation in the parieto-occipital regions on CT in its early stages. MRI is more sensitive than CT for detection of PRES. It is seen as T2/FLAIR hyperintensity on MR, predominately within white matter with involvement of the subcortical U-fibers, and less pronounced scattered cortical involvement. The parietal and occipital lobes are the most commonly affected regions of the brain, with less common involvement of the frontal and temporal lobes, cerebellum, deep gray nuclei, and the brainstem; typically, these latter regions are seen with advanced disease.

Asymmetric bilateral hemispheric involvement is a characteristic finding, while unilateral findings are seen in 2% of cases. The T2/FLAIR hyperintensity in PRES is usually due to vasogenic edema, although areas of infarction (11% to 26%) and hemorrhage (15%) can be seen. Diffusion-weighted imaging in PRES is useful in determining patient prognosis, as patients with complicated PRES manifested as areas of cytotoxic edema are often left with residual neurologic deficits.

References: Bartynski WS. Posterior reversible encephalopathy syndrome, part 1: fundamental imaging and clinical features. *AJNR Am J Neuroradiol* 2008;29:1036–1042.

Bartynski WS, Boardman MD. Distinct patterns and lesion distribution in posterior reversible encephalopathy syndrome. *AJNR Am J Neuroradiol* 2007;28:1320–1327.

Bartynski WS, Tan HP, Boardman JF, et al. Posterior reversible encephalopathy syndrome after solid organ transplantation. *AJNR Am J Neuroradiol* 2008;29:924–930.

Casey SO, Sampaio RC, Michel E, et al. Posterior reversible encephalopathy syndrome: utility of fluid-attenuated inversion recovery MR imaging in the detection of cortical and subcortical lesions. *AJNR Am J Neuroradiol* 2000;21:1199–1206.

Mckinney AM, Short J, Charles L, et al. Posterior reversible encephalopathy syndrome: incidence of atypical regions of involvement and imaging findings. *AJR Am J Roentgenol* 2007;189:904–912.

7a **Answer B.** Acute hyperammonemic encephalopathy.

7b **Answer A.** GI bleeding.

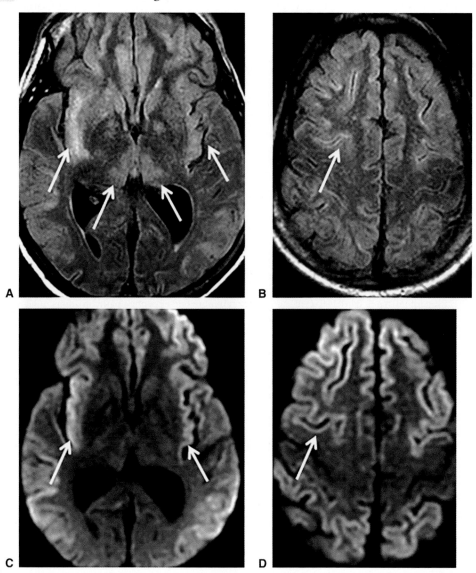

Imaging Findings: There is FLAIR hyperintensity (A and B) and restricted diffusion seen in bilateral insular, parieto-occipital, and frontal cortices (C and D). There is FLAIR hyperintensity seen in bilateral thalamus (A).

Discussion: Acute hyperammonemia in adults is commonly caused by hepatic dysfunction and portosystemic shunt surgery, often triggered by infection, gastrointestinal bleeding, and metabolic disturbances. Other etiologies include drugs (sodium valproate or chemotherapy), infections, multiple myeloma, and transplants.

When hepatic capability for ammonia metabolism is overwhelmed, elimination happens in the brain, kidneys, and skeletal muscle. In astrocytes, ammonia and glutamate are metabolized into glutamine, with subsequent increase in cellular osmolarity and resultant cellular swelling. Inflammatory cascades, various metabolic pathways, and apoptosis are triggered with lactate elevation, loss of cerebral autoregulation, and edema.

The typical imaging abnormality is bilateral symmetrical insular and cingulate gyrus T2 hyperintensity. The rest of the cortex can also be involved to variable extent but generally asymmetrically. Most of the signal abnormality shows diffusion restriction. In severe cases, there can be involvement of the subcortical white matter, deep nuclei, and brainstem. The extent of imaging abnormality generally correlates with the degree of hyperammonemia. These changes are potentially reversible with correction of hyperammonemia. Otherwise, atrophy ensues in involved regions. With severe hyperammonemia, brain edema and herniations ensue and can be fatal. Spectroscopy shows reduced choline, reduced myoinositol, and increased glutamine/glutamate (2.2 to 2.4 ppm in short TE spectrum). In cases of underlying liver disease, increase T1 signal can be seen in globus pallidi, subthalamic regions, and midbrain.

Differential considerations:

Transient postictal change: generally localized and not diffuse and bilateral.
Diffuse ischemic injury: preferential involvement of insula is unlikely.
Creutzfeldt-Jakob disease: subacute presentation. Diffusion restriction is
    irreversible.

References: Hepatic Encephalopathy | Radiology Reference Article | Radiopaedia.org. Accessed June 29, 2016. http://radiopaedia.org/articles/hepatic-encephalopathy

U-King-Im JM, Yu E, Bartlett E, et al. Acute hyperammonemic encephalopathy in adults: imaging findings. *AJNR Am J Neuroradiol* 2011;32(2):413–418. doi: 10.3174/ajnr.A2290

8a **Answer D.** Hypoglycemic injury. This is a case of neonatal hypoglycemic injury. Preferential parieto-occipital cortical involvement is the key imaging feature here. The distribution of abnormality in this case is not entirely typical for hypoxic ischemic injury. Mitochondrial disorder is unlikely to manifest at the time of birth.

8b **Answer A.** Increased incidence in preterm infants, large for age infants, and infants born to diabetic mothers.

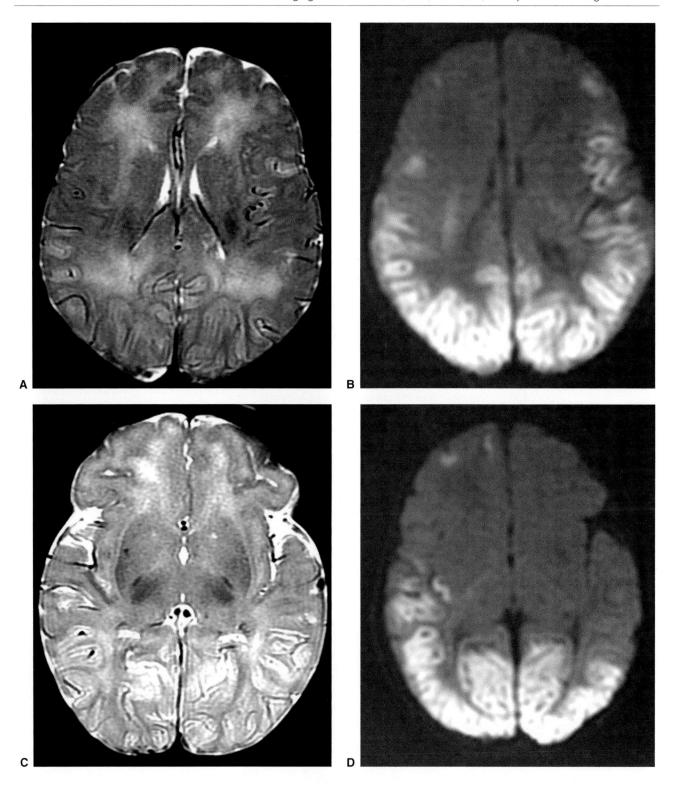

Imaging Findings: There is extensive bilateral T2 hyperintensity involving parietoccipital cortices with corresponding restricted diffusion.

Discussion: Hypoglycemia affects intracellular energy production. Accumulation of excitatory neurotransmitter (aspartate) also appears to contribute to neuronal injury.

Hypoglycemia in adults:
Commonly seen in diabetic patients and can occur as a complication of insulin therapy. Blood glucose level <70 mg/dL is considered hypoglycemia.

Changes are usually bilateral, though asymmetric.

Three imaging patterns have been described:

1. Predominant gray matter involvement affecting the cortex, neostriatum, and hippocampi
2. Predominant white matter involvement affecting periventricular white matter, internal capsule, and splenium of corpus callosum
3. Mixed pattern, involving both gray matter and white matter

Thalami, brainstem, and cerebellum are characteristically spared.

Neonatal hypoglycemia:

Glucose levels below 36 mg/dL is considered hypoglycemia.

Neonatal hypoglycemic encephalopathy shows predilection for occipital and parietal cortices; the exact reason is unclear. Remaining cerebral hemispheres, white matter and deep gray nuclei, can also be involved. Contrary to adult hypoglycemic injury, thalamic and cerebellar involvement can occasionally be seen.

Differential Diagnosis: The most important differential consideration is hypoxic encephalopathy, either alone or in combination with hypoglycemia. Predominantly parieto-occipital abnormality favors hypoglycemic injury. If there is diffuse involvement, it is difficult to exclude hypoxia or a combined insult.

MRI is much more sensitive than CT in detection of lesions. Lesions are typically hyperintense on T2 images and iso- to hypointense on T1 images and show diffusion restriction. Diffusion findings are the earliest to appear and may predict clinical outcome. Contrast enhancement is absent to minimal.

In milder degree of hypoglycemia, some of the abnormality, especially white matter abnormality, can be reversible. Otherwise, sequelae are encephalomalacia and atrophy.

References: Bathla G, Policeni B, Agarwal A. Neuroimaging in patients with abnormal blood glucose levels. *AJNR Am J Neuroradiol* 2014;35(5):833–840. doi: 10.3174/ajnr.A3486

Ma JH, Kim YJ, Yoo WJ, et al. MR imaging of hypoglycemic encephalopathy: lesion distribution and prognosis prediction by diffusion-weighted imaging. *Neuroradiology* 2009;51(10):641–649. doi: 10.1007/s00234-009-0544-5

9 **Answer B.** Hypoxic–ischemic encephalopathy. Most likely diagnosis given recent history of cardiac arrest s/p CPR. The signal changes seen in the caudate, putamen, and within the scattered foci of the cortical ribbon are most compatible with this diagnosis.

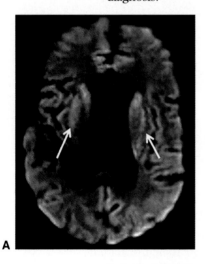 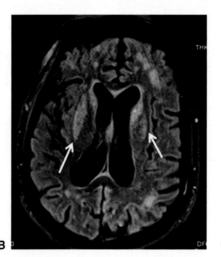 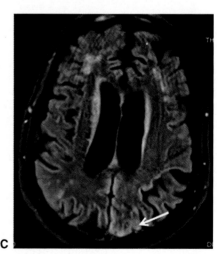

A   B   C

Imaging Findings: Restricted diffusion seen in the caudate nucleus and putamen with corresponding FLAIR hyperintense signal; in addition, FLAIR hyperintensity is seen in the left parieto-occipital cortex.

Discussion: Hypoxic ischemic encephalopathy (HIE).

HIE is characterized by injury to high energy demand CNS structures as a result of a hypoxic ischemic event such as a cardiac arrest, respiratory depression such as seen with opioid overdoses, strangulation, or drowning.

The regions most typically involved are the brain watershed areas that are susceptible to vascular compromise or high energy demand gray matter structures. These latter structures include cerebral cortical ribbon, basal ganglia, hippocampi, and ultimately thalamus and cerebellum.

On CT, there are diffuse effacement of gray and white matter differentiation and hypoattenuation involving the deep gray matter structures, and in severe cases, there may be reversal of gray and white matter relative attenuation properties with the white matter appearing higher attenuation compared to the gray matter structures. This pattern can also be seen in advanced cerebral edema sparing the brainstem and cerebellum, namely, the "white cerebellum sign" because of diffuse supratentorial hypoattenuation resulting in relative cerebellar/brainstem hyperattenuation.

On MRI, there may be varying degrees of restricted diffusion within the involved gray matter structures, based on the severity of insult and corresponding T2 hyperintensity seen within these structures. In delayed phases, there may be postanoxic delayed leukoencephalopathy and generalized volume loss.

Differential diagnosis: While many systemic and metabolic conditions can have overlapping features, the clinical history is key for making the diagnosis of HIE.

- CO poisoning: Characteristic involvement of the globus pallidus. Predisposed toward basal ganglia with involvement of cerebral cortex in more advanced cases.
- Methanol and cyanic poisoning: Characteristic putaminal necrosis. White matter edema may also be seen with methanol.
- Hypoglycemia: Very similar pattern of involvement with severe hypoglycemia, although thalamus may be spared. Mild hypoglycemia may show often reversible preferential white matter involvement with T2 prolongation seen in the splenium, internal capsule, and corona radiata.
- Creutzfeldt-Jakob disease: A prion-mediated neurodegenerative fatal condition. Characteristic pattern of thalamic pulvinar involvement, resulting in the hockey stick sign, is seen.
- Extrapontine myelinolysis: Typically seen in conjunction with central pontine involvement. Rarely although may occur in isolation. The cortical involvement however is characteristically insular. Cerebellar involvement may also be seen.

Reference: Hegde AN, Mohan S, Lath N, et al. Differential diagnosis for bilateral abnormalities of the basal ganglia and thalamus. *Radiographics* 2011;31(1):5–30.

9 Spine Trauma and Degeneration

GAURAV JINDAL • PRACHI DUBEY • RAFEEQUE BHADELIA

QUESTIONS

1 Patient s/p MVA.

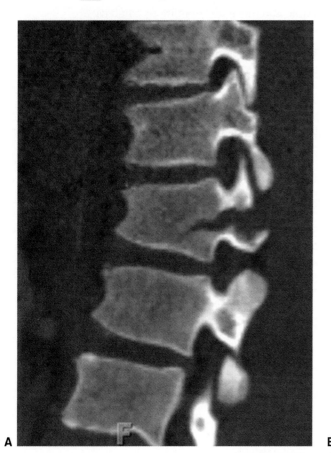
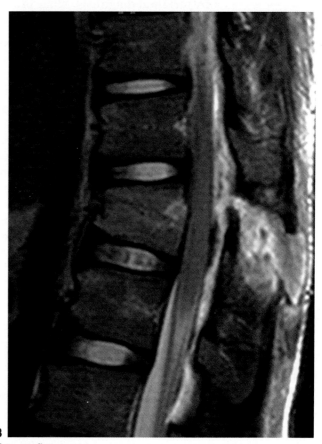

Images courtesy of Dr. Nafi Aygun

1a What is the best description for the pattern of injury shown?

    A. Chance fracture

    B. Compression fracture

    C. Burst fracture

    D. Avulsion fracture

1b Which of the following is associated with the above injury?

    A. Mechanically stable injury without any associated injuries

    B. Most patients have significant neurologic injury.

    C. Commonly associated with visceral injuries

    D. Extreme hyperextension resulting in dorsal soft tissue injury

2 A 50-year-old woman with acute midthoracic back pain presented to the ER. An MRI was performed with intravenous contrast; key images are shown below.

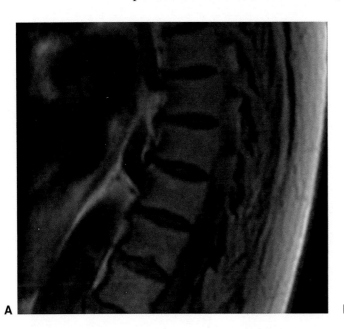

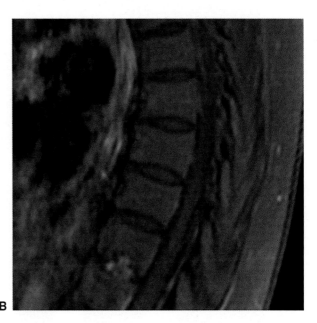

A   B

2a Further clinical workup did not reveal any signs of symptoms to suggest infection. What is the most likely diagnosis?

    A. Acute Schmorl node

    B. Discitis/osteomyelitis

    C. Disc metastasis

    D. Intraosseous hemangioma

2b Which of the following disorders is associated with the above condition in younger individuals?

    A. Mucopolysaccharidoses

    B. Ankylosing spondylitis

    C. Scheuermann disease

    D. Renal osteodystrophy

3 A 34-year-old male presents with pain in lower neck after a weight-lifting accident in the gym. There was focal tenderness on palpation in the lower cervical spine on examination. The patient was neurologically intact. A radiograph of the cervical spine was performed, provided below.

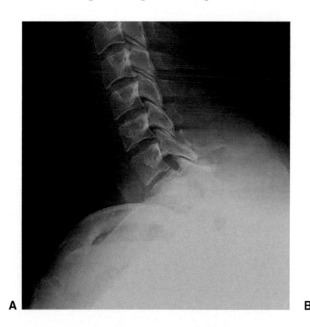

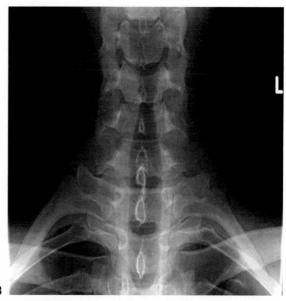

A

B

What is the most likely diagnosis?

A. Muscular strain with neck spasm
B. Possible facet fracture, CT is recommended.
C. Clay shoveler's fracture
D. Normal study

4 Key images from MRI performed for evaluation of back pain in the setting of fall are provided below.

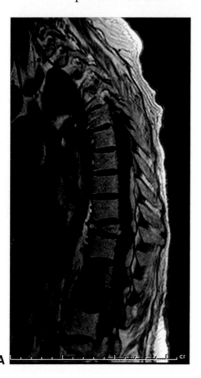

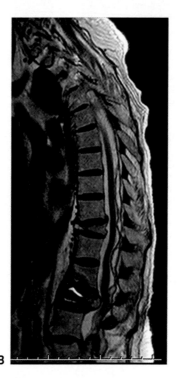

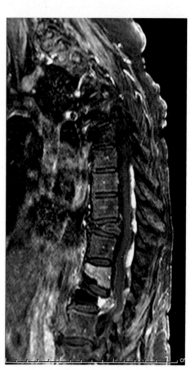

A   B   C

4a What is the most likely diagnosis?

    A. Osteomyelitis with epidural phlegmon/abscess

    B. Metastatic disease

    C. Compression fracture and epidural hematoma

    D. Epidural lipomatosis

4b Which of the following is correct regarding the above entity?

    A. Urgent neurosurgery consultation

    B. Check inflammatory markers.

    C. Get follow-up MRI in 6 weeks.

    D. Obtain bone scan.

5 Regarding the following images, select the best option.

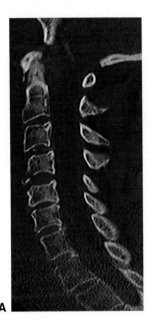 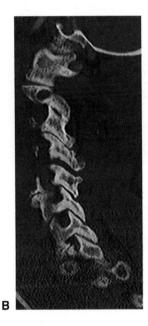 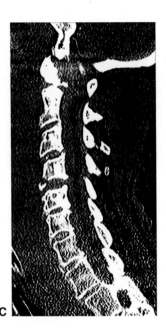

A   B   C

    A. Flexion teardrop fracture

    B. Extension teardrop fracture

    C. Anterior disc ossification

    D. Lytic endplate metastasis

6 Patient presents with trauma.

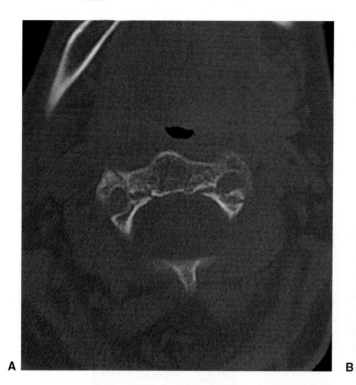

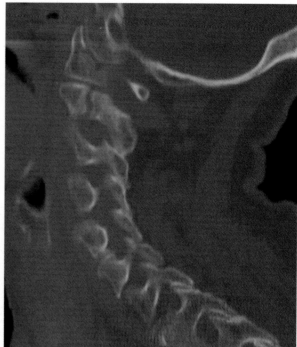

A

B

6a What is the hallmark of the above injury?

    A. Bilateral C2 pars interarticularis fractures
    B. C1 anterior ring fracture
    C. Atlanto-occipital disassociation
    D. Bilateral perched facets

6b Which additional imaging investigation is warranted in this patient?

    A. CT angiogram of the neck
    B. CT angiogram of the head
    C. MRI brain without contrast
    D. CT neck soft tissues with contrast

7 A 27-year-old male with motor vehicle accident, key images are shown below.

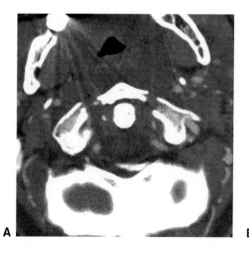

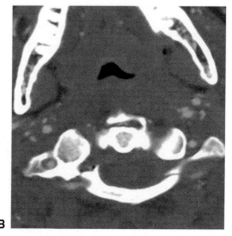

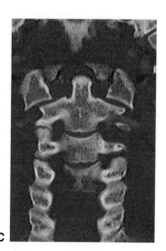

A

B

C

7a What is the most common mechanism of injury to cause the fracture shown?

    A. Hyperextension
    B. Hyperflexion
    C. Rotation
    D. Axial loading

7b Which of the following C1 fractures is considered most unstable?

    A. Isolated anterior arch fracture
    B. Isolated posterior arch fracture
    C. Burst fracture with intact transverse ligament
    D. Burst fracture with disruption of transverse ligament

8 Which of the following is shown on the image below?

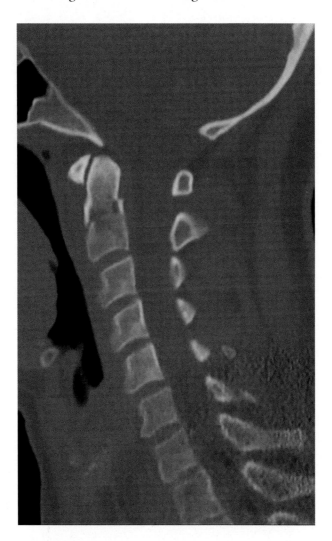

    A. Os odontoideum
    B. Type 1 odontoid fracture
    C. Type 2 odontoid fracture
    D. Type 3 odontoid fracture

9   A 75-year-old postmenopausal women with severe lower back pain had an MRI evaluation. Key images are shown below.

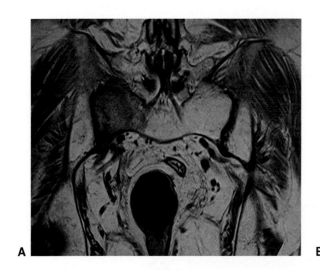

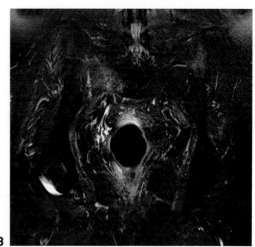

A   B

What is the most likely diagnosis?

A. Plasmacytoma
B. Metastatic disease
C. Sacroiliitis
D. Sacral insufficiency fracture

10   What is the most likely cause for cervical cord abnormality in this patient?

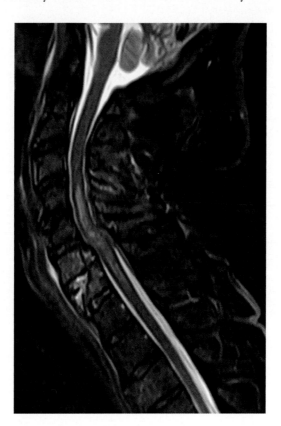

A. Cord infarction
B. Cord contusion
C. Chronic compressive myelopathy
D. Infiltrative astrocytoma

11 A 72-year-old female with history of breast cancer presents with neck pain.

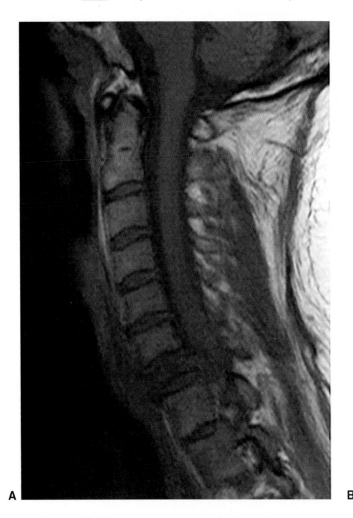

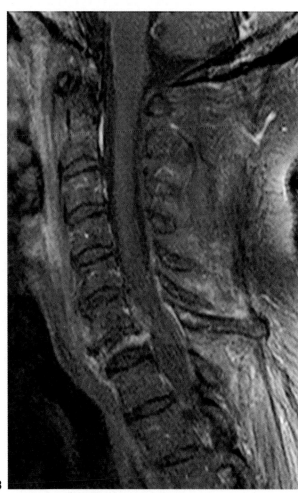

A

B

11a Which of the following is the most likely diagnosis for the images shown above?

    A. Benign osteoporotic compression fracture

    B. Osteomyelitis

    C. Acute traumatic fracture

    D. Pathologic compression fracture

11b Which of the following features favors the diagnosis of a benign compression fracture?

    A. Marrow replacement

    B. Marrow enhancement

    C. Prevertebral soft tissue edema

    D. Fluid-filled cleft on T2-weighted images

12 A 65-year-old male with low back pain and lower extremity radiculopathy undergoes an MRI for further evaluation. Key images from MRI are shown below.

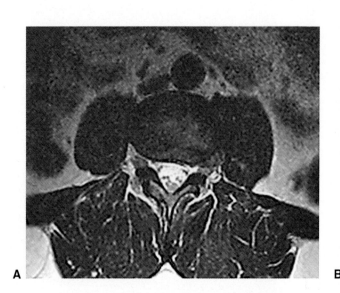

A

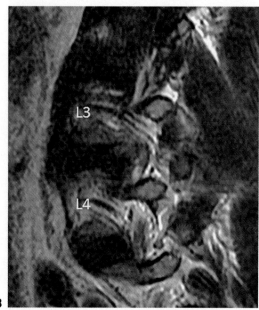

B

12a Based on the above images, which nerve root might explain patient's symptoms?

    A. Left L3
    B. Left L4
    C. Right L3
    D. Right L4

12b What is the best term to describe the anatomic location of the abnormality?

    A. Left L3 lateral recess
    B. Left L4 lateral recess
    C. Left L3 extraforaminal zone
    D. Left L4 extraforaminal zone

13

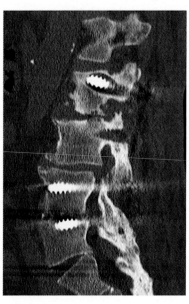

A

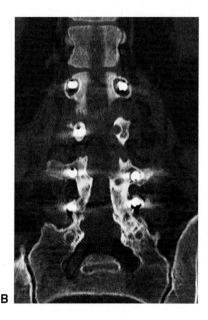

B

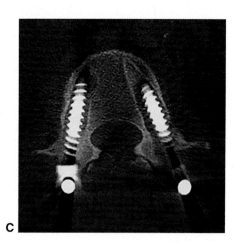

C

13a Which of the following findings can suggest screw loosening in patients with fusion hardware?

   A. Sclerosis around the screw margin
   B. >1 mm lucency around the screw margin
   C. >2 mm lucency around the screw margin
   D. Presence of any lucency around the screw margin

13b What is an indication of possible motion across the fused levels?

   A. Presence of premineralized osteoid formation
   B. Centrally interrupted trabeculation
   C. Accelerated osteophytosis across facet joints
   D. Bridging osseous matrix

14 A 65-year-old female had recent kyphoplasty. What abnormality is noted on this CT?

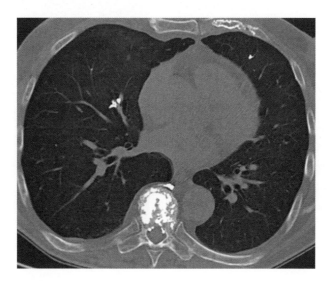

   A. Cement embolism
   B. Calcified granulomas
   C. Aspiration
   D. Chronic calcified pulmonary embolism

ANSWERS AND EXPLANATIONS

1a **Answer A.** Chance fracture.

1b **Answer C.** Commonly associated with visceral injuries.

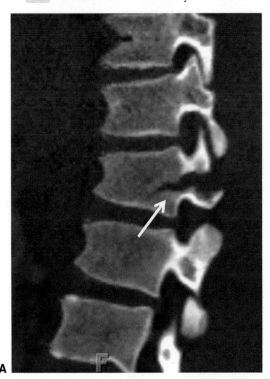
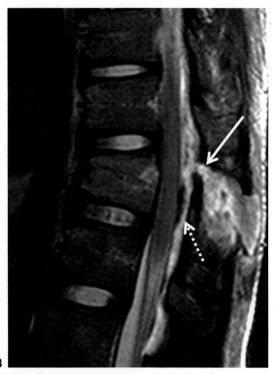

Images courtesy of Dr. Nafi Aygun

Imaging Findings: Sagittal CT image shows a transverse fracture through the vertebral body and pedicle, (arrow A). Sagittal T2 weighed MRI shows disruption of the ligamentum flavum, (arrow B), adjacent interspinous edema and widening. Note there is also a dorsal epidural hematoma, (dotted arrow).

Discussion: Chance fracture is an unstable injury characterized by horizontal splitting of the spinal canal resulting from a flexion distraction mechanism. It may involve the osseous and/or discoligamentous complex. It is most commonly seen at the thoracolumbar junction. On radiographs, distraction of the posterior elements results in an "empty body" sign on frontal view due to displacement of the spinous process from its normal position. On CT, a transverse split of the spinal column is seen as a fracture line through the posterior elements often with extension into the vertebral body.

Anterosuperior compression fractures of the vertebral body are also commonly associated. Burst vertebral fracture morphology may also be seen (Chance–burst fracture).

MRI can better delineate posterior ligamentous complex injury as well as identify any cord damage. Although mechanically unstable, patients seldom have neurologic deficits at presentation. Intra-abdominal injuries especially involving the bowel and mesentery have been reported in up to 40% of cases and must be closely sought in patients with a Chance-type fracture.

References: Bernstein MP, Mirvis SE, Shanmuganathan K. Chance-type fractures of the thoracolumbar spine: imaging analysis in 53 patients. *AJR Am J Roentgenol* 2006;187(4):859–868.

Dane B, Bernstein MP. Imaging of spine trauma. *Semin Roentgenol* 2016;51(3):180–202.

2a **Answer A.** Acute Schmorl node. This study shows endplate edema involving the central and posterior aspect with corresponding enhancement. Note relatively rounded nodular morphology invaginating along the endplates on the pre- and postcontrast T1w sequences, typical for Schmorl node formation. Often, the appearance can be indistinguishable on imaging from discitis/osteomyelitis especially early in the disease course, and therefore, interpretation in the clinical context is very important.

2b **Answer C.** Scheuermann disease. A condition of abnormal kyphosis typically seen in the thoracic spine in the prepubertal age group, it has been associated with multiple endplate Schmorl node formation. The other conditions also have skeletal manifestations, but none of them have a specific predisposition toward Schmorl node formation.

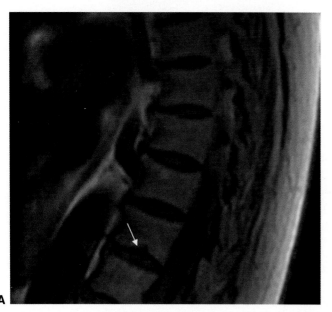 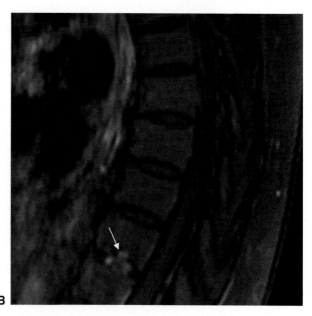

A   B

Imaging Findings: Sagittal pre (A) and post contrast T1w image (B) shows herniation of disc material through the inferior endplate (arrow A) with corresponding enhancement (arrow B). This is compatible with acute Schmorl node formation.

Discussion: Schmorl nodes are disc herniations into the endplates, either into the weakened cartilaginous endplates or within the subchondral bone. The weakened zones provide least resistance to expansion of the nucleus pulposus especially in younger individuals with intact annulus fibrosis. The herniated material typically comprises the nucleus pulposus with associated degenerative or inflammatory response. In the chronic phases, there is characteristic sclerosis along the abutting vertebral spongiosa; however, this is absent in the acute stage often making the diagnosis challenging especially overlapping with features of discitis/osteomyelitis. The majority of these lesions are asymptomatic; however, occasionally patients can present with pain. These are conservatively managed with symptomatic treatment.

References: Grivé E, Rovira A, Capellades J, et al. Radiologic findings in two cases of acute Schmörl's nodes. *AJNR Am J Neuroradiol* 1999;20(9):1717–1721.

Wagner AL, Murtagh FR, Arrington JA, et al. Relationship of Schmorl's nodes to vertebral body endplate fractures and acute endplate disk extrusions. *AJNR Am J Neuroradiol* 2000;21(2):276–281.

3 **Answer C.** Clay shoveler's fracture. There is a fracture of C7 spinous process. The facets are intact.

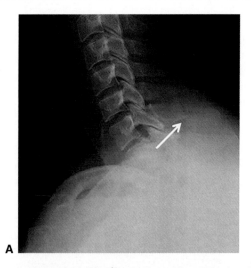
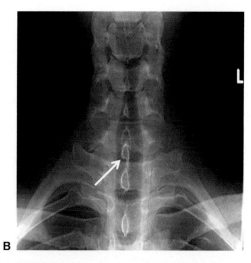

Imaging Findings: Lateral cervical radiograph: Oblique fracture of C7 spinous process. AP radiograph demonstrates double spinous process of C7 due to inferior displacement of fracture fragment.

Discussion: Clay shoveler's fracture. This is an avulsion fracture of the spinous process, most commonly C7. It can result from both hyperflexion and hyperextension injury as well as direct trauma to the spinous processes. It is mostly seen on x-ray/CT as an oblique fracture of the spinous process midway between the tip and lamina with posterior–inferior displacement of distal fracture fragment. On frontal radiograph, displaced fracture fragment appears as double spinous process of the involved vertebra. Management is mostly conservative as this injury in isolation is neurologically stable.

Reference: Posthuma de Boer J, van Wulfften Palthe AF, Stadhouder A, et al. The Clay Shoveler's fracture: a case report and review of the literature. *J Emerg Med* 2016;51(3):292–297.

4a **Answer C.**   Compression fracture and epidural hematoma.

4b **Answer A.**   Urgent neurosurgery consultation.

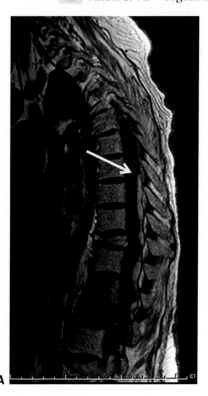
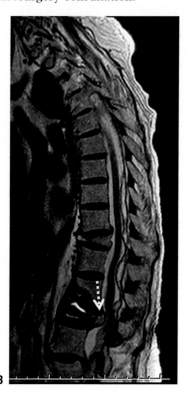
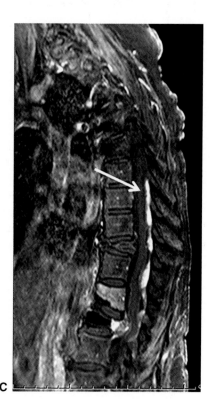

Imaging Findings: Sagittal T1, sagittal T2, and sagittal T1w fat-saturated postcontrast images demonstrate abnormal T1 and T2 hyperintense collection in the posterior epidural space (solid arrow A, B, and C). Note acute disc herniation (dotted arrow, B) with hemorrhage/edema within the herniated disc. Acute compression fracture of L2, postvertebroplasty changes in L3, and a chronic compression fracture of T12 are also seen.

Discussion: Spinal epidural hematoma. Hemorrhage in the spinal epidural space may be traumatic or nontraumatic in etiology. MRI is the most sensitive imaging modality for detection. MR signal depends on age of hemorrhage. Acute blood is isointense on T1 and hyperintense on T2w images, whereas in the subacute stage, methemoglobin results in T1 high signal as seen in the case above. Fat-saturated sequences differentiate it from epidural lipomatosis, and administration of gadolinium helps differentiate from enhancing epidural abnormalities including epidural phlegmon and neoplastic etiologies such as lymphoma and metastases.

Spinal epidural hematomas can result in devastating neurologic outcomes if unrecognized. Symptomatic patients often require urgent decompression to preserve neurologic function.

References: Al-Mutair A, Bednar DA. Spinal epidural hematoma. *J Am Acad Orthop Surg* 2010;18(8):494–502.

Braun P, et al. MRI findings in spinal subdural and epidural hematomas. *Eur J Radiol* 2007;64(1):119–125.

5   **Answers A.**   Flexion teardrop fracture.

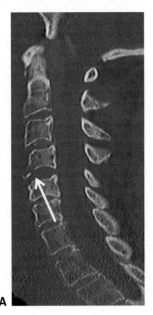 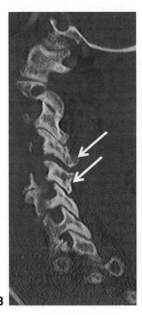 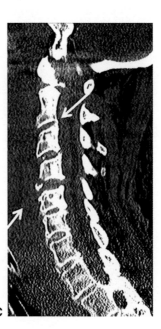

Imaging Findings: Multiple sagittal images of the cervical spine demonstrate a triangular bone fragment (solid arrow A) at the anteroinferior C4 vertebral body, along with widening of interspinous distance, widened facet joint (solid arrow B), as well as widened C4–C5 disc space suggestive of a three-column injury.

There is severe prevertebral soft tissue swelling (C). Also note the epidural hematoma spanning the entire cervical canal best seen on image C.

Discussion: Flexion teardrop fracture results from severe hyperflexion and axial compression injury of the cervical spine such as diving head first into a shallow pool. "Teardrop" refers to the triangular shape of the bone fragment at the anteroinferior (more common) or posteroinferior angle of the vertebral body typically C5/C6.

Hyperflexion injury results in disruption of the posterior ligaments with progressive injury resulting in posterior longitudinal ligament and discal disruption from posterior to anterior. Fracture of the anterior vertebral body completes the three-column injury.

These injuries are often associated with retropulsion of the posterior vertebral body fragment resulting in mass effect on the anterior spinal cord. Additional vertebral body and posterior element fractures are often seen.

It is important to recognize subtle signs of posterior ligamentous disruption on CT imaging especially in patients in a cervical collar. Look for widened interspinous distance, incongruity or widening of facet joints, and asymmetric widening of the disc in addition to osseous injuries. Lastly, attention should always be paid to the prevertebral and epidural soft tissues to detect any obvious hemorrhage such as in the case shown.

References: Bari D, Bernstein MP. Imaging of spine trauma. *Semin Roentgenol* 2016;51(3):180–202.

Kim KS, Chen HH, Russell EJ, et al. Flexion teardrop fracture of the cervical spine: radiographic characteristics. *AJR Am J Roentgenol* 1989;152(2):319–326.

6a **Answer A.** Bilateral C2 pars interarticularis fractures. Bilateral C2 pars interarticularis fractures, often described as "hangman's fracture."

6b **Answer A.** CT angiogram of the neck. Extension through bilateral transverse foramen is seen, indicating need for CTA or MRA neck for assessment of potential vertebral artery injury.

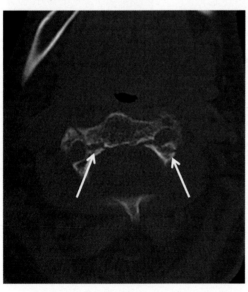
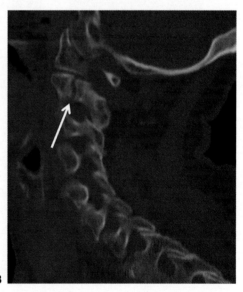

A   B

Imaging Findings: There is a linear fracture seen along bilateral C2 pars interarticularis (A and B). Note that the fracture margin extends into the transverse foramen. Therefore, a CTA or MRA neck to evaluate for potential vertebral artery injury is necessary (A).

Discussion: Hangman's fracture or traumatic bilateral pars interarticularis fractures of C2. It is typically seen with hyperextension and distraction such as with hanging; however, it may result from both hyperflexion and hyperextension injury.

There are three types based on extent of translation and angulation (Effendi classification):

Type 1: Minimal translation (<2 mm, no angulation)
Type 2: Anterior translation with anterior angulation of more than 11 degrees
Type 2A: Severe angulation without anterior translation
Type 3: Bilateral fracture dislocation

Look for associated fractures of odontoid and C1. Although classically described as pars fractures, any part of the C2 ring including posterior vertebral body, pedicles, and laminae may be involved.

References: Dane B, Bernstein MP. Imaging of spine trauma. *Semin Roentgenol* 2016;51(3):180–202.

David D, Letzing M, Sliker CW, et al. Multidetector CT of blunt cervical spine trauma in adults. *Radiographics* 2014;34(7):1842–1865.

7a **Answer D.** Axial loading.

7b **Answer D.** Burst fracture with disruption of transverse ligament.

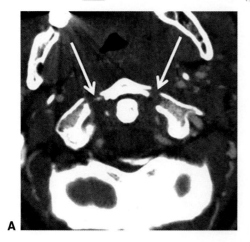
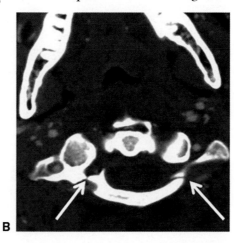
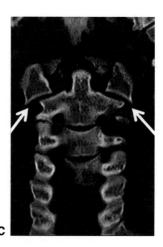

A   B   C

Imaging Findings: Images A and B show fractures through anterior and posterior arch of C1. Coronal image through the cervical spine demonstrates offset of the lateral masses of C1 and C2.

Discussion: Jefferson fracture. Burst fracture of C1 (Atlas) resulting from axial loading injury. C1 is a ring-shaped vertebra that comprises anterior arch, posterior arch, and two lateral masses, which articulate superiorly with occipital condyles and inferiorly with lateral masses of C2. The classic Jefferson fracture is a 4-part fracture with four fractures, two involving junction of anterior arch with the lateral masses and two fractures at the junction of posterior arch and lateral masses. Isolated arch fractures or lateral mass fractures may also occur.

Most patients remain neurologically intact. Clinical management often depends on integrity of the transverse atlantal ligament, which is instrumental in preserving atlantoaxial stability. This can be assessed directly with MRI. On open mouth view radiographs or coronal CT, sum of lateral displacement of lateral masses of C1 over C2 exceeding 7 mm is considered as a sign of transverse ligament injury (rule of Spence).

Congenital fusion anomalies of the anterior or posterior arch may mimic fractures but can be differentiated by their well-corticated edges.

References: Dane B, Bernstein MP. Imaging of spine trauma. *Semin Roentgenol* 2016;51(3):180–202.

Dreizin D, Letzing M, Sliker CW, et al. Multidetector CT of blunt cervical spine trauma in adults. *Radiographics* 2014;34(7):1842–1865.

8 **Answer C.**   Type 2 odontoid fracture. There is a fracture at the base of the dens without extension of the fracture line into the body of C2, compatible with a type 2 odontoid fracture.

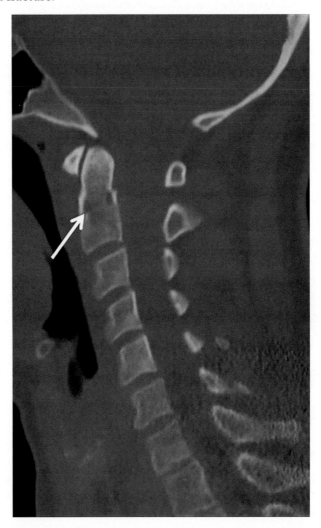

Imaging Findings: Top left sagittal CT image through the cervical spine demonstrates a nondisplaced fracture through the base of the odontoid process. Top right coronal CT image shows no extension of the fracture line into the body of C2, compatible with type 2 odontoid fracture.

Discussion: Odontoid fracture is the most common fracture of C2. They may result from hyperflexion or hyperextension injuries. It is common in the elderly even with low-energy trauma.

Types of odontoid fracture:

Type 1: Avulsion fracture of the alar ligament involving the tip of odontoid
Type 2: Fracture through base of dens; usually unstable
Type 3: Fracture through base of dens with extension into body of C2

Differential Diagnosis: It is important to differentiate odontoid fractures from common variants at this location.

Os odontoideum: Well-corticated ossicle in association with a hypoplastic odontoid process, often accompanied by hypertrophy of C1 anterior arch.
Ossiculum terminale: Small well-corticated bone just superior to the odontoid tip with a normal-appearing den.

References: Dreizin D, Letzing M, Sliker CW, et al. Multidetector CT of blunt cervical spine trauma in adults. *Radiographics* 2014;34(7):1842–1865.

Munera F, Rivas LA, Nunez DB Jr, et al. Imaging evaluation of adult spinal injuries: emphasis on multidetector CT in cervical spine trauma. *Radiology* 2012;263(3):645–660.

9 **Answer D.** Sacral insufficiency fracture. This is the most likely diagnosis in view of the morphology, location, and patient demographics.

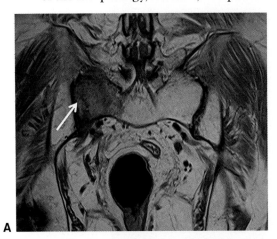 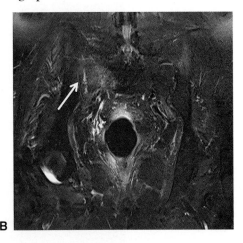

Imaging Findings: Coronal T1w image demonstrates focal area of marrow signal abnormality with T1 hypointense band (A). STIR image of the pelvis makes the marrow edema more conspicuous (B). Fracture line is seen as a bright line parallel to the sacroiliac joint (B).

Discussion: Sacral insufficiency fracture (SIF). An insufficiency fracture results from normal stress on a weakened/osteopenic bone most commonly secondary to osteoporosis or metabolic bone disease. Sacral insufficiency fracture is a relatively underdiagnosed cause of severe back pain especially in the elderly. MRI is almost 100% sensitive in detecting these fractures. Although classically described as an H-shaped fracture with vertical fractures of bilateral sacral ala and horizontal fracture through the body (Honda sign on bone scintigraphy), unilateral fractures are common.

The most conspicuous imaging finding is detection of marrow edema. The fracture lines itself may be seen as dark bands on both T1- and T2-weighted images. If fluid filled, fracture lines can appear T2 bright. Although not as sensitive, CT imaging reveals these fractures as sclerotic bands lateral to the neural foramina and parallel to the sacroiliac joints. Interruption of the anterior sacral cortex may be seen in some cases.

It is imperative to scrutinize the sacral ala on MR images of the lumbar spine as well as on CT of abdomen images to recognize unsuspected cases of this entity. Treatment is mostly conservative with bedrest and pain control. Role of sacroplasty (akin to vertebroplasty) remains under evaluation.

References: Diel J, Ortiz O, Losada RA, et al. The sacrum: pathologic spectrum, multimodality imaging, and subspecialty approach. *Radiographics* 2001;21:83–104.

Lyders EM, Whitlow CT, Baker MD, et al. Imaging and treatment of sacral insufficiency fractures. *AJNR Am J Neuroradiol* 2010;31(2):201–210.

10 **Answer B.** Cord contusion. Although cord signal changes can be seen with any of the entities given as choices in this question, the presence of an acute fracture and expansion of the cord is most consistent with cord contusion in this patient. A T*GRE sequence can performed to assess for potential blood products.

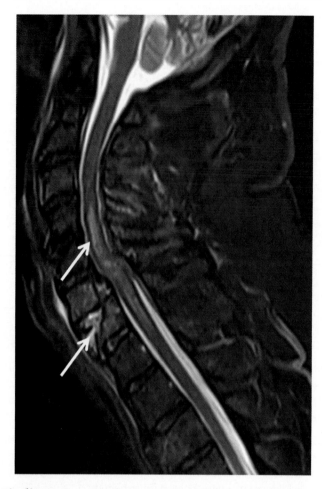

Imaging Findings: Sagittal T2w image reveals fractures of C6 and C7 vertebral bodies with retropulsion of the posterior cortex of C6 resulting in spinal cord injury.

Discussion: Spinal cord contusion or spinal cord injury (SCI) is among the most devastating sequelae of blunt spinal trauma. Preexisting spinal canal narrowing, either congenital or secondary to spondylosis, increases the likelihood of cord trauma.

MRI is well suited for depicting spinal cord injury. Five basic patterns of cord injury have been described with MRI. These include

Cord swelling: Increased cord diameter without signal alteration.
Cord edema: Swelling of the cord at the site of injury with increased T2 signal.
Cord contusion: T2 isointense/hypointense foci with surrounding edema.
Cord hemorrhage: T2 hypointensity with surrounding rim of high signal.
    Increased T1 signal is typically not seen in the acute phase but may be
    detected after 3 days once methemoglobin starts to form.
Cord transection: Very rare with blunt trauma.

The sensitivity for depicting intramedullary hemorrhage can be enhanced by obtaining T2* images.

In terms of clinical outcome, cord swelling and edema are associated with better neurologic recovery compared to cord contusion and hemorrhage.

Although imaging findings may revert to normal in patients with cord edema, those with cord hemorrhage often progress to myelomalacia.

Progressive posttraumatic myelomalacic myelopathy is an uncommon sequel of spinal cord injury seen in <2% cases. It manifest with myelomalacic changes/cyst formation noncontiguous to site of initial trauma.

Subacute progressive ascending myelopathy (SPAM) is another rare sequel of SCI. Patients present with ascending neurologic deficit within 3 weeks of initial injury. MRI demonstrates abnormal T2 signal and edema spanning at least 4 segments proximal to the site of injury.

References: Goldberg AL, Kershah SM. Advances in imaging of vertebral and spinal cord injury. *J Spinal Cord Med* 2010;33(2):105–116.

Mahmood NS, Kadavigere R, Ramesh AK, et al. Magnetic resonance imaging in acute cervical spinal cord injury: a correlative study on spinal cord changes and 1 month motor recovery. *Spinal Cord* 2008;46:791–797.

11a **Answer D.** Pathologic compression fracture. Note the soft tissue component in the epidural space, enhancing vertebral body, and lack of abutting disc enhancement. This appearance in the setting of breast cancer is compatible with a metastatic disease–related pathologic compression fracture.

11b **Answer D.** Fluid-filled cleft on T2-weighted images. This finding has been associated with benign osteoporotic compression fractures.

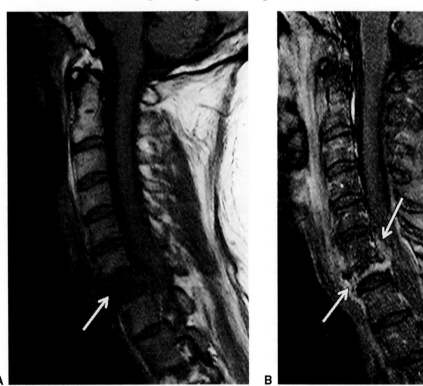

A   B

Imaging Findings: Sagittal T1-weighted precontrast image (left) demonstrates flattened C7 vertebral body with diffuse marrow replacement and convex posterior border. Postcontrast T1 w image depicts diffuse marrow enhancement as well as enhancing ventral epidural soft tissue component. Findings are compatible with pathologic compression fracture.

Discussion: Vertebra plana refers to the morphologic appearance of a flattened vertebral body with normal adjacent disc spaces. It can be secondary to benign etiologies such as osteoporosis, trauma, infection, as well as malignant causes including metastatic disease, lymphoma, and myeloma. In the pediatric population, eosinophilic granuloma is the most common cause of vertebra plana.

Differentiating benign from malignant causes is not always straightforward. Some of the imaging features that favor a benign etiology include

Presence of fracture line resulting from trabecular compression seen as dark bands on T1-/T2-weighted images
Fluid-filled cleft on T2w images
Preserved normal marrow signal
Preserved posterior contour of the vertebral body
Absence of an associated soft tissue mass

Pathologic compression fractures often demonstrate marrow replacement, convex bulging of the posterior vertebral body secondary to an intraosseous mass, absence of fracture lines (as normal trabeculae are replaced by infiltrating tumor), presence of enhancing prevertebral or epidural soft tissue mass, and marrow signal abnormality extending into posterior elements.

Presence of enhancement within the vertebral body may be seen in both benign and malignant compression fractures.

References: Baur A, Stäbler A, Arbogast S, et al. Acute osteoporotic and neoplastic vertebral compression fractures: fluid sign at MR imaging. *Radiology* 2002;225(3):730–735.

Jung HS, Jee WH, McCauley TR, et al. Discrimination of metastatic from acute osteoporotic compression spinal fractures with MR imaging. *Radiographics* 2003;23(1):179–187.

12a **Answer A.** Left L3. The images show soft tissue density in the left L3–L4 extraforaminal zone. This is compatible with an extraforaminal disc protrusion encroaching on the exiting left L3 nerve root.

12b **Answer C.** Left L3 extraforaminal zone. The disc protrusion involves the proximal extraforaminal zone abutting the exiting left L3 nerve root. Note that the traversing left L4 nerve root in the lateral recess or subarticular zone is not involved in this case.

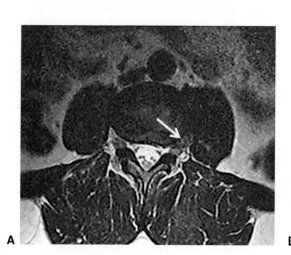

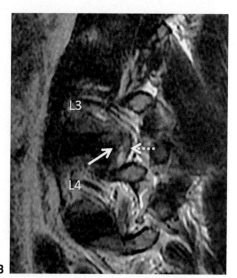

A   B

Imaging Findings: There is a small disc protrusion involving the left extraforaminal zone (solid arrow A and B) that abuts the exiting L3 nerve root (dotted arrow L3). The traversing L4 nerve root seen in the lateral recess (also known as subarticular zone bounded laterally by the medial margin of the pedicle) is completely spared.

Discussion: This case refers to usage of the lumbar disc nomenclature version 2.0, employed to standardize the reporting of lumbar spine degenerative abnormalities. The term disc "herniation" is reserved for displacement of disc material beyond the edges of vertebral apophysis in a focal or localized fashion (<25%

of disc circumference). This is in contrast to a bulge that extends >25% of disc circumference. The following types of herniations can be present:

- Disc protrusion: A type of herniation where the distance between the edges of the herniated disc material is less than the distance between the edges of the base (at the site of connection with the disc of origin).
- Disc extrusion: A type of herniation where the distance between the edges of the herniated disc material is more than the distance between the edges of the base in at least any one plane (note that the measurement for base and herniated disc edges must be made on the same plane). If there is no continuity between the extruded disc material and disc of origin, this latter subtype of extrusion is referred to as a "sequestered" disc.

The reader is encouraged to read the following reference for other details related to terminology in lumbar spine degenerative disease reporting.

Reference: Fardon DF, Williams AL, Dohring EJ, et al. Lumbar disc nomenclature: version 2.0: recommendations of the combined task forces of the North American Spine Society, the American Society of Spine Radiology and the American Society of Neuroradiology. *Spine J* 2014;14(11):2525-2545.

13a **Answer C.** >2 mm lucency around the screw margin. This is indicative of screw loosening, which may occur because of abnormal motion or infection that may lead to hardware failure.

13b **Answer B.** Centrally interrupted trabeculation. These can be seen with abnormal motion across the fused segment and may result in loosening of hardware.

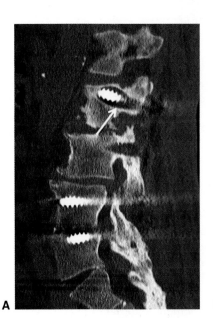
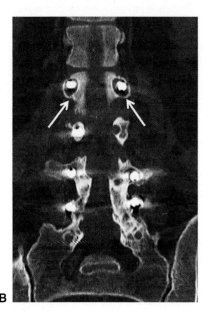
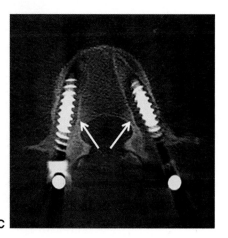

A   B   C

Imaging Findings: There is a lucency surrounding the screw tract that is >2 mm, suggestive of screw loosening.

Discussion: Loosening of hardware is an indication of potential hardware failure and abnormal motion across the fused segments. It may be seen as an enlarging lucency around the screw tract or a lucency of >2 mm surrounding it. This can lead to hardware fracture, subsidence (collapse of the cage devices through the endplate), or migration.

Postoperative CT and MR remain a cornerstone for assessment of hardware integrity and degree of anatomic fusion. Typically, osseous fusion can be identified on CT in the form of osseous trabeculae bridging across the fused segments. Disruption of this trabeculation is an indication of abnormal motion and may result in hardware failure. Formation of a pseudoarthrosis and infection are other etiologies for hardware failure, which can be evaluated on both CT and MRI. MRI is particularly sensitive to detection of infection, arachnoiditis, or postoperative fibrosis. In addition, recurrent disc herniations, abnormal stress on the facet articulations, and worsening listhesis can be detected.

Reference: Malhotra A, Kalra VB, Wu X, et al. Imaging of lumbar spinal surgery complications. *Insights Imaging* 2015;6(6):579–590.

14 Answer A. Cement embolism. There are curvilinear branching hyperdensities in the pulmonary vasculature. Note there is cement material in the perivertebral venous plexus. Although the other entities can be associated with pulmonary calcifications, the morphology and clinical scenario are most compatible with cement embolism.

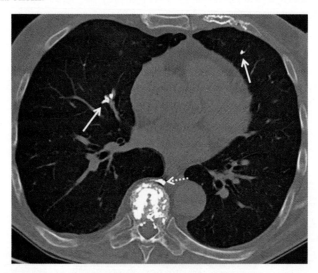

Imaging Findings: There are branching hyperdensities (arrows) that are seen in the setting of recent kyphoplasty with presence of cement in the perivertebral venous plexus (dotted arrow) most compatible with cement embolism.

Discussion: Percutaneous vertebral kyphoplasty and vertebroplasty are techniques used for vertebral augmentation and treatment of painful compression fractures. Vertebroplasty was first employed using a transpedicular approach to introduce cement (polymethylmethacrylate [PMMA]) into the affected vertebra. Subsequently, this technique was modified using a balloon kyphoplasty approach that employs inflation of balloon to expand the compression fracture and create a void for cement injection. These interventions have been found to aid correction of loss of vertebral body height, angular kyphosis, pain, and overall functional state.

Although rare, serious complications such as extrusion of cement material in the spinal canal or neural foramina resulting in cord compression or nerve root compression or venous infiltration resulting in pulmonary embolism as seen in this case may occur.

Reference: Yaltirik K, Ashour AM, Reis CR, et al. Vertebral augmentation by kyphoplasty and vertebroplasty: 8 years experience outcomes and complications. *J Craniovertebr Junction Spine* 2016;7(3):153–160.

10 Spine Infection, Inflammation, and Demyelination

DAVID B. KHATAMI • PRITESH MEHTA • PRACHI DUBEY • YU-MING CHANG •
RAFEEQUE BHADELIA

QUESTIONS

1 A 50-year-old female with back pain, fevers, and chills presented to the ER.
A contrast-enhanced CT was performed. Key image is shown below.

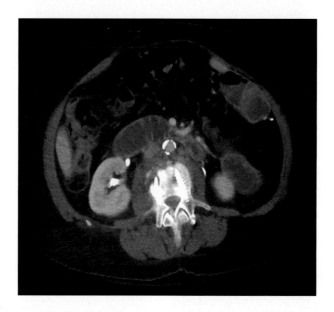

1a Which of the following can be a possible explanation for the patient's symptoms?

A. Mechanical small bowel obstruction
B. Lumbar fusion hardware infection
C. Pyelonephritis
D. Ruptured viscus with abscess formation

To further assess the abnormality, an MRI of the lumbar spine was performed. Key image is shown below.

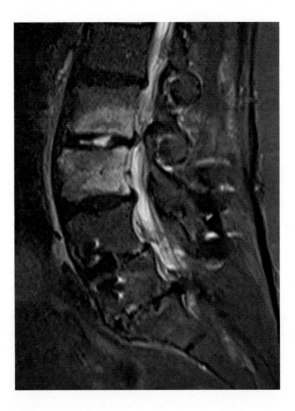

1b   What is the diagnosis?

    A. Discitis/osteomyelitis
    B. Modic type 1 endplate changes
    C. Metastasis
    D. Inflammatory spondylitis

2   A 42-year-old male with seizures was found down and brought to the ER.

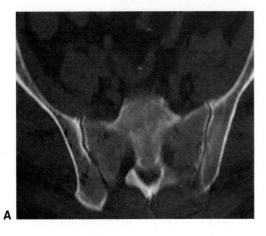
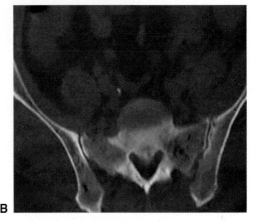

2a Which of the following imaging features seen on this image is highly concerning and warrants further evaluation?

A. Sacroiliac joint sclerosis
B. Intraosseous gas
C. Surrounding soft tissue stranding
D. Osteophytosis

Additional workup included an MRI with contrast. Key images are provided below.

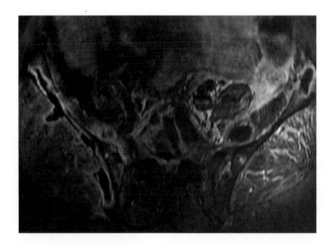

2b What is the most likely diagnosis?

A. Multifocal bone infarction
B. Intraosseous pneumatocysts
C. Metastasis
D. Emphysematous osteomyelitis

3 A 47-year-old female presented with chronic back pain and right thigh pain. An MRI was performed. Key images are shown below.

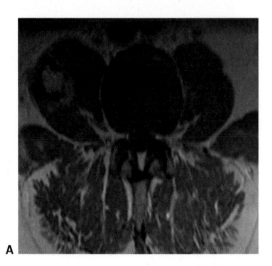

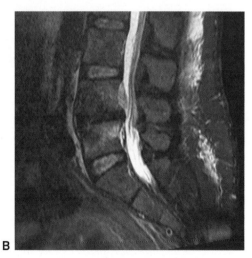

A   B

3a   What is the most likely diagnosis?

    A. Metastases with right psoas involvement
    B. Discitis/osteomyelitis with a right psoas abscess
    C. Modic type 1 endplate changes and right psoas hematoma
    D. Retroperitoneal fibrosis and secondary endplate changes

3b   What is the most common pathology in the iliopsoas compartment?

    A. Primary neoplasm (liposarcoma, fibrosarcoma)
    B. Retroperitoneal hematoma
    C. Abscess
    D. Retroperitoneal fibrosis

4   A 54-year-old male presents with low-grade fever, sweats, low back pain, and possible new cardiac murmur.

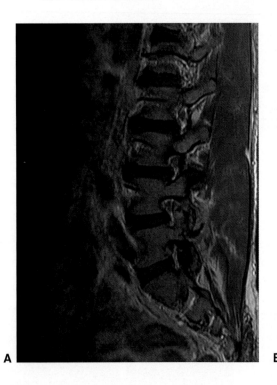
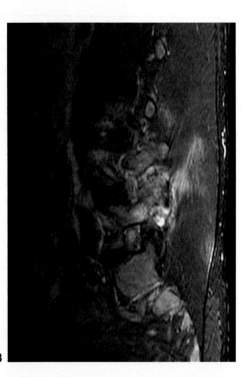

A   B

4a   What is the most likely diagnosis in the current clinical scenario?

    A. Rheumatoid arthritis
    B. Metastasis
    C. Facet joint septic arthritis
    D. Modic type 1 degenerative changes

4b   Which of the following is the most common organism associated with this entity?

    A. *Staphylococcus aureus*
    B. Streptococcus
    C. *Clostridium difficile*
    D. *E. coli*

5   A 61-year-old male, newly immigrated from Brazil presents with focal back tenderness, weakness, and low-grade fever.

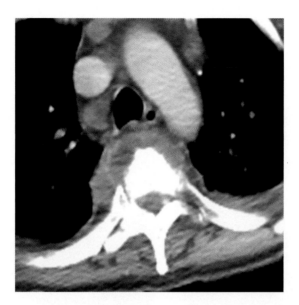

5a   A CT of the chest was performed with contrast; key finding is shown above. What is the next best step?

A. Bone scan
B. MRI of the spine
C. Antibiotics
D. Surgery

5b

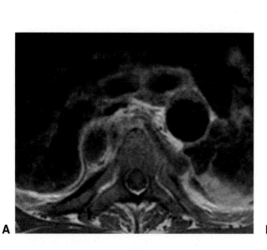

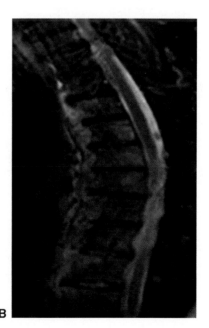

A   B

What is the most likely diagnosis?

A. Pyogenic osteomyelitis
B. Tuberculous spondylitis
C. Metastasis
D. Modic type 1 changes

6 A 63-year-old male with history of meningitis/encephalitis presenting with 3 days of progressive numbness and weakness. An MRI of the lumbar spine was performed; key images are shown below.

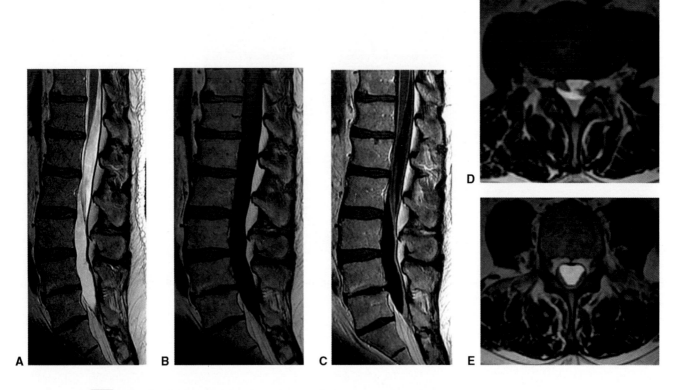

6a Which of the following key abnormalities is noted on these images?

A. Nerve root clumping
B. Normal enhancement
C. Subdural hemorrhage
D. All of the above

6b Which of the following is most likely to result in arachnoiditis?

A. Tumor
B. Surgery
C. Demyelination
D. Advanced degenerative change

7   A 39-year-old man recently recovered from an upper respiratory tract infection presents with bilateral lower extremity weakness and difficulty breathing. An MRI with contrast was performed. Key images are shown below.

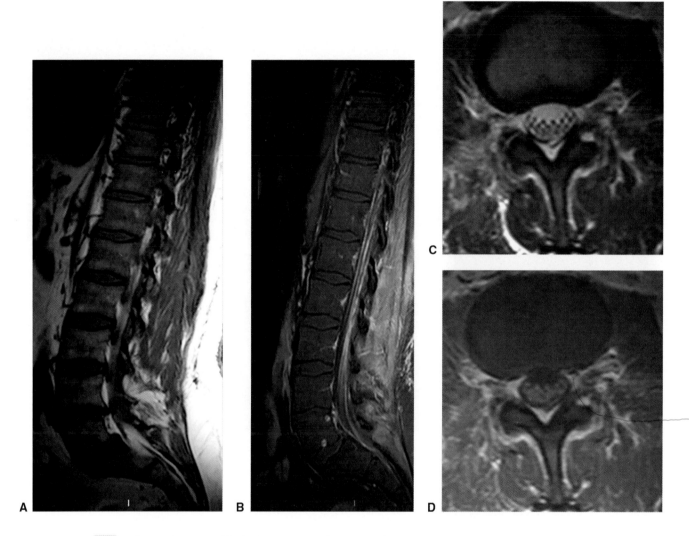

7a   What is the most likely diagnosis in the given clinical scenario?

    A. Lymphoma

    B. Metastasis

    C. Guillain-Barre syndrome

    D. Transverse myelitis

7b   Which of the following best describes the underlying pathophysiology for the above entity?

    A. Autoimmune demyelination

    B. Bacterial infection

    C. Drop metastases

    D. Granulomatous inflammation

8 A 59-year-old woman presenting with new sensory changes in bilateral arms. Patient had a previous similar episode that spontaneously resolved 6 months ago. An MRI was performed; key images are below.

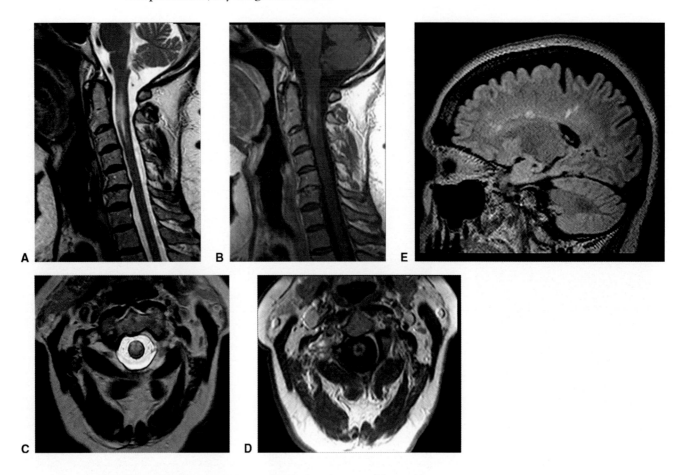

8a What is the most likely diagnosis?

A. Multiple sclerosis
B. Transverse myelitis
C. Guillain-Barre syndrome
D. Glioma

8b Which of the following imaging features is compatible with dissemination in space for multiple sclerosis?

A. Presence of enhancement
B. Simultaneous periventricular and cord lesions
C. Involvement of the dorsal column cervical cord
D. Multiple lesions perpendicular to the callososeptal junction

9   A 43-year-old woman with long-standing wrist pain presents with waxing and waning neck pain. Key images are shown below.

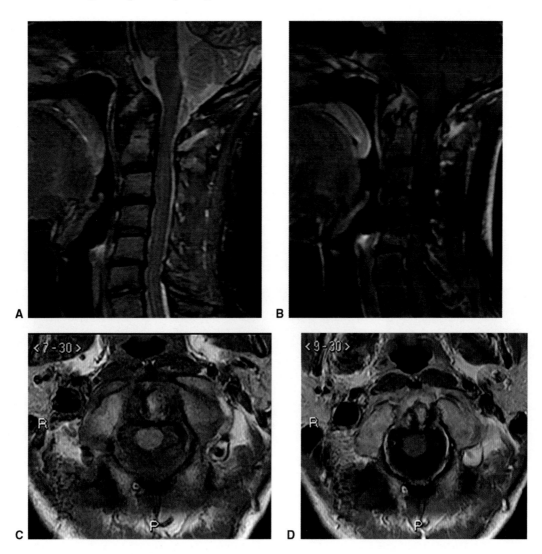

9a   Which of the following inflammatory disorders is classically associated with involvement of the atlantoaxial joint?

A. Osteoarthritis
B. Rheumatoid arthritis
C. Juvenile idiopathic arthritis
D. Ankylosing spondylitis

9b   Advanced rheumatoid arthritis of the cervical spine is associated with which of the following imaging features?

A. Abscess formation
B. Osteophyte formation
C. C1–C2 subluxation
D. Calcification

10 A 54-year-old man presenting with progressive sensory loss and urinary incontinence. An MRI of cervical spine was performed with contrast. Key images are shown below.

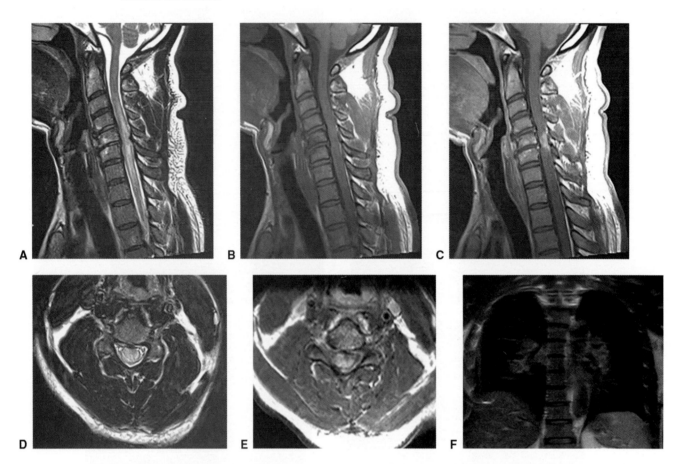

10a What abnormality is incidentally found on the coronal localizer images for this cervicothoracic spine MRI (image F)?

A. Pneumothorax
B. Aortic dissection
C. Hilar lymphadenopathy
D. Liver mass

10b What is the most likely diagnosis?

A. Metastasis
B. Lymphoma
C. Tuberculosis
D. Sarcoidosis

11 A 32-year-old woman presenting with 1 week history of gait instability and ataxia.
Key images from MRI are shown below.

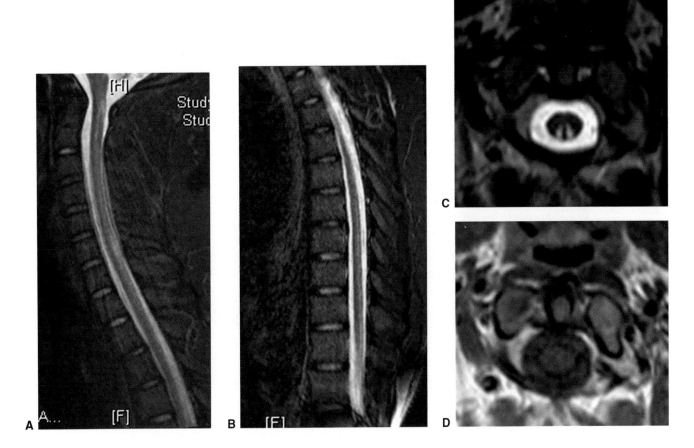

11a Which of the following best describes the anatomic location of this abnormality?

A. Lateral columns
B. Dorsal columns
C. Posterior horn cells
D. Anterior horn cells

11b Which of the following best describes the function of dorsal columns?

A. Motor—skeletal muscle
B. Sensory—pain
C. Sensory—crude touch
D. Sensory—fine touch, vibration, proprioception

12 A 15-year-old male with distal extremity motor weakness and foot deformity. An MRI was performed; key images are shown below.

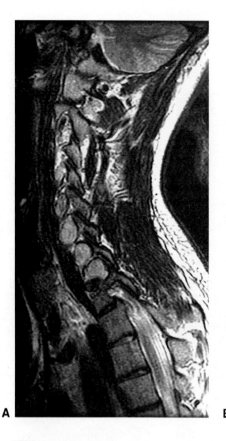

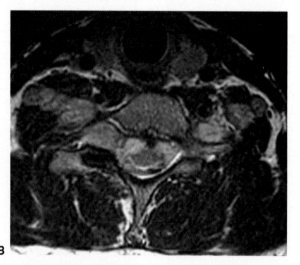

12a Which of the following clinical information is useful in understanding the above changes?

A. Family history
B. Recent international travel
C. Recent URI
D. Underlying primary malignancy

12b Further workup revealed decreased nerve conduction velocity, and contrast-enhanced MRI shows no corresponding abnormal enhancement (images not shown). The most likely diagnosis is:

A. Amyloid polyneuropathy
B. Neurosarcoid
C. Charcot Marie tooth disease
D. Lymphoma

13 A 50-year-old male with reduced range of motion, low back pain, and chronic compression fracture noted on radiograph (not shown). An MRI was performed; key images shown below.

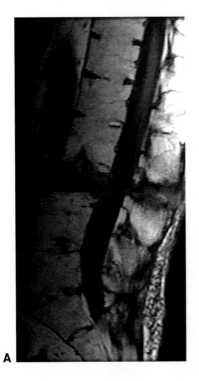

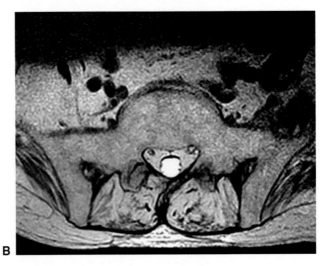

13a Based on the above images, which of the following serum abnormalities can be seen in this patient?

    A. RF positivity

    B. ANA positivity

    C. CRP elevation

    D. Leukocytosis

13b What is the most likely diagnosis?

    A. Rheumatoid arthritis

    B. Ankylosing spondylitis

    C. Discitis/osteomyelitis

    D. Psoriatic arthritis

14   A 25-year-old female presented with rapidly progressive lower extremity weakness
and incontinence. An MRI was performed; key image is shown below.

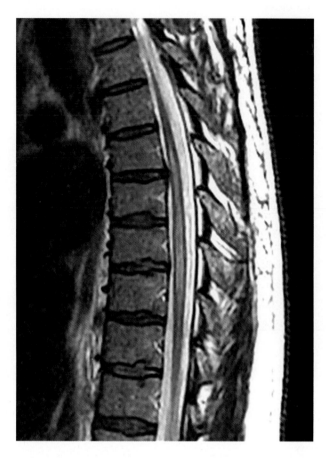

Which of the following imaging features differentiates this condition from multiple
sclerosis?

A. Longitudinally extensive nature
B. Thoracic cord involvement
C. Central cord involvement
D. Lack of cord expansion

15 A 52-year-old male presents with known discitis/osteomyelitis, on IV antibiotics, now with worsening bilateral lower extremity weakness. Key images from MRI are shown below.

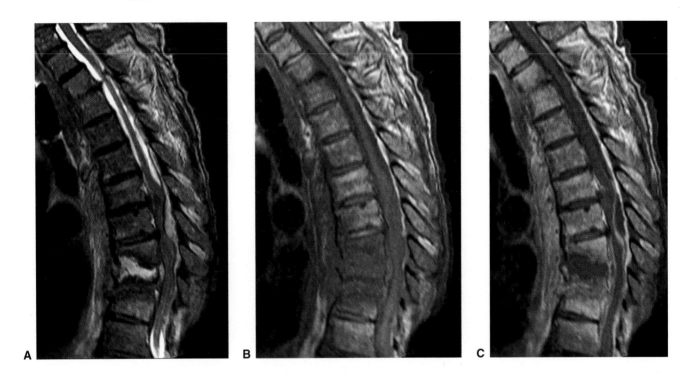

A   B   C

What is the next best step in management?

A. Biopsy with culture and sensitivity
B. Urgent neurosurgical consultation
C. IV steroid administration
D. Continued follow-up

ANSWERS AND EXPLANATIONS

1a **Answer B.** Lumbar fusion hardware infection. Note the soft tissue thickening seen in the right psoas muscle and lucency surrounding the tip of the right pedicle screw.

1b **Answer A.** Discitis/osteomyelitis. This is at the level of hardware as noted on CT and likely to be secondary to hardware infection.

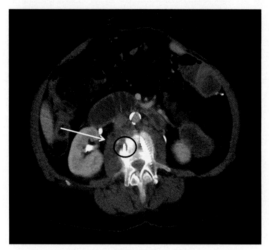

Figure 1

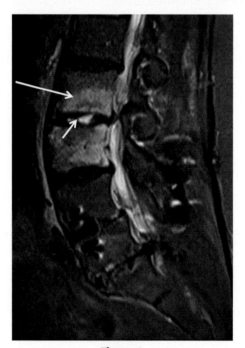

Figure 2

Imaging Findings: Figure 1. CT demonstrates soft tissue thickening surrounding the right psoas muscle (arrow in A) and a lucency along the tip of the right pedicle screw (black circle in A), concerning for infection.

Figure 2. Sagittal STIR images demonstrate edema in the L2 and L3 vertebral bodies (long arrow in A) and within the disc space (short arrow in A), concerning for discitis/osteomyelitis.

Discussion: Discitis/osteomyelitis with hardware infection. This can be seen in the early postoperative phase, usually 1 to 4 weeks following surgery. The aseptic enhancement sometimes seen along the posterior disc or within the nerve root early on is typically reactive in nature and can be a diagnostic pitfall. Edema and enhancement may also be seen in the vertebral body and disc space in asymptomatic patients early in the postoperative course. Therefore, clinical presentation is key to better understanding early postoperative changes.

Presence of osseous erosive changes, soft tissue abscess, or phlegmon formation increases the sensitivity of MRI to hardware infection. The causes of infection may be intraoperative seeding, hematogenous seeding, or metal fretting. The risk of management includes antibiotics and surgical removal of the infected hardware.

References: Malhotra A, Kalra VB, Wu X, et al. Imaging of lumbar spinal surgery complications. *Insights Imaging* 2015;6(6):579-590.

Viola RW, King HA. Delayed infection after elective spinal instrumentation and fusion: a retrospective analysis of eight cases. *Spine* 1997;22(20):P2444-P2450.

2a **Answer B.**   Intraosseous gas. Presence of intraosseous gas raises concern for emphysematous osteomyelitis, particularly given lack of contiguity with the joint space.

2b **Answer D.**   Emphysematous osteomyelitis. The abnormal enhancement and intraosseous collections are concerning for emphysematous osteomyelitis.

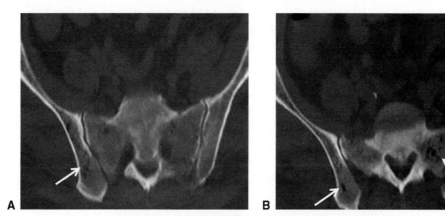

Figure 1

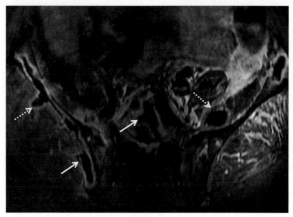

Figure 2

Imaging Findings: Figure 1. Noncontrast CT scan through the pelvis demonstrates intraosseous gas (arrows).

Figure 2. Postcontrast fat-suppressed axial T1w image shows abnormal soft tissue enhancement and multifocal intraosseous (solid arrows) and intramuscular abscesses (dotted arrows). The constellation of findings is concerning for emphysematous osteomyelitis.

Discussion: Emphysematous osteomyelitis is a rare but severe infection that is characterized by presence of intraosseous gas. The intraosseous gas seen with this entity is not in the typical distribution abutting the endplates as seen with degenerative disease and can involve both the axial and appendicular skeletons. Anaerobic organisms such as *Fusobacterium necrophorum* and *Clostridium septicum* and gram-negative Enterobacteriaceae family are typically implicated as common causative organisms. These patients commonly have other comorbidities such as diabetes or malignancy predisposing to this infection. Nearly every bone can be affected; however, most cases affect the vertebra, sacrum, and long bones.

Differential Diagnosis: Bone infarction, which usually presents as a serpentine contour of infarction with peripheral enhancement; however, soft tissue involvement will not be seen with this condition as noted in the presented case. Bony infarction is usually associated with steroids, sickle cell disease, pancreatitis, vasculitis, emboli, and caisson disease. Degenerative intraosseous pneumatocysts can be considered; however, those are usually abutting the sacroiliac joint and will also not have associated soft tissue changes.

References: Chen JLY, Huang YS. Emphysematous osteomyelitis of spine. *QJM* 2016;109(6):427–428.

Larson J, Muhlbauer J, Wigger T, et al. Emphysematous osteomyelitis. *Lancet Infect Dis* 2015;15(4):486.

3a **Answer B.** Discitis/osteomyelitis with a right psoas abscess. There is edema and enhancement involving the endplates of L4 and L5 is suggestive of an infectious process with a focal right psoas abscess. Paravertebral psoas abscesses should prompt a careful search for spinal infections. Infection and abscess formation in the iliopsoas is typically due to spread of infection from contiguous structures, most commonly bone, kidney, bowel, and appendix.

3b **Answer B.** Retroperitoneal hematoma. Iliopsoas is the most common site for a spontaneous retroperitoneal hemorrhage either secondary to anticoagulation or a bleeding diathesis. The MR appearance of the hematoma is variable, depending on the age of the hematoma.

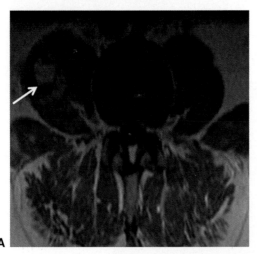
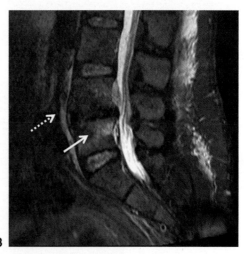

A   B

Imaging Findings: Postcontrast axial images through the lumbar spine demonstrate collection within the right psoas muscle concerning for a soft tissue phlegmon/developing abscess (A).

On the sagittal STIR, marrow edema is seen within L4 and L5 vertebral bodies and mild edema along anterior disc and prevertebral soft tissues (dotted arrow). Also note that preexisting Modic type 2/3 (type 2, yellow marrow conversion, and type 3, subchondral sclerosis) endplate changes can often partially obscure the presence of edema. These findings are consistent with discitis/osteomyelitis with right psoas involvement.

Discussion: Infection and abscess formation in the iliopsoas are typically secondary to spread of infection from contiguous structures. Common bowel sources of an iliopsoas infection include diverticulitis, Crohn disease, and appendicitis. Renal sources include pyelonephritis or renal/perirenal abscess. It is important to look for secondary features of infection such as fat stranding, blurring of the fat planes, and ectopic gas.

Primary infection is rare unless the patient is immunocompromised or a user of intravenous drugs, in which case the infection is usually due to *Staphylococcus aureus* and mixed gram-negative organisms. Primary neoplasms such as liposarcoma, fibrosarcoma, or hemangiopericytoma rarely originate from the iliopsoas compartment. A psoas abscess can lead to significant morbidity and mortality. Risk factors include advanced age, bacteremia, and inadequate treatment.

Differential Diagnosis: The most common differential diagnoses are hematoma, which can have a variable appearance dependent on the age of the hematoma. Neoplasms such as lymphoma, melanoma, or metastasis can be considered and may involve the psoas compartment.

References: Chern CH, Hu SC. Psoas abscess: making an early diagnosis in the ED. *Am J Emerg Med* 1997;15(1):83–88.

Muckley T, Schutz T, Kirschner M, et al. Psoas abscess: the spine as a primary source of infection. *Spine* 2003;28(6):E106–E113.

4a **Answer C.** Facet joint septic arthritis. Postcontrast T1 and STIR images demonstrate a small collection and increased STIR signal abnormality within the L4–L5 facet joint, consistent with septic facet joint.

4b **Answer A.** *Staphylococcus aureus. Staphylococcus aureus* is the offending organism in a majority of the cases. The next most common organism is Streptococcus.

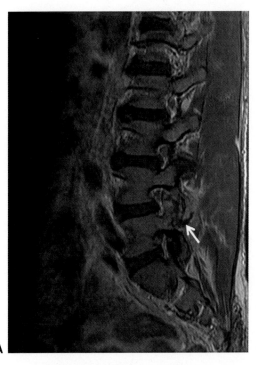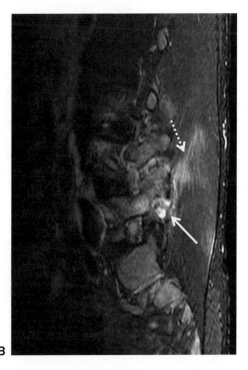

A   B

Imaging Findings: Sagittal postcontrast T1w imaging demonstrates a nonenhancing fluid collection seen along the inferior aspect of the L4–L5 facet joint (A). Sagittal STIR demonstrates marrow and periarticular soft tissue edema (solid arrow, B) and paraspinal muscular edema (dotted arrow). Findings are suggestive of septic facet arthritis in the given clinical scenario.

Discussion: The most common cause is hematogenous contamination. Otherwise, infection can be acquired through direct inoculation from penetrating trauma, surgical intervention, or diagnostic procedures such as facet joint injections. It is also important to consider pelvic sources such as diverticulitis/appendicitis, or IBD. Predisposing factors include immunosuppression, IVDU, and diabetes. Secondary complications to be aware of are epidural extension of infection resulting in cord compression and neuroforaminal narrowing. Intrathecal spread of infection could lead to meningitis/arachnoiditis.

Differential Diagnosis: Facet joint osteoarthritis and rheumatoid arthritis. Particularly, facet joint synovial cyst can often exist in the setting of advanced degenerative changes and pedicle stress reaction. This creates a diagnostic dilemma because of morphologic overlap with septic arthritis; however, findings such as rim enhancement and clinical features of infection favor septic arthritis.

References: Heenan SD, Britton J. Septic arthritis in a lumbar facet joint: a rare cause of an epidural abscess. *Neuroradiology* 1995;37:462–464.

Michel-Batot C, Dintinger H. A particular form of septic arthritis: septic arthritis of the facet joint. *Joint Bone Spine* 2008;75(1):78–83.

5a **Answer B.** MRI of the spine. Given the patient's symptoms and paraspinal soft tissue thickening, it is important to determine intrathecal involvement. An MRI will also provide superior soft tissue detail and asses for osseous involvement.

5b **Answer B.** Tuberculous spondylitis. Tuberculous spondylitis (TS) often presents with hyperintense marrow, disc, phlegmon/abscess on the STIR, and marrow enhancement. There is usually sparing of the intervertebral disc.

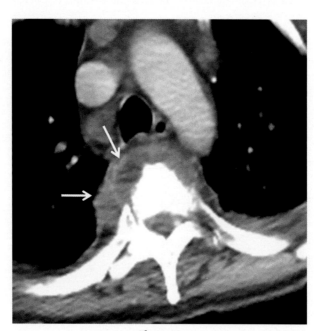

Figure 1

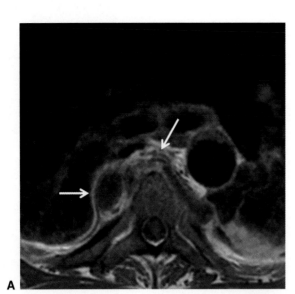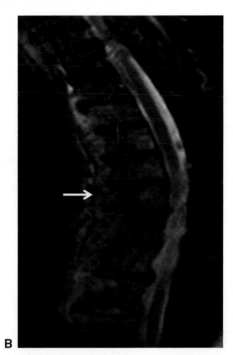

Figure 2

Imaging Findings: Figure 1. Postcontrast axial CT scan through the aortic arch demonstrates paraspinal soft tissue thickening.

Figure 2. Axial postcontrast T1s images shows paravertebral abscess and enhancement (A). Sagittal STIR shows subligamentous phlegmon seen along the anterior cortices (B).

Discussion: Tuberculous spondylitis, otherwise known as Pott disease, is one of the oldest known diseases. An inoculum is initially introduced along an anterior vertebral body with spread through lymphatics, commonly from pulmonary origin. It can be distinguished from pyogenic osteomyelitis where the initial infection is in the subchondral bone adjacent to the endplate and the intervertebral discs are typically affected. Furthermore, tuberculous spondylitis is more common in the thoracic spine, likely given its proximity to the pulmonary source. Current treatment modalities are highly effective against TS, particularly in the absence of severe deformity or neurologic deficit. Early diagnosis is essential to prevent significant morbidity due to progressive bone destruction, kyphotic deformity, and risk of developing paraplegia.

Differential Diagnosis: Differential diagnosis includes fungal osteomyelitis and brucellar spondylitis, both of which may be indistinguishable from tuberculous spondylitis.

References: Kilzilbash QF, Seaworth BJ. Multi-drug resistant tuberculous spondylitis. *Ann Thorac Med* 2016;11(4):233-236.

Smith AS, Weinstein MA, Mizushima A, et al. MR imaging characteristics of tuberculous spondylitis vs vertebral osteomyelitis. *AJNR Am J Neuroradiol* 1989;10:619-625.

6a **Answer A.** Nerve root clumping. The images demonstrates nerve root clumping and abnormal enhancement that is often associated with arachnoiditis. This is caused by irritation and inflammation of the arachnoid matter resulting in abnormal adhesions of the nerve roots to each other and to the surface of the thecal sac.

6b **Answer B.** Surgery. Historically, arachnoiditis has been associated with trauma and infection. In modern times, however, lumbar spine surgery is the most common cause.

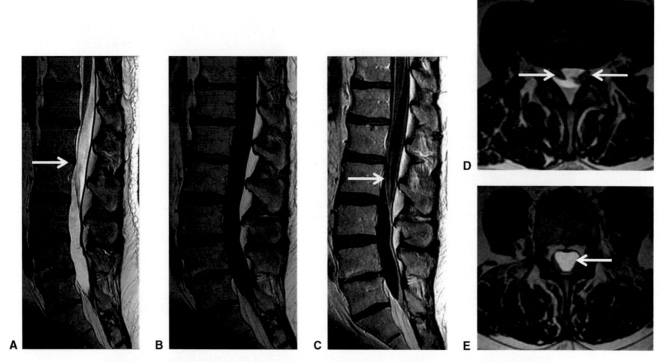

Imaging Findings: Sagittal T2 and pre- and postcontrast T1w images (A–C) and two axial T2WI (D, E) of the lumbar spine show abnormal clumping and enhancement of the cauda equina nerve roots. On the more inferior axial image (E), the nerve roots are adherent to the posterior wall of the thecal sac, giving the impression of absent nerve roots, the so-called empty sac sign.

Discussion: Arachnoiditis is caused by any process that causes inflammation of the arachnoid layer such as infection, trauma, hemorrhage, or intrathecal injection of some substances. It often results in chronic irreversible clumping and tethering of the nerve roots to each other or the surface of the thecal sac. It can occur anywhere along the spine, but is most commonly observed in the lumbar spine with distinctive appearance of the cauda equina nerve roots. Arachnoiditis can also result in the formation of loculated CSF collections that are trapped as a result of adhesions. Restriction of movement and clumping of the nerve roots and leptomeningeal inflammation may present as back or leg pain or less commonly other neurologic deficits such as paresis, paresthesia, or loss of bowel/bladder control. In some cases, the inflammatory changes can calcify leading to "arachnoiditis ossificans." No effective treatment is available. Differential diagnosis includes severe spinal stenosis, carcinomatous meningitis, and some intradural masses.

References: Delamarter RB, et al. Diagnosis of lumbar arachnoiditis by magnetic resonance imaging. *Spine* 1990;15(4):304–310.

Ross JS, et al. MR imaging of lumbar arachnoiditis. *AJR Am J Roentgenol* 1987;149:1025–1032.

7a **Answer C.** Guillain-Barre syndrome. Ascending weakness shortly after a viral illness with imaging features of smooth diffuse nerve root thickening and enhancement is highly suggestive of acute inflammatory demyelinating polyradiculoneuropathy (AIDP) or Guillain-Barre syndrome.

7b **Answer A.** Autoimmune demyelination. The pathologic mechanism for Guillain-Barre syndrome is thought to be autoimmune and related to cross-reactive antibodies against myelin; hence, the effectiveness of plasma exchange or intravenous immunoglobulin (IVIG) as treatment strategies.

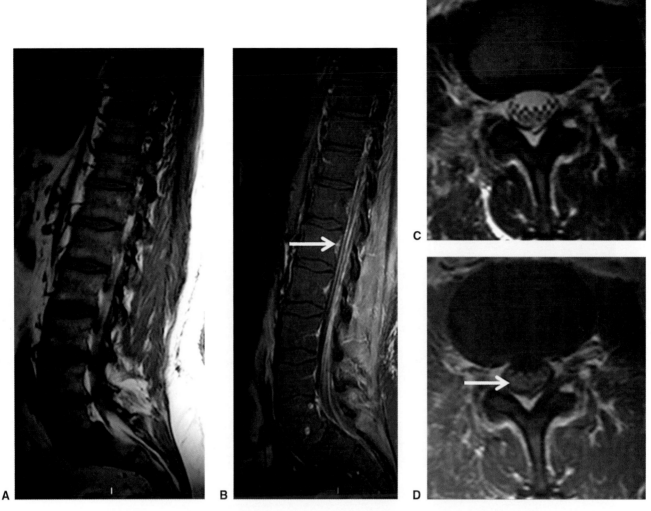

Imaging Findings: Sagittal pre- (A) and postcontrast (B) T1WI of the lumbar spine show smooth enhancement of the cauda equina nerve roots. Axial T2WI (C) and postcontrast T1WI (D) of the cauda equina show slight thickening and avid enhancement of all visualized nerve roots.

Discussion: Acute inflammatory demyelinating polyradiculoneuropathy (AIDP) or Guillain-Barre syndrome is an autoimmune demyelinating disease that is often triggered by circulating antibodies to a recent infection (most commonly respiratory or gastrointestinal). The affected individuals are typically children or young adults without a gender predilection. The disease presents as ascending weakness and can involve the respiratory muscles and the cranial nerves. In addition to supportive care, plasma exchange and IVIG have been found to be effective therapies. However, the disease has a variable course, and, depending on severity, full recovery might take weeks or months. In a minority of cases, the disease may become chronic. In some severe cases, death has been reported.

On imaging of the spine, the most common presentation is mild smooth thickening and enhancement of multiple cauda equina nerve roots and pial enhancement of the conus medullaris. The morphology and signal intensity of the spinal cord are preserved. Although nerve root enhancement is not specific to Guillain-Barre, enhancement of only the anterior nerve roots is strongly suggestive of this disease.

Differential Diagnosis: The imaging differential diagnosis includes lymphoma, metastatic disease, infection, chronic polyneuropathies, postradiation effects, etc. Clinical history and lumbar puncture provide valuable information for narrowing the differential spectrum.

References: Byun WM, et al. Guillain-Barre syndrome: MR imaging findings of the spine in eight patients. *Radiology* 1998;208:137–141.

Yuki N, Hartung HP. Guillain-Barre syndrome. *N Engl J Med* 2012;366:2294–2304.

8a **Answer A.** Multiple sclerosis. There are multifocal brain and cord lesions along with an enhancing lesion in the cervical cord, compatible with multiple sclerosis with evidence of dissemination in space (DIS) and time (DIT).

8b **Answer B.** Simultaneous periventricular and cord lesions. Periventricular and infratentorial or cord lesions are classified as DIS. Although presence of enhancing or new lesion is classified as DIT, it is not a criterion for DIS.

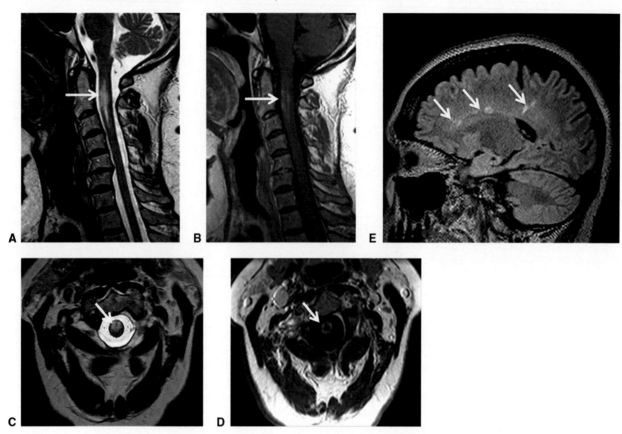

Imaging Findings: Sagittal and axial T2WI (A, C) and postcontrast sagittal and axial T1WI (B, D) of the cervical spine demonstrate short-segment mildly expansile cord signal abnormality with superimposed ill-defined rim enhancement. Brain MRI of the same patient demonstrates multiple periventricular white matter FLAIR hyperintense foci, some of which are oriented perpendicular (E). These findings are consistent with multiple sclerosis.

Discussion: Multiple sclerosis is a demyelinating disease of the central nervous system. The clinical and imaging criteria for diagnosis revolve around the concept of dissemination of lesions in time and space. The disease typically affects young females more than males, and prognosis depends on the subtype. Clinically the disease manifests as muscle weakness/paralysis, paresthesia, gait disturbance, diplopia, and bladder/bowel dysfunction.

The classic MR features of multiple sclerosis plaques when it involves the spine are one or more focal T2 hyperintense lesions that typically involve less than half the cross-sectional area of the cord and are less than two vertebral segments in length. The lesions are typically peripheral and asymmetric and may or may not enhance. Simultaneous presence of brain lesions with evidence of DIS and DIT is highly suggestive of MS. The appearance of the spine lesions alone, however, is nonspecific and often requires correlation with clinical history, lumbar puncture, and brain imaging to arrive at the correct diagnosis.

Differential Diagnosis: The differential diagnosis includes neuromyelitis optica, interamedullary neoplasms, subacute infarction, and infection such as syphilis.

Reference: Filippi M, Rocca M. MR imaging of multiple sclerosis. *Radiology* 2011;259:659–681.

9a **Answer B.** Rheumatoid arthritis. Rheumatoid disease in the axial skeleton typically manifests in the atlantoaxial joint (C1–C2). Osteoarthritis is a degenerative, rather than primary, inflammatory process that often affects the uncovertebral and facet joints at multiple levels. Juvenile idiopathic arthritis and ankylosing spondylitis are associated with bony overgrowth and fusion at multiple levels.

9b **Answer C.** C1–C2 subluxation. Rheumatoid arthritis is a purely erosive inflammatory arthropathy. In advanced cases, erosive changes at the atlantoaxial joint and ligamentous laxity from chronic inflammation result in atlantoaxial subluxation and impaction.

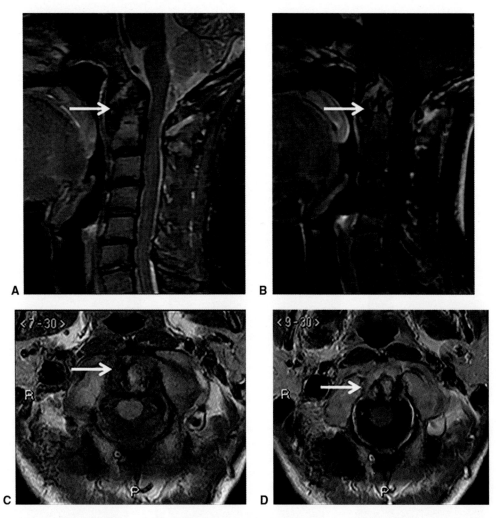

Imaging Findings: Sagittal STIR (A) and sagittal postcontrast (B) T1WI of the cervical spine and axial pre- (C) and postcontrast (D) images at C1–C2 demonstrate enhancing soft tissue centered at the atlantoaxial joint. Although no definite erosions are identified, the enhancing soft tissue likely represents early pannus formation in this patient with confirmed long-standing rheumatoid arthritis and no history of trauma.

Discussion: Rheumatoid arthritis of the axial skeleton most frequently affects the atlantoaxial (C1–C2) articulation. In advanced disease, extensive inflammatory pannus results in erosion of the odontoid process and the facet joints and ligamentous instability, leading to atlantoaxial subluxation or impaction. The inflammatory pannus is mass-like and by direct extension or through erosion/ subluxation can lead to spinal canal compromise and cord compression.

On MR imaging, the rheumatoid pannus often shows heterogeneous high and low signal on T2WI and avid enhancement. Erosions appear as defects along the cortex of the bone with adjacent fluid signal on T2WI. Reactive marrow edema is often present in the affected bone. Radiography (plain films or CT) is more sensitive for detecting erosions, whereas MRI is superior in identifying inflammatory pannus and marrow edema, which typically precede frank erosions.

Generally, the imaging features have to be combined with clinical information (patient demographics, anatomic distribution and time course of disease, and laboratory tests) to arrive at the correct diagnosis.

Differential Diagnosis: The imaging features of rheumatoid arthritis can mimic infection and other seronegative spondyloarthropathies. Correlation with clinical features and involvement of other joints is essential for accurate diagnosis.

References: Jurik AG. Imaging the spine in arthritis—a pictorial review. *Insights Imaging* 2011;2:177–191.

Sommer OF, et al. Rheumatoid arthritis: a practical guide to state-of-the-art imaging, image interpretation, and clinical implications. *Radiographics* 2005;25:381–398.

10a **Answer C.** Hilar lymphadenopathy. The localizer images captured bilateral hilar lymphadenopathy that was subsequently verified on chest CT.

10b **Answer D.** Sarcoidosis. Although metastatic disease, infection, and lymphoma are on the differential, the combination of these imaging features and right paratracheal and bilateral hilar lymphadenopathy strongly favors sarcoidosis.

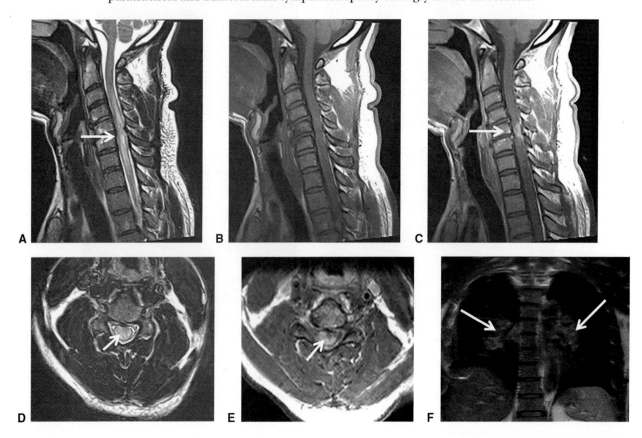

Imaging Findings: Sagittal T2WI (A) and sagittal pre- (B) and postcontrast (C) T1WI of the cervical spine and axial T2WI (D) and postcontrast T1WI (E) at C5–C6 demonstrate cord edema from C3 to T1 and superimposed mild cord expansion and nodular intramedullary enhancement centered at C5–C6 that involves the periphery of the cord more than the center. The coronal localizer images are notable for bilateral hilar lymphadenopathy (F).

Discussion: Sarcoidosis typically affects young adults (20 to 40), and although the systemic disease has a female predominance, spinal sarcoidosis has a male predilection. Imaging evidence of CNS involvement in sarcoidosis is relatively uncommon (<10%), and spinal intramedullary sarcoidosis is even less common (<1%). The pathology of sarcoidosis is noncaseating granuloma formation in multiple organ systems. A wide spectrum of nonspecific imaging features have contributed to its reputation as one of the "great mimickers."

Sarcoidosis of the spine can manifest as a combination of leptomeningeal and intramedullary mass-like enhancement. When intramedullary lesions are present, the cord often appears expanded with focal or diffuse T2 hyperintense signal and variable superimposed nodular intramedullary enhancement that favors the periphery of the cord. This is likely due to spread of leptomeningeal inflammation through perivascular spaces into the cord.

Clinical symptoms are variable and include a combination of weakness, paresthesia, and bladder/bowel dysfunction. Corticosteroids and immunosuppressive agents are the mainstay of therapy.

Differential Diagnosis: The differential diagnosis for intramedullary lesions of sarcoidosis includes intramedullary neoplasms, lymphoma, subacute infarction, multiple sclerosis, and transverse myelitis. The differential diagnosis for leptomeningeal involvement includes infection, including tuberculosis and lymphoma.

References: Ginat DT, et al. Magnetic resonance imaging of neurosarcoidosis. *J Clin Imaging Sci* 2011;1:15.

Sohn M, et al. Spinal cord neurosarcoidosis. *Am J Med Sci* 2014;347:195–198.

11a **Answer B.**   Dorsal columns. The region of signal abnormality sharply delineated by presence of T2 hyperintense signal on the axial images corresponds to the dorsal/posterior columns of the spinal cord.

11b **Answer D.**   Sensory—fine touch, vibration, proprioception. The dorsal column medial lemniscus (DCML) system is responsible for transmission of fine touch, vibration, and proprioception sensory input to the brain.

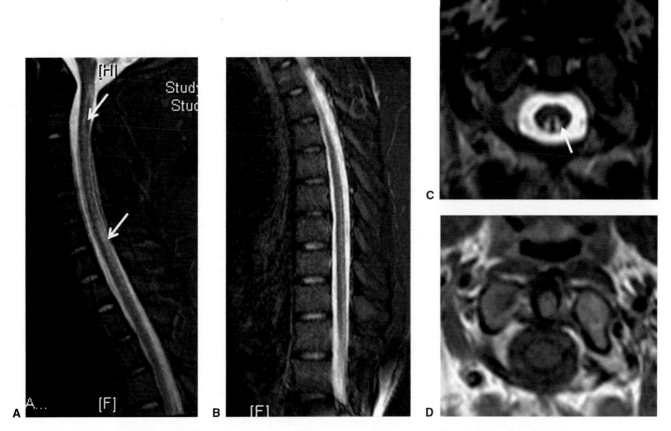

Imaging Findings: Midsagittal STIR images of the cervical and thoracic spine (A, B) and representative axial T2 and postcontrast T1WI (C, D) show nonenhancing signal abnormality in the posterior portion for the entire spinal cord that is limited to the dorsal columns.

Discussion: Subacute combined degeneration, generally attributed to vitamin B_{12} deficiency, results in selective demyelination of the dorsal and sometimes lateral columns of the spinal cord. The presenting symptoms are paresthesia in hands and feet and gait ataxia.

The imaging abnormalities initially manifest in the upper thoracic cord, but can progress to involve the entire length of the cord and are bilateral. The "inverted V sign" on axial T2WI of the spinal cord represents bilateral high signal in the dorsal columns. On sagittal T2/STIR images, the abnormal high signal involves a long segment and although ill defined spares the anterior half of the cord. Enhancement is usually absent. If diagnosed early, the abnormalities resolve and neurologic function improves after correction of B_{12} deficiency.

Differential Diagnosis: The imaging differential diagnosis for subacute combined degeneration includes B_{12} deficiency, either due to inadequate intake or malabsorption or indirectly as a result of copper deficiency or nitrous oxide anesthesia. Additionally, infections such as syphilis, herpes, or HIV may also have a similar imaging appearance.

Reference: Ravina B, et al. MR findings in subacute combined degeneration of the spinal cord. A case of reversible cervical myelopathy. *AJR Am J Roentgenol* 2000;74(3):863–865.

12a **Answer A.** Family history. There is diffuse fusiform enlargement of nerve roots. Many hereditary polyneuropathies can explain the imaging findings and clinical features in this patient. Therefore, a careful clinical history is extremely important.

12b **Answer C.** Charcot Marie tooth disease. The imaging and clinical features are most compatible with Charcot-Marie-Tooth disease, one of the hereditary motor and sensory neuropathy.

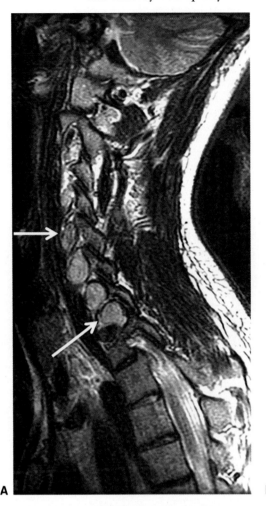

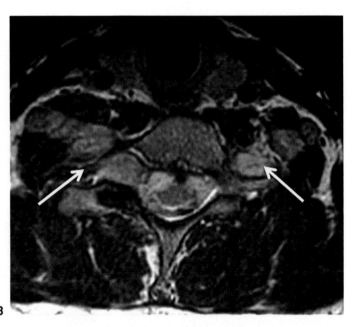

A   B

Imaging findings: There is fusiform enlargement of nerve roots with mild intrinsic T2 hyperintensity seen bilaterally in the cervical spine (A and B). Reported lack of contrast enhancement argues against plexiform neurofibromatosis. In the younger age group as in this patient, this finding is most consistent with Charcot-Marie-Tooth disease.

Discussion: Charcot-Marie-Tooth disease (CMT) is an autosomal dominant hereditary motor and sensory neuropathy characterized by distal muscle weakness, foot deformities, decreased nerve conduction velocity, and typical onion bulb hypertrophy noted on pathology. On imaging, there is fusiform enlargement of nerve roots diffusely and variable minimal to no enhancement.

Differential Diagnosis: There may be cranial nerve involvement associated with CMT, although not as commonly as, with chronic inflammatory demyelinating polyneuropathy (CIDP), which is a differential diagnosis. Overall clinical features, EMG findings, and family history help differentiation with CIDP. Other etiologies such as plexiform neurofibromas, neurosarcoidosis, lymphoma, amyloid polyneuropathy, or inflammatory demyelinating polyneuropathies may also have varying degrees of nerve enlargement; however, many of these also have relatively more enhancement.

References: Aho TR, Wallace RC, Pitt AM, et al. Charcot-Marie-Tooth disease: extensive cranial nerve involvement on CT and MR imaging. *AJNR Am J Neuroradiol* 2004;25(3):494–497.

De Smet K, De Maeseneer M, Talebian Yazdi A, et al. MRI in hypertrophic mono- and polyneuropathies. *AJNR Am J Neuroradiol* 2004;25(3):494–497.

13a **Answer C.** CRP elevation. This is likely ankylosing spondylitis, with presence of fusing syndesmophytes, bilateral sacroiliac joint fusion, and a chronic fracture involving L3 vertebral body. Although nonspecific, CRP has been found to be elevated in AS. Because this is a seronegative spondyloarthropathy, the RF factor is absent. ANA is seen with lupus, and there is no evidence of infection to suggest leukocytosis.

13b **Answer B.** Ankylosing spondylitis.

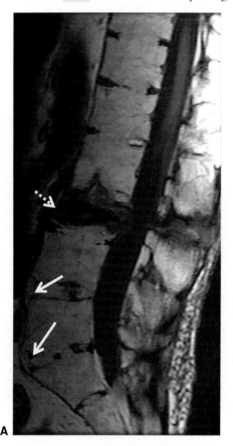

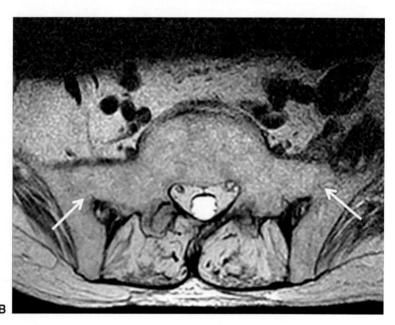

Imaging Findings: Fusing thin smooth syndesmophytes (A) and fusion of bilateral sacroiliac joints (B) are seen on sagittal and axial T1w images. Note a chronic compression fracture of L3 (dotted arrow, A). These findings are compatible with ankylosing spondylitis.

Discussion: Ankylosing spondylitis (AS) is a debilitating seronegative spondyloarthropathy, characterized by early onset of symmetric, bilateral sacroiliac joint inflammation. Early in the course of disease, there is subchondral bone resorption along the iliac side of the joint with joint space widening and reactive sclerosis. Later in the course of disease, the joint space is completely ankylosed. The hallmark of vertebral column involvement is formation of fusing syndesmophytes that result from ossification within the outer fibers of the disc annulus fibrosis. Extensive syndesmophyte formation results in fusion across the disc space and an undulating spinal contour, namely, the bamboo spine. The fused spine is rigid and prone to fractures and, as seen in this case, therefore should be suspected in AS patients with acute worsening of pain.

Differential Diagnosis: The differential diagnosis is spondylosis deformans due to prominent osteophyte formation; however, those degenerative bony spurs typically arise slightly removed from disc space. Diffuse idiopathic skeletal hyperostosis is typically thick with flowing pattern of ossification along the anterior longitudinal ligament. Additionally, the sacroiliitis is not seen with these latter entities.

Reference: Ostergaard M, Lambert RG. Imaging in ankylosing spondylitis. *Ther Adv Musculoskelet Dis* 2012;4(4):301–311.

14 **Answer A.**   Longitudinally extensive nature. The lesion in the thoracic cord spans more than three vertebral segments. Such involvement is relatively unusual with multiple sclerosis.

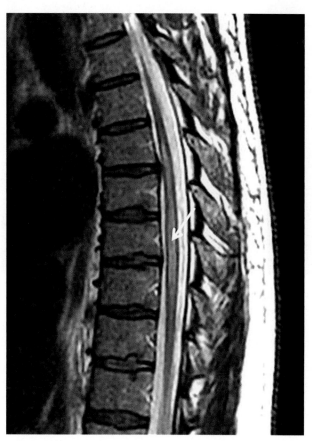

Imaging Findings: There is extensive intrinsic T2 hyperintensity within the thoracic cord spanning greater than three vertebral segments, compatible with longitudinally extensive transverse myelitis (LETM).

Discussion: Longitudinally extensive transverse myelitis (LETM) is characterized by intrinsic cord signal intensity abnormality that spans more than three vertebral segments with greater than two-thirds cord cross-section involved. There may be associated cord expansion and variable degree of enhancement.

Differential Diagnosis: This pattern of abnormality has wide differential considerations, such as demyelinating conditions, collagen vascular disorders, paraneoplastic, radiation changes, and infectious myelitis. Vascular abnormalities including dural AV fistula and cord infarct can also result in such signal changes. Idiopathic TM is a diagnosis of exclusion and accounts for 15% to 30% of acute cases. Clinically, these patients can present with motor, sensory, and autonomic dysfunction. Clinical course and management of LETM rely on the underlying cause. The idiopathic TM prognosis is variable ranging from completely recovery to severe disability.

References: Choi KH, Lee KS, Chung SO, et al. Idiopathic transverse myelitis: MR characteristics. *AJNR Am J Neuroradiol* 1996;17(6):1151–1160.

Mirbagheri S, Eckart Sorte D, Zamora CA, et al. Evaluation and management of longitudinally extensive transverse myelitis: a guide for radiologists. *Clin Radiol* 2016;71(10):960–971.

15 **Answer B.** Urgent neurosurgical consultation. There is discitis/osteomyelitis and epidural abscess causing cord compression. Urgent neurosurgical consultation is therefore necessary.

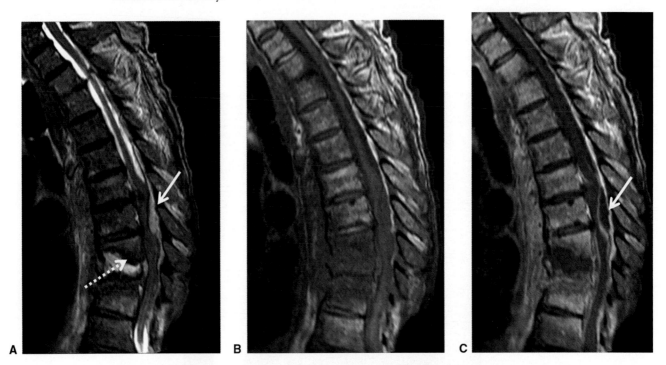

Imaging Findings: There is a posterior epidural fluid collection with rim enhancement, seen on sagittal T2 (A) and postcontrast sagittal T1w image (C). Note presence of edema and fluid in the disc space and vertebral body (dotted arrow, A). Findings are compatible with discitis/osteomyelitis with epidural abscess.

Discussion: Epidural abscess is a nontraumatic spinal cord emergency. The neurologic deficits are severe and in the absence of timely intervention can become permanent. These can result from hematogenous inoculation or direct contiguous spread from discitis osteomyelitis. The most common causative organism is *Staphylococcus aureus*. Other etiologies include *Streptococcus, E. coli,* or *Pseudomonas*. IV drug use and immunocompromised state are underlying risk factors.

The neurologic deficits are largely due to extrinsic compression from the epidural abscess; occasionally, this may be accompanied by a thrombophlebitis contributing to neurologic compromise. Therefore, urgent neurosurgical consultation for decompression and drainage is warranted for these patients. IV antibiotic alone will not help with the spinal cord decompression.

Reference: Flanagan EP, Pittock SJ. Diagnosis and management of spinal cord emergencies. *Handb Clin Neurol* 2017;140:319–335.

11

Spine Neoplasms, Spine and Neck Vascular Diseases

JONATHAN YOUNGSUK KIM • ARCHANA SIDDALINGAPPA •
LIDIA MAYUMI NAGAE • RAFAEL ROJAS • PRACHI DUBEY • RAFEEQUE BHADELIA

QUESTIONS

1 A 52-year-old man presents with progressive lower back pain.

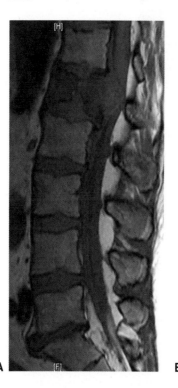
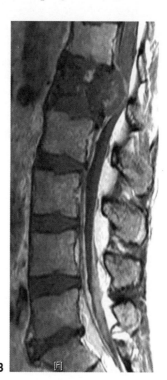
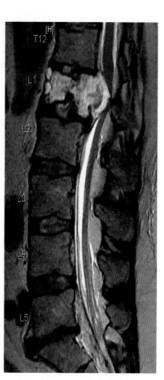

What is the most likely diagnosis?

A. Hemangioma

B. Osteomyelitis

C. Neoplasm

D. Aneurysmal bone cyst

2 Which of the following lesions is the most common malignancy of the spine?

    A. Chondrosarcoma

    B. Chordoma

    C. Metastasis

    D. Osteosarcoma

3 A 72-year-old woman presenting with right lower extremity weakness.

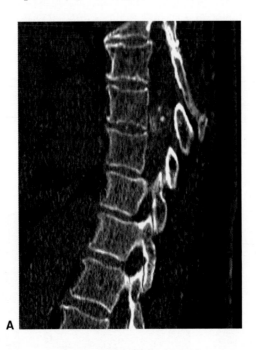

A

3a What is the next best step in evaluation?

    A. No further evaluation

    B. CT with contrast

    C. MRI with contrast

    D. MRI without contrast

An MRI with contrast was performed. Key images are shown below:

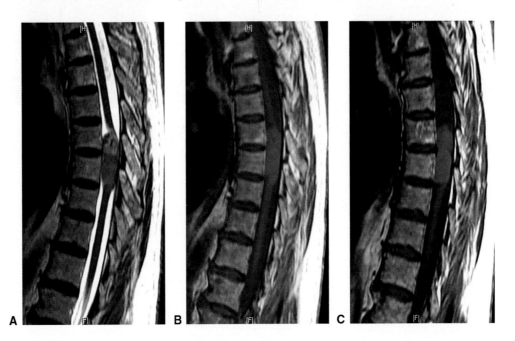

A   B   C

3b What is the most likely diagnosis?

    A. Meningioma

    B. Metastasis

    C. Schwannoma

    D. Paraganglioma

4 A 35-year-old man presents with lower back pain and lower extremity radiculopathy.

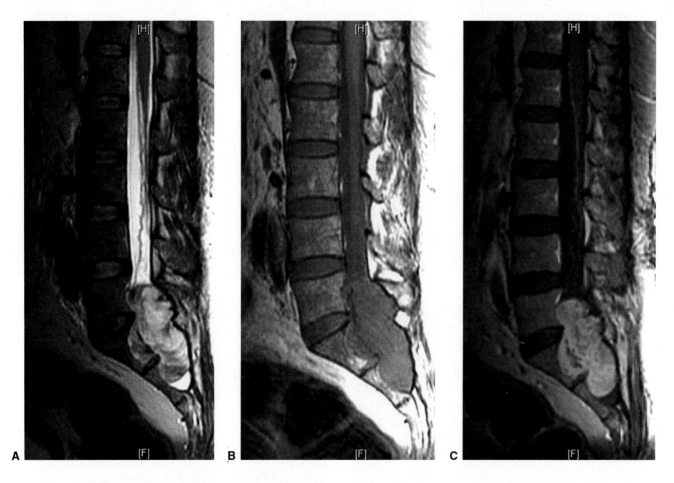

4a What is the most likely diagnosis?

    A. Meningioma

    B. Schwannoma

    C. Myxopapillary ependymoma

    D. Chordoma

4b Which of the following anatomic location best characterizes this lesion?

    A. Intradural, extramedullary

    B. Intramedullary

    C. Extradural

    D. Presacral

5 A 26-year-old woman presents with severe neck pain.

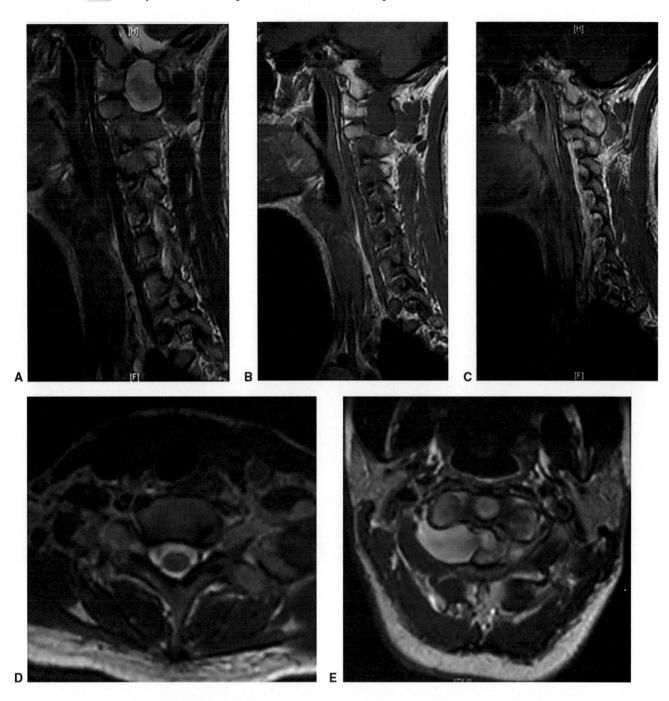

5a What is the most likely diagnosis?

    A. Meningioma

    B. Abscess

    C. Nerve sheath tumor

    D. Perineural root sleeve cyst

5b Multiple cutaneous lesions are also seen. Which of the following is the most likely underlying disorder?

    A. Tuberous sclerosis

    B. Neurofibromatosis type 1

    C. Neurofibromatosis type 2

    D. Von Hippel-Lindau syndrome

6   A 55-year-old man presenting with lower back pain.

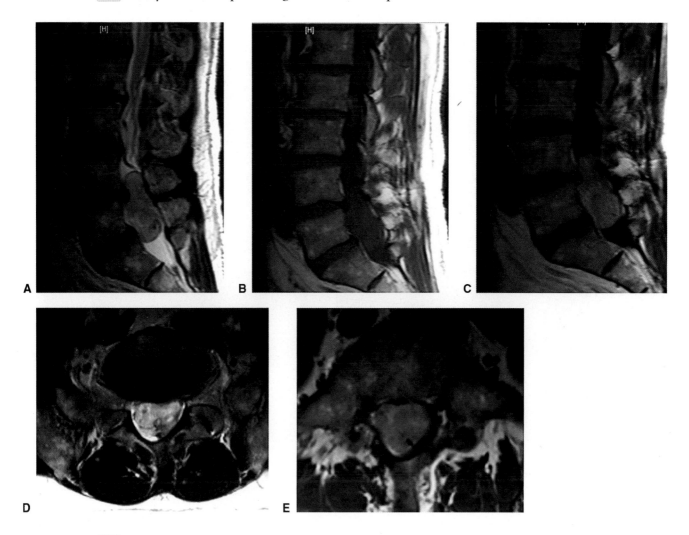

6a   What imaging finding is seen in this case that suggests a specific diagnosis?

A. Cap sign
B. Flow voids
C. Target sign
D. Curtain sign

6b   Given the imaging findings, what is the most likely diagnosis?

A. Lymphoma
B. Hematoma
C. Meningioma
D. Paraganglioma

7 A 15-year-old male presents with back pain. Key images are shown below:

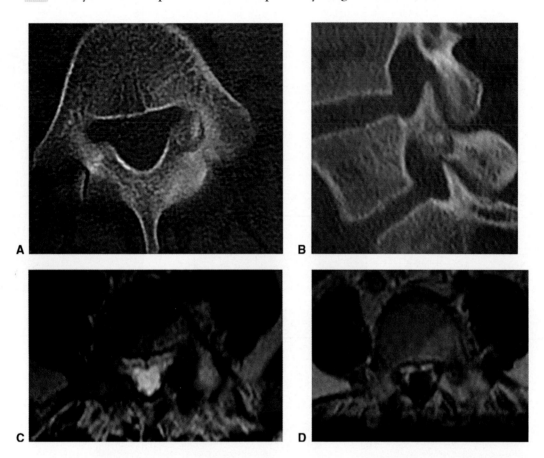

7a What is the most likely etiology of this lesion?

    A. Traumatic
    B. Infectious
    C. Benign tumor
    D. Malignant tumor

7b Which of the following is a typical clinical presentation seen with this entity?

    A. Sports injury
    B. Night pain relieved with aspirin
    C. Intravenous drug use
    D. Known primary malignancy

8   A 67-year-old male presents with severe lower extremity weakness and urinary incontinence. Key images from an MRI are shown below:

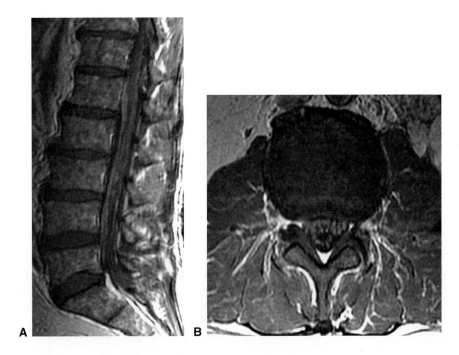

A   B

8a   What is the salient imaging finding seen in this patient?

   A. Nerve root enhancement and thickening
   B. Phlegmon and inflammation
   C. Endplate cortical erosion
   D. Vertical fracture of the vertebral body

8b   What is the most likely diagnosis?

   A. Campylobacter viral infection with GI symptoms
   B. Leptomeningeal metastasis
   C. Demyelinating disease
   D. Arachnoiditis

9   Key images from an MRI performed for evaluation of a spinal mass are shown below.

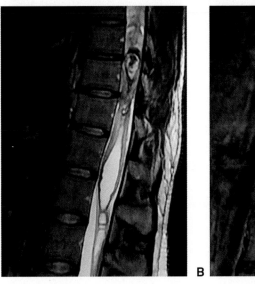 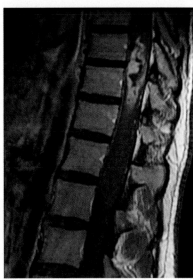

A   B

9a   What is the most likely diagnosis?

    A. Hemangioblastoma
    B. Meningioma
    C. Metastasis
    D. Astrocytoma

9b   Which of the following imaging features is characteristically associated with this entity?

    A. Cyst with a nodule
    B. Syringohydromyelia
    C. Infiltrative and enhancing mass
    D. Marginal cysts and peripheral hemorrhage

10   A 30-year-old male presents with gait ataxia and upper extremity motor weakness. Key images from an MRI are shown below:

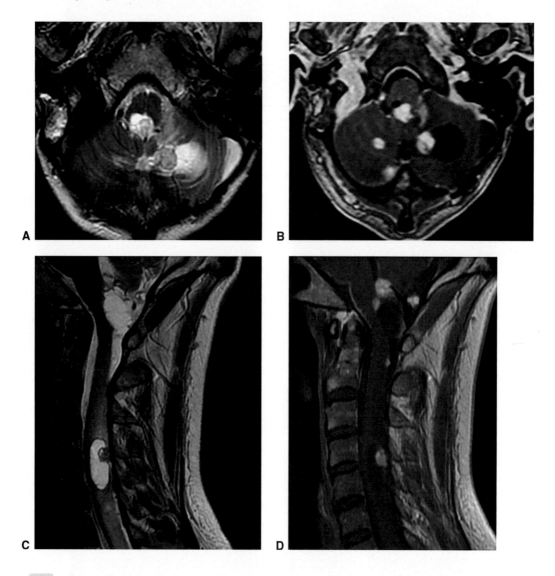

10a What is the most likely cause for the brain findings?

    A. Congenital
    B. Inherited
    C. Acquired
    D. Cannot be determined

10b What is the most likely diagnosis?

    A. Pilocytic astrocytoma

    B. Medulloblastoma

    C. Hemangioblastoma

    D. Ependymoma

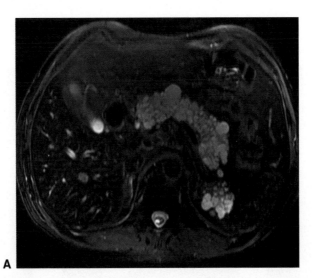

A

10c Based on additional findings shown above, what is the associated syndrome?

    A. Tuberous sclerosis

    B. Sturge-Weber

    C. Von Hippel-Lindau syndrome

    D. Neurofibromatosis 2

11 A 30-year-old female presents with carotidynia. Key image is shown below.

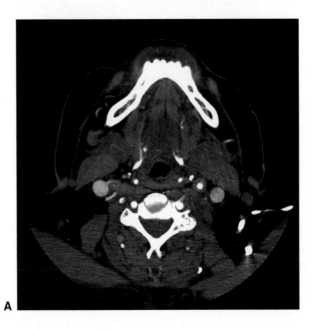

A

11a What is the most likely diagnosis?

    A. Kawasaki syndrome

    B. Deep venous thrombosis

    C. Septic thrombophlebitis

    D. Takayasu arteritis

11b Which of the following vessel wall layers are typically involved with this entity?

    A. Intima

    B. Media

    C. Adventitia

    D. Panarteritis

12 A 40-year-old male presents with neck pain, gait disturbances, and paresthesias. An MRI with contrast was performed. Key images are shown below.

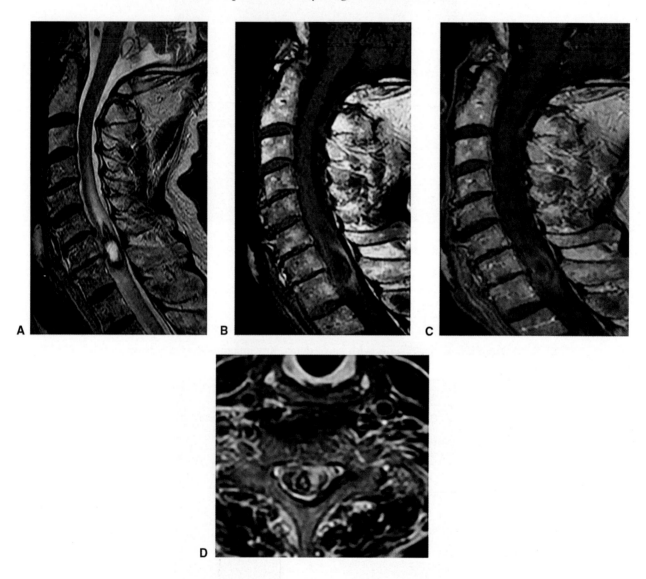

12a What is the most likely diagnosis?

    A. Hemangioblastoma

    B. Meningioma

    C. Astrocytoma

    D. Ependymoma

12b Which of the following imaging findings is a characteristic feature of this entity?

    A. Cyst with a nodule

    B. Marginal cysts and peripheral hemorrhage

    C. Enhancing mass

    D. Syringohydromyelia

13 A 62-year-old female presents with a history of chronic back pain, exacerbated after fall. A CT, followed by an MRI of the spine, was performed. Key images are shown below:

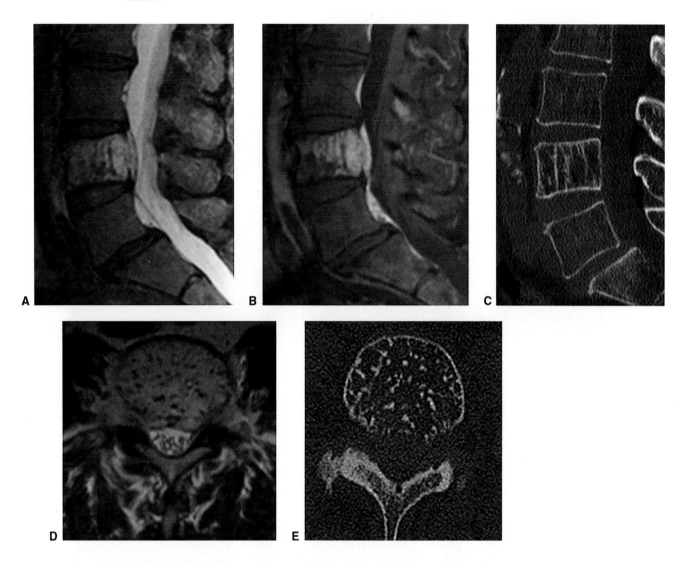

13a Which of the following imaging features are characteristically seen with this entity?

A. Rugger jersey spine
B. Bullet shaped vertebra
C. Polka-dot appearance
D. Picture frame vertebra

13b What is the most likely diagnosis?

A. Typical osseous hemangioma
B. Aggressive spinal hemangioma
C. Osteopoikilosis
D. Multiple myeloma

14 A 50-year-old male presents with severe upper thoracic pain. Key images from an MRI are shown below.

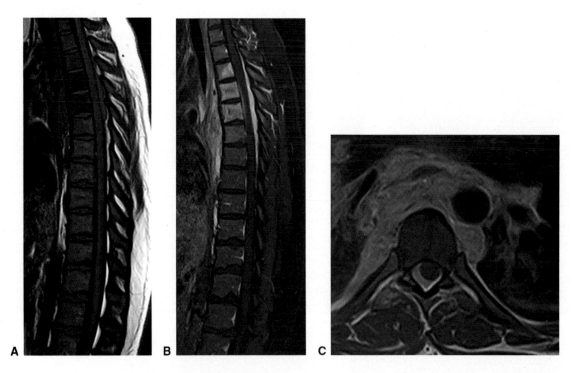

What is the most likely diagnosis?

A. Discitis/osteomyelitis with abscess
B. Aortitis with reactive osseous sclerosis
C. Lymphoma with soft tissue component
D. Aggressive hemangioma with soft tissue component

15 A 36-year-old male presents with a genetic syndrome and increasing neck pain. Key images from CT and MRI are shown below.

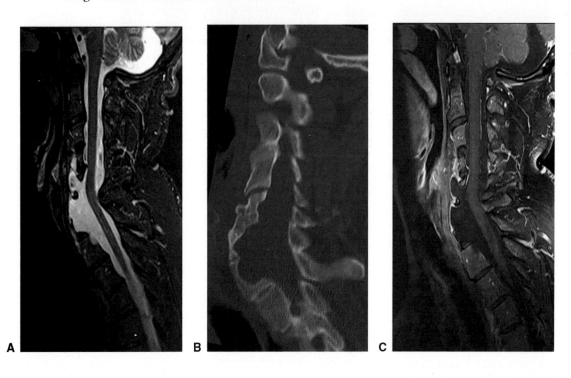

15a Which of the following processes would you favor in the bone?

    A. Neoplastic

    B. Congenital with segmentation anomaly

    C. Long-standing process with bone remodeling

    D. Postsurgical changes

15b What is the most likely diagnosis?

    A. Butterfly vertebrae

    B. Dural ectasia

    C. Diastematomyelia

    D. Arachnoid cyst

16 A 60-year-old male presents with gait imbalance and progressive motor weakness. An MRI was performed, and key images are shown below:

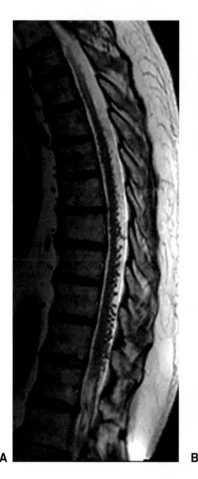
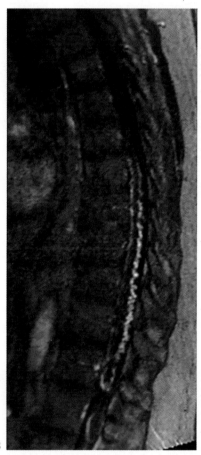
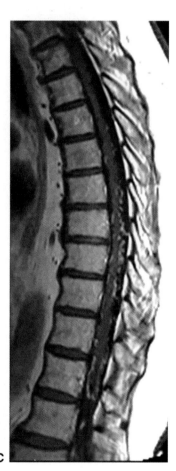

A   B   C

16a What is the most likely diagnosis?

    A. Leptomeningeal metastasis

    B. Dural AV fistula

    C. Intramedullary AVM

    D. Diffuse arachnoiditis

16b Which of the following conditions may result from the above abnormality?

    A. Intraspinal arachnoid cysts because of adhesions

    B. Intracranial CSF dissemination of metastasis

    C. Myelopathy secondary to venous congestion

    D. Cord infarction because of radiculomedullary artery thrombosis

17   Key images from an MRA neck performed for evaluation of dizziness are shown below. There is reported history of an abnormal neck Doppler evaluation.

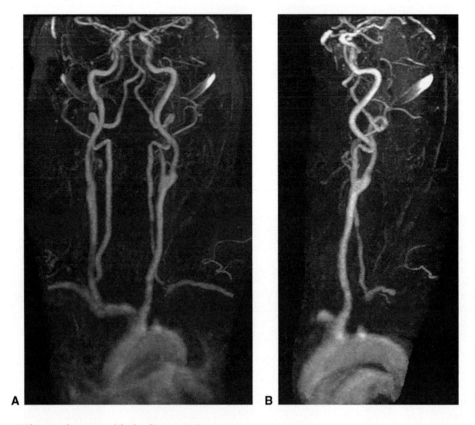

A   B

What is the most likely diagnosis?

A. Vertebral artery dissection
B. Severe atherosclerotic vertebral stenosis
C. Fibromuscular Dysplasia
D. Subclavian steal syndrome

18   A 55-year-old diabetic patient develops acute-onset sensory deficits in the postoperative period following surgery for toe amputation.

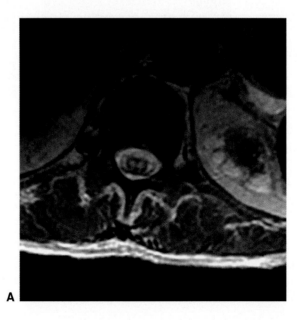

A

18a What is the most likely diagnosis in the current clinical scenario?

    A. Central cord infarction because of severe hypotension
    B. Anterior cord infarction secondary to embolic event
    C. Nitrous oxide–induced myelopathy
    D. Demyelinating disease

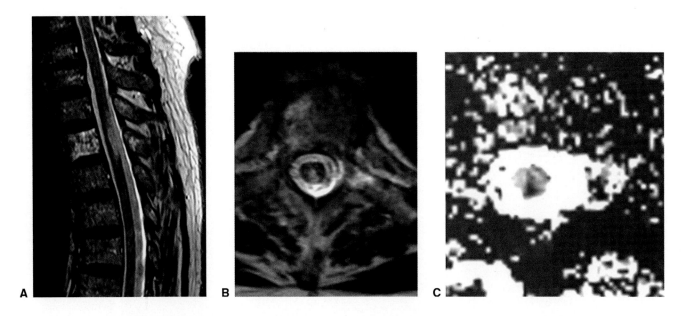

18b This is a different patient with acute-onset deficit in vibration and proprioception. MRI key images are shown above. What is the most likely diagnosis?

    A. Central cord infarction
    B. Anterior cord infarction
    C. Posterior cord infarction
    D. Vascular malformation

ANSWERS AND EXPLANATIONS

1 **Answer C.** Neoplasm. There is an expansile vertebral body mass that extends into the anterior epidural space, most likely neoplastic in etiology.

2 **Answer C.** Metastasis.

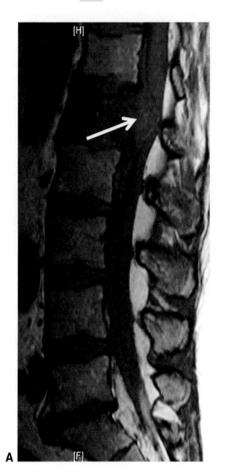
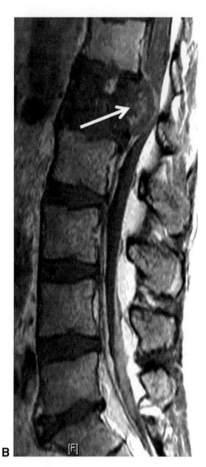
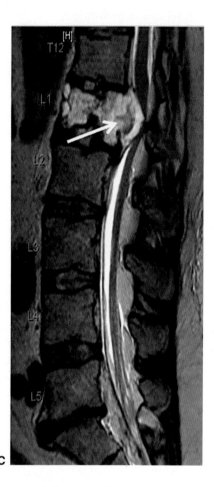

A   B   C

Imaging Findings: Images demonstrate a pathologic compression deformity of the L1 vertebral body with a highly T2 hyperintense (C), T1 hypointense (A), and mildly enhancing lesion (B), replacing the entirety of the vertebral body with epidural extension and resultant cord compression.

Discussion: Metastatic disease, myeloma, and lymphoproliferative tumors are the most common malignant spinal tumors. These usually present with multiple lesions. In case of solitary lesions, one must consider lesions such as plasmacytoma, Ewing sarcoma and chordoma. Chordoma, although quite rare, remains the most common primary malignancy of spine in adults after lymphoproliferative lesions and myeloma. It arises from cells of the primitive notochord and thus can arise from the bone anywhere in the axial skeleton from Rathke pouch to the coccyx. Cases typically are most common in the sacrococcygeal region followed by the clivus and then the vertebral bodies. Though chordomas are locally aggressive, they metastasize relatively infrequently, roughly 15% of the time. Chordomas are treated with surgical resection and radiation therapy with gross total resection having a better prognosis.

Differential Diagnosis: Unfortunately, the imaging appearance of chordoma can be quite nonspecific and the differential would include metastasis, lymphoproliferative disorder/plasmacytoma, chondrosarcoma, and giant cell tumor.

References: Ha AS, Chew FS. Imaging of sacral masses: self-assessment module. *AJR Am J Roentgenol* 2010;195:S32–S36.

Murphey MD, Andrews CL, Flemming DJ, et al. From the archives of the AFIP. Primary tumors of the spine: radiologic pathologic correlation. *Radiographics* 1996;16:1131–1158.

Nishiguchi T, Mochizuki K, Ohsawa M, et al. Differentiating benign notochordal cell tumors from chordomas: radiographic features on MRI, CT, and tomography. *AJR Am J Roentgenol* 2011;196:644–650.

3a **Answer C.** MRI with contrast. Although a partially calcified mass of the spinal canal is clearly evident on the CT images, MRI with contrast is indicated for further evaluation given superior soft tissue contrast and also to evaluate the relationship of the mass to the spinal cord.

3b **Answer A.** Meningioma. All choices are reasonable differential etiologies, however given intradural, extramedullary location, well-defined borders, broad-based dural attachment, calcifications, and relatively homogenous enhancement, meningioma is most likely. Meningioma is overall the second most common intradural, extramedullary lesion in the spine, with the thoracic spine being the most common location.

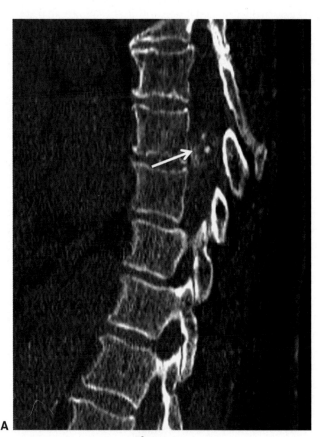

Figure 1

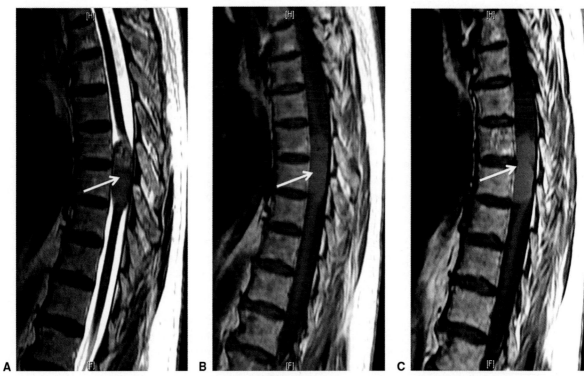

Figure 2

Imaging Findings: Figure 1. This figure shows a sagittal CT of the thoracic spine demonstrating a partially calcified lesion within the spinal canal at the midthoracic level.

Figure 2. This figure shows sagittal T2, T1, and T1 postcontrast images demonstrating a T1 and T2 intermediate intradural extramedullary lesion with areas of low signal corresponding to calcification, a broad-based dural attachment, and relatively homogenous postcontrast enhancement. There is significant displacement and compression of the adjacent spinal cord.

Discussion: Spinal meningioma is the second most common intradural extramedullary spinal neoplasm after schwannoma and is more common in women and elderly. Extradural or mixed location is possible, though much less common. Within the spine, meningioma is most common in the thoracic spine, followed by the cervical spine, and is rarely seen in the lumbosacral spine.

Most lesions are isolated, and when multiple lesions are seen, neurofibromatosis type 2 should be suspected. Imaging findings are generally identical to intracranial meningioma, with a dural-based, homogeneously enhancing lesion with calcifications being common. Like within the intracranial compartment, a dural tail and adjacent hyperostosis can be seen, though less common. Total surgical resection is generally curative, and recurrence is uncommon.

Differential Diagnosis: The primary differential etiology is nerve sheath tumor, though other possibilities include other intradural extramedullary lesions such as ependymoma or metastasis.

References: De Verdelhan O, Haegelen C, Carsin-Nicol B, et al. MR imaging features of spinal schwannomas and meningiomas. *J Neuroradiol* 2005;32:42–49.

Lee JW, Lee IS, Choi KU, et al. CT and MRI findings of calcified spinal meningiomas: correlation with pathological findings. *Skeletal Radiol* 2010;39:345–352.

4a **Answer C.** Myxopapillary ependymoma. This is the most common intradural extramedullary lesion of the cauda equina/filum terminale and is thus the most likely diagnosis in this case. Though imaging findings are nonspecific, hemorrhagic component and calcification, shown here, are commonly seen in myxopapillary ependymoma.

4b **Answer A.** Intradural, extramedullary. The lesion in question is intradural, extramedullary in location, which is most common for myxopapillary ependymoma. The other locations are possible, but far less likely.

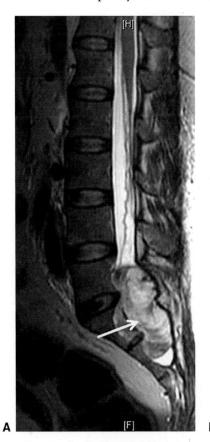
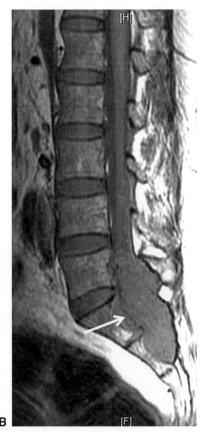
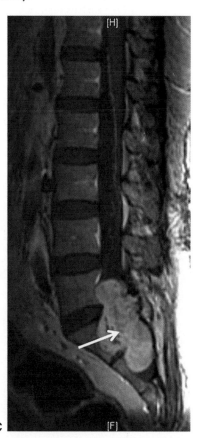

A   B   C

Imaging Findings: Images demonstrate a large, lobulated T2 hyperintense (A), largely homogeneously enhancing (C), intradural extramedullary mass at the lumbosacral junction. There are areas of low T2 signal suggesting hemorrhage and calcification, respectively. There is scalloping of the adjacent posterior vertebral bodies (A–C).

Discussion: Myxopapillary ependymoma is a low-grade variant of ependymoma that is limited to the conus medullaris/filum terminale and is also the most common malignancy in this location in adults. This variant has a younger age of presentation in the 30s as compared to other ependymoma subtypes and demonstrates a slight male predominance.

Differential Diagnosis: Imaging features can be difficult to distinguish from other lesions such as schwannoma or paraganglioma in the intradural location. Depending on the level of involvement, it can also be difficult to distinguish between other entities such as chordoma or giant cell tumor. However, hemorrhage is more common in myxopapillary ependymoma. As a low-grade tumor, outcomes are generally good with total surgical resection. However, in a minority of cases, the lesion can disseminate through CSF and multiple lesions can be seen.

References: Abul-Kasim K, Thurnher MM, McKeever P, et al. Intradural spinal tumors: current classification and MRI features. *Neuroradiology* 2008;50:301–314.

Ha AS, Chew FS. Imaging of sacral masses: self-assessment module. *AJR Am J Roentgenol* 2010;195:S32–S36.

Shors SM, Jones TA, Jhaveri MD, et al. Myxopapillary ependymoma of the sacrum. *Radiographics* 2006;26:S111–S116.

Wippold FJ, Smirniotopoulos JG, Moran CJ, et al. MR imaging of myxopapillary ependymoma: findings and value to determine extent of tumor and its relation to intraspinal structures. *AJR Am J Roentgenol* 1995;165:1263–1267.

5a **Answer C.** Nerve sheath tumor. Well-circumscribed T2 hyperintense mass centered in the neural foramen with bony expansion is most consistent with a diagnosis of nerve sheath tumor. Based on appearance, it would be impossible to distinguish between neurofibroma and Meningioma is a reasonable differential diagnosis, though is the second most common intradural extramedullary spinal lesion behind nerve sheath tumors. Abscess is unlikely given the lack of a clear source and lack of surrounding inflammatory change. Perineural root sleeve cyst is also excluded as this lesion demonstrates enhancement.

5b **Answer B.** Neurofibromatosis type 1. Given the presence of a likely nerve sheath tumor and cutaneous lesion the patient most likely has neurofibromatosis type 1. Neurofibromatosis type 2 lacks the cutaneous lesions and is associated with intracranial schwannomas as well as meningioma and spinal ependymoma.

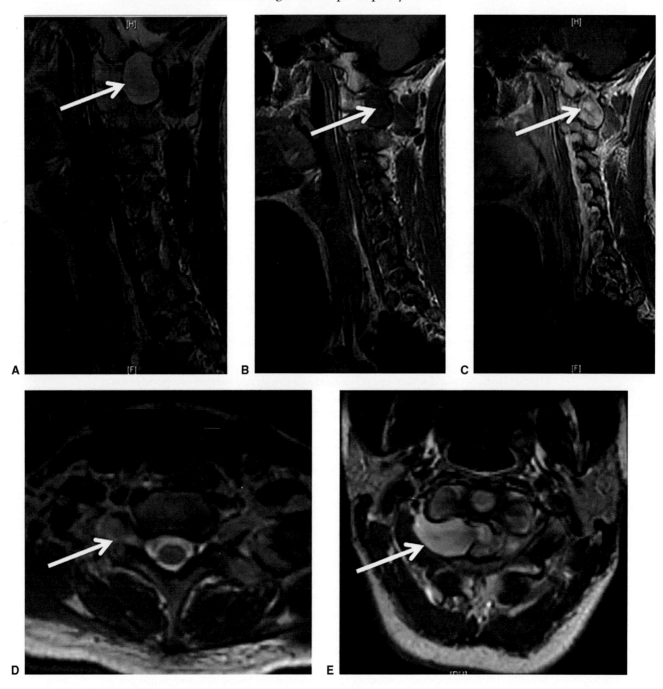

Imaging Findings: Images demonstrate a well-circumscribed, lobulated T2 hyperintense lesion, (arrow A) with heterogeneous enhancement, (arrow B and C) centered in the right C1–C2 neural foramen (arrow D and E).

Discussion: Nerve sheath tumors are benign neoplasms and constitute the most common primary intradural extramedullary spinal lesion. Purely extradural or mixed intradural and extradural location can be seen but is less common. Nerve sheath tumors include both schwannoma and neurofibroma, though these entities largely cannot be distinguished from one another by imaging characteristics alone. Nerve sheath tumors typically arise from the dorsal root ganglion, and thus affected patients present more often with pain rather than weakness.

Neurofibromas have an association with neurofibromatosis type 1 and multiple lesions are common. Neurofibromas tend to grow encasing a nerve root and sometimes a target sign suggesting this can be seen, though this is nonspecific and can also be seen in schwannoma. Although neurofibromas are a benign lesion, a minority (~10%) can undergo malignant transformation into neurofibrosarcoma.

Spinal schwannomas have an association with neurofibromatosis type 2. When present, hemorrhage and cystic degeneration is a more common finding in schwannoma rather than neurofibroma and may suggest toward a specific diagnosis, though these can be seen in both entities. As compared to neurofibroma, schwannomas almost never undergo malignant degeneration.

For either lesion, surgical excision is considered curative, though recurrence is more common when these lesions occur in the background of neurofibromatosis type 1/2.

References: Abul-Kasim K, Thurnher MM, McKeever P, et al. Intradural spinal tumors: current classification and MRI features. *Neuroradiology* 2008;50:301–314.

De Verdelhan O, Haegelen C, Carsin-Nicol B, et al. MR imaging features of spinal schwannomas and meningiomas. *J Neuroradiol* 2005;32:42–49.

Mautner VF, Tatagiba M, Lindenau M, et al. Spinal tumors in patients with neurofibromatosis type 2: MR imaging study of frequency, multiplicity, and variety. *AJR Am J Roentgenol* 1995;165:951–955.

6a **Answer B.** Flow voids. Scattered flow voids are seen especially on the sagittal T2 sequence, which is suggestive of paraganglioma. Cap sign refers to a rim of T2 hypointensity or susceptibility artifact denoting hemorrhage, which is nonspecific and can be seen in both ependymoma and paraganglioma. The target sign refers to a targetoid appearance of neurofibroma on T2 imaging with a bright rim and dark core. Curtain sign refers to the appearance of a vertebral body lesion with anterior epidural extension, which causes a bilobed uplifting of the posterior longitudinal ligament.

6b **Answer D.** Paraganglioma. The presence of flow voids in this case is most suggestive of paraganglioma.

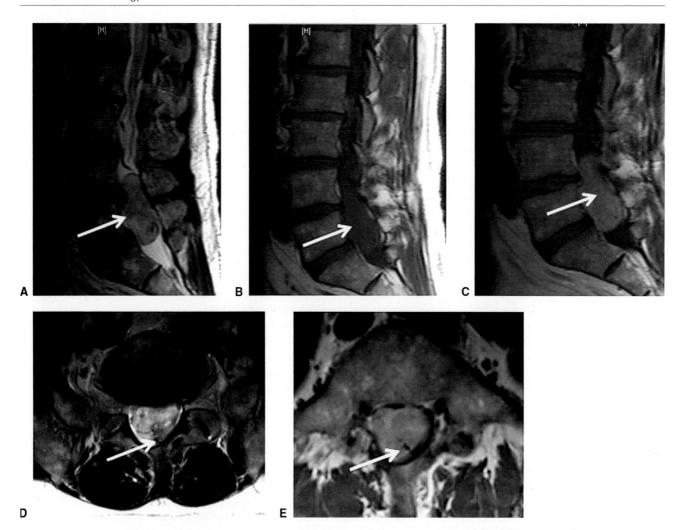

Imaging Findings: Images demonstrate a relatively well-defined, homogeneously enhancing, extramedullary, intradural mass centered at the level of L5. Axial T2 images demonstrate scattered, punctate areas of low signal suggestive of flow voids (arrow in D and E).

Discussion: Spinal paraganglioma is a neuroendocrine tumor, which is histologically identical to paraganglioma at any other site, and can occur at any location where there are paraganglion cells such as the adrenal gland (pheochromocytoma), paravertebral station, and head and neck (glomus tumors).

Spinal paraganglioma is rare, with most cases of paraganglioma being adrenal in origin and the majority of extra-adrenal cases being located in the head and neck. Despite its rarity, paraganglioma should be considered in the differential along with the more common entities of schwannoma or ependymoma as outcomes are dependent on totality of surgical resection and as these tumors are considered insensitive to radiation therapy. However, complete surgical resection is usually curative, and recurrence after resection is uncommon (<5%).

Differential Diagnosis: Includes schwannoma, neurofibroma, ependymoma, and meningioma.

References: Mishra T, Goel NA, Goel AH. Primary paraganglioma of the spine: a clinicopathological study of eight cases. *J Craniovertebr Junction Spine* 2014;5:20–24.

Sahdev A, Sohaib A, Monson JP, et al. CT and MR imaging of unusual locations of extra-adrenal paragangliomas (pheochromocytomas). *Eur Radiol* 2005;15:85–92.

Sundgren P, Annertz M, Englund E, et al. Paragangliomas of the spinal canal. *Neuroradiology* 1999;41:788–794.

7a **Answer C.** Benign tumor. Nidus with surrounding edema is classic appearance of osteoid osteoma, a benign tumor.

7b **Answer B.** Night pain relieved with aspirin. Patients with osteoid osteoma present with night pain relieved by aspirin, NSAIDs. Some patients have scoliosis related to muscle spasm.

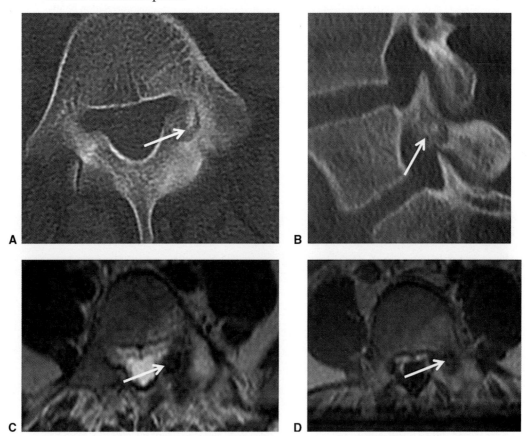

Imaging Findings: Axial and sagittal CT images at L5 demonstrate a central nidus with variable amount of ossification. The nidus measures <1.5 cm. There is dense sclerosis around the tumor (A and B). Axial T2 (C) and postcontrast T1 axial (D) images demonstrate a rounded T2 hypointense nidus with surrounding T2 hyperintense edema and enhancing reactive zone.

Discussion: Osteoid osteoma is a benign osteoid-producing tumor. It is an important cause of painful scoliosis in a child or young adult. The most common symptom is night pain relieved by aspirin or other NSAIDs. The majority of the lesions are found in the lumbar spine. The best diagnostic feature is a small radiolucent tumor nidus with surrounding sclerosis. The nidus is typically <1.5 cm; the larger lesions are called osteoblastoma. The surrounding sclerosis represents reactive edema because of prostaglandin release and can be hyperintense on T2 with contrast enhancement. The nidus can show variable T2 signal but typically demonstrate avid and rapid enhancement. Complete resection of the nidus is curative in most cases. Other treatment options include thermo-/photocoagulation.

Differential Diagnoses: osteoblastoma (similar to osteoid osteoma, but larger than 1.5 cm and expansile) and stress fracture (fracture line rather than a rounded nidus, and pain related to activity). Osteomyelitis (sequestrum or focal abscess can mimic nidus but tend to be irregular shape; usually adjacent osseous erosion or destruction is present). Ewing sarcoma (no nidus, centered in the vertebral body, with diffuse surrounding edema).

References: Assoun J, et al. Osteoid osteoma: MR imaging versus CT. *Radiology* 1994;191(1):217–223.

Chai JW, et al. Radiologic diagnosis of osteoid osteoma: from simple to challenging findings. *Radiographics* 2010;30(3):737–749. Erratum in: *Radiographics* 2010;30(4):1156.

Greenspan A. Benign bone-forming lesions: osteoma, osteoid osteoma, and osteoblastoma. Clinical, imaging, pathologic, and differential considerations. *Skeletal Radiol* 1993;22(7):485–500.

Woods ER, et al. Reactive soft-tissue mass associated with osteoid osteoma: correlation of MR imaging features with pathologic findings. *Radiology* 1993;186(1):221–225.

8a **Answer A.** Nerve root enhancement and thickening.

8b **Answer B.** Leptomeningeal metastasis. This should be the most likely diagnosis given the nodular enhancing and thickened appearance of nerve roots.

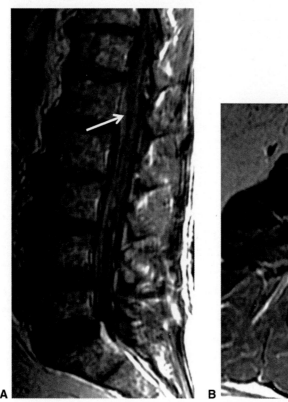

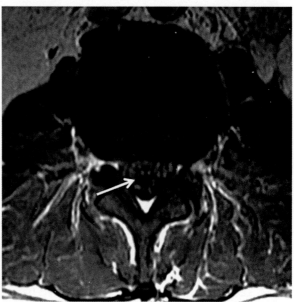

A   B

Imaging Findings: T1 sagittal and axial postcontrast images demonstrate thickening and diffuse enhancement of the cauda equine nerve roots with nodular enhancing foci (A and B). Note diffusely abnormal marrow signal compatible with osseous metastatic disease.

Discussion: Metastases from central nervous system malignancies generally occur at a younger age and include medulloblastoma, choroid plexus neoplasms, glioblastoma, and ependymoma, among other entities. In adults, the most common non-CNS solid tumors to present with leptomeningeal metastasis are lung and breast cancer, although lymphoma can also have such presentation. MRI with contrast is the imaging modality of choice, demonstrating thickened nerve roots with enhancing nodules on the spinal cord, nerve roots, or cauda equina, with a "sugar-coating" appearance of the spinal cord. Cord edema may be seen if there is an intramedullary component.

Differential Diagnosis: Differential diagnosis for diffuse nodular enhancement (sugar coating) include arachnoiditis and Guillain-Barré syndrome. Arachnoiditis will demonstrate clumping of nerve roots, "empty sac sign," and often history of prior surgery. Guillain-Barré syndrome tends to show smooth pial enhancement of the cauda equina and conus medullaris in a patient with a history of recent viral illness.

References: Brant WE, Helms CA. *Fundamentals of diagnostic radiology*. Philadelphia, PA: Lippincott Williams & Wilkins, 2006. ISBN: 0781765188.

Grossman RI, Yousem DM. *Neuroradiology, the requisites*. Mosby Inc., 2003.

Soderlund KA, Smith AB, Rushing EJ, et al. Radiologic-pathologic correlation of pediatric and adolescent spinal neoplasms: Part 2, Intradural extramedullary spinal neoplasms. *AJR Am J Roentgenol* 2012;198(1):44–51.

9a **Answer D.**   Astrocytoma. There is a mass with adjacent cysts and demonstrating strong enhancement, compatible with infiltrative astrocytoma.

9b **Answer C.**   Infiltrative and enhancing mass. This feature strongly supports the diagnosis of an infiltrative astrocytoma.

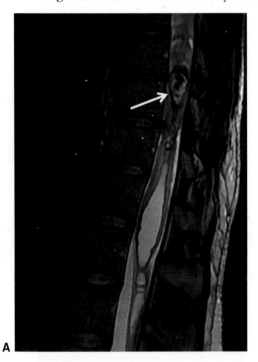 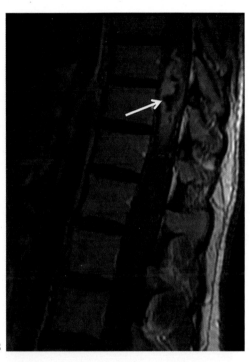

A   B

Imaging Findings: T2 and T1 postcontrast sagittal images demonstrate a long-segment infiltrative mass with cord expansion and adjacent cysts (A and B). Postcontrast images demonstrate strong enhancement of the solid mass with nonenhancing cystic component (B). There is small amount of intratumoral hemorrhage (A, low T2 signal).

Discussion: Infiltrative astrocytomas of the spinal cord are the second most common spinal cord tumor in adults and most common spinal cord tumor in children. Astrocytomas are typically long multisegment intramedullary masses approximately 4 to 7 vertebral body segments in length. The most common location is the thoracic cord. Occasionally, there can be involvement of the entire spinal cord (holocord). In contrast to cord ependymomas, a cleavage plane is not present in most spinal astrocytomas. There is diffuse cord expansion, with eccentric location of the tumor within the spinal cord. There is extensive peritumoral edema. Intratumoral and peritumoral cysts are less common. Hemorrhage is uncommon and is more commonly seen with ependymomas.

Differential Diagnosis: The main differential diagnosis is spinal ependymoma. Ependymomas are more common in adults, are typically central in location, and occasionally demonstrate a hemorrhagic cap and larger polar and intratumoral cysts.

References: Brant WE, Helms CA. *Fundamentals of diagnostic radiology*. Philadelphia, PA: Lippincott Williams & Wilkins, 2007. ISBN: 0781761352.

Koeller KK, Rosenblum RS, Morrison AL. Neoplasms of the spinal cord and filum terminale: radiologic-pathologic correlation. *Radiographics* 2000;20(6):1721–1749.

Smith AB, Soderlund KA, Rushing EJ, et al. Radiologic-pathologic correlation of pediatric and adolescent spinal neoplasms: Part 1, intramedullary spinal neoplasms. *AJR Am J Roentgenol* 2012;198(1):34–43.

10a **Answer B.** Inherited. Multiple tumors are seen demonstrating cyst and a nodule, compatible with hemangioblastomas. These are associated with von Hippel-Lindau, an inherited syndrome.

10b **Answer C.** Hemangioblastoma. This typically demonstrates a cyst and a mural nodule. Additional feature not seen on these images includes flow voids.

10c **Answer C.** Von Hippel-Lindau syndrome. Both intracranial and spinal involvement of hemangioblastomas are seen with VHL.

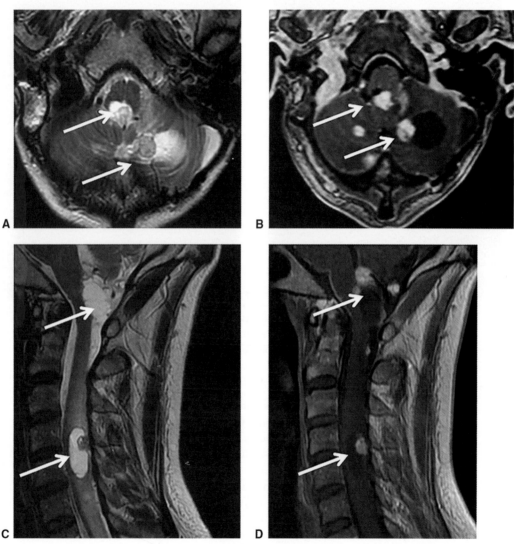

Figure 1

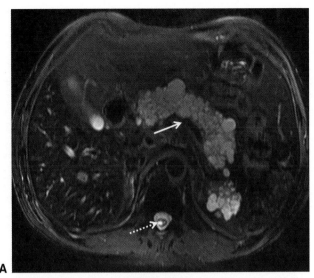

A

Figure 2

Imaging Findings: Figure 1. Axial T2 and T1 postcontrast images demonstrate multiple cysts with mural nodules within the posterior fossa (A, B). T2w (C) and T1 postcontrast (D) images demonstrate a C4–C5 cystic lesion with a peripherally located mural nodule. There is adjacent peritumoral edema. An additional small enhancing nodule is seen posterior to C2 spinal cord.

Figure 2. Axial T2 of the pancreas demonstrates numerous pancreatic cysts. Note another small cystic focus in the spinal cord seen on the same image (dotted arrow), suggestive of hemangioblastoma.

Discussion: Hemangioblastomas are WHO grade 1 highly vascular tumors. Approximately 25% to 40% of hemangioblastomas occur in patients with von Hippel-Lindau (VHL), an autosomal dominant disease caused by chromosome 3p mutation. Patients with VHL have 2 or more CNS hemangioblastomas or 1 hemangioblastoma in addition to visceral lesion or retinal hemorrhage. Hemangioblastomas typically occur in young to middle-aged adults but earlier in patients with VHL. Spinal hemangioblastoma accounts for 3% to 13% of spinal cord tumors. The tumor usually demonstrates a cyst with a highly vascular mural nodule. Cysts are presumably part of the tumor and should be resected.

Differential Diagnosis: Differential diagnoses include metastasis (sold, rather than cyst and nodule), ependymoma (usually contain hemosiderin caps and peritumoral cysts along the cranial and caudal aspect), infiltrative astrocytoma (eccentric lesions that are long segments), and, for the posterior fossa, pilocystic astrocytoma (cyst with nodule but in children) and medulloblastoma (solid and restricted diffusion).

References: Grossman RI, Yousem DM. *Neuroradiology, the requisites.* Philadelphia, PA: Mosby Inc., 2003.

Ho VB, Smirniotopoulos JG, Murphy FM, et al. Radiologic-pathologic correlation: hemangioblastoma. *AJNR Am J Neuroradiol* 1992;13(5):1343-1352.

Slater A, Moore NR, Huson SM. The natural history of cerebellar hemangioblastomas in von Hippel-Lindau disease. *AJNR Am J Neuroradiol* 2003;24(8):1570-1574.

11a **Answer D.**   Takayasu arteritis. There is a soft tissue collar surrounding the left carotid artery and near complete occlusion of the right carotid artery with marked circumferential soft tissue thickening. This is most compatible with Takayasu arteritis (TA).

11b **Answer D.**   Panarteritis. TA is a panarteritis involving all three layers of vessel wall, typically beginning with adventitia with subsequent extension into media and intima.

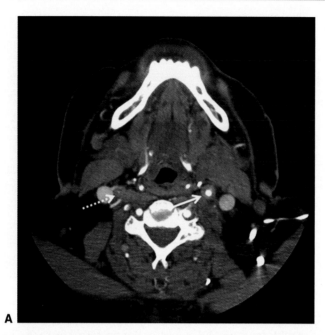

A

Imaging Findings: There is thick soft tissue collar circumferentially present around the left internal carotid artery (solid arrow). Note string like narrowing of the right ICA (dotted arrow).

Discussion: Takayasu arteritis is a chronic vascular inflammation characterized by panarteritis involvement spanning all three layers of the vessel wall, involving aorta and its major branches. Pulmonary artery involvement may also be seen.

The disease can affect a wide age range from adolescents to older adults; however, it is more common in younger females. Clinically, these patients can present with carotid tenderness and neurologic symptoms such as transient ischemic attacks and hypertension. There may be constitutional symptoms of chronic inflammation such as fever, weight loss, and fatigue.

CTA, MRA, and catheter angiogram can be performed for diagnosis. The typical imaging features include vessel wall thickening, calcification, luminal narrowing/stenosis, and occlusion or aneurysmal dilation. Management relies upon steroid, immunosuppression, surgical bypass, and angioplasty.

References: Khandelwal N, Kalra N, Garg MK, et al. Multidetector CT angiography in Takayasu arteritis. *Eur J Radiol* 2011;77(2):369-374.

Sueyoshi E, Sakamoto I, Uetani M. MRI of Takayasu's arteritis: typical appearances and complications. *AJR Am J Roentgenol* 2006;187(6):W569-W575.

12a **Answer D.** Ependymoma. Hemangioblastoma usually shows cyst with an enhancing nodule and flow voids. Astrocytoma is eccentric in location and is more infiltrative with cord expansion. Meningioma tends to occur more commonly in the extramedullary compartment.

12b **Answer B.** Marginal cysts and peripheral hemorrhage. The latter is also known as the hemosiderin cap; both are strongly associated with an ependymoma.

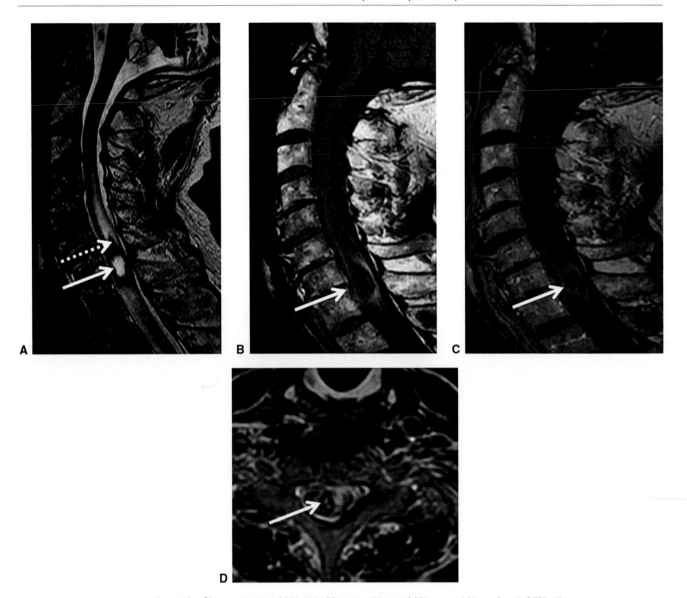

Imaging Findings: Sagittal T2 (A), T1 pre (B), and T1 post (C) and axial T2 (D) images demonstrate an intramedullary mass with intratumoral cyst (solid arrow, A) and peripheral hemosiderin rim (dotted arrow, A). There is peripheral cord edema with cord expansion and mild peripheral enhancement (C). Findings are most compatible with an ependymoma.

Discussion: Spinal ependymomas are the most common intramedullary neoplasm in adults and typically presents within fourth decade of life. Ependymomas arise from central canal or cell rests along the filum. Most intramedullary ependymomas are WHO grade II or III (anaplastic), whereas myxopapillary ependymomas are typically grade I lesions. The cervical cord is the most common site of involvement, although it could occur anywhere along the spinal cord. The common features seen with ependymomas include central location within the spinal cord with symmetric cord expansion, marginal and nontumoral cysts, and peritumoral edema. Peripheral hemorrhage is commonly associated with this lesion, leading to the "cap sign," which is a hypointense T2 rim seen with ependymoma and some other tumors such as hemangioblastoma and paraganglioma.

Differential Diagnosis: The main differential diagnosis is an infiltrative astrocytoma, more commonly in children, usually eccentric in location and spanning a longer cord segment. Hemorrhage is uncommon with astrocytoma, although can be seen occasionally.

References: Kahan H, Sklar EM, Post MJ, et al. MR characteristics of histopathologic subtypes of spinal ependymoma. *AJNR Am J Neuroradiol* 1996;17(1):143–150.

Koeller KK, Rosenblum RS, Morrison AL. Neoplasms of the spinal cord and filum terminale: radiologic-pathologic correlation. *Radiographics* 2000;20(6):1721–1749.

Smith AB, Soderlund KA, Rushing EJ, et al. Radiologic-pathologic correlation of pediatric and adolescent spinal neoplasms: Part 1, intramedullary spinal neoplasms. *AJR Am J Roentgenol* 2012;198(1):34–43.

13a **Answers C.** Polka dot appearance. This is an appearance seen with a hemangioma.

13b **Answer B.** Aggressive spinal hemangioma. This case shows a vertebral hemangioma (VH) with aggressive features as is evident with the soft tissue component. This was treated with transarterial embolization.

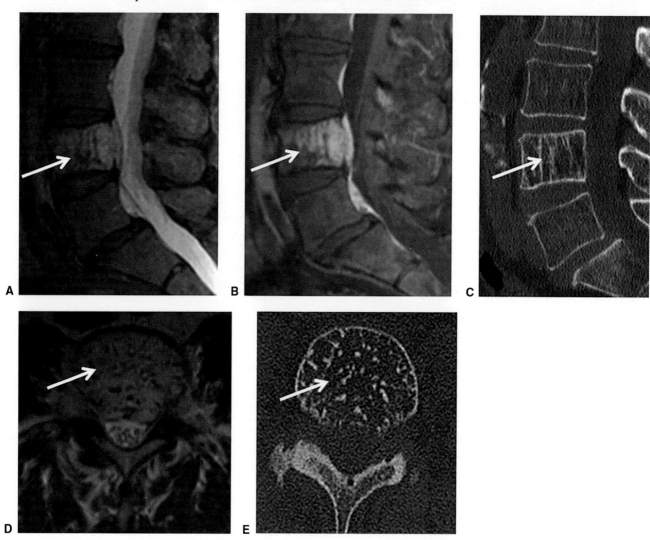

Imaging Findings: Axial CT and MRI, (D and E), demonstrate the typical polka-dot appearance. Sagittal CT, (C) demonstrates coarse vertical trabeculae with edema shown on STIR sequence, (A) and avid enhancement on T1 postcontrast images, (B). In addition, expansion and extension into the epidural spaces are seen, narrowing the spinal canal and conferring aggressive behavior to the lesion. These findings are diagnostic of aggressive VH.

Discussion: Aggressive vertebral hemangioma. Radiologically, VHs are classified as typical, atypical, and aggressive. The typical hemangiomas contain fat and mild hyperintense signal on STIR (because of the vascular component of the lesion) and variable degrees of postcontrast enhancement. The higher intensity of the latter two features suggestive of a more active behavior, with predominant vascular component of the lesion, could potentially evolve to aggressive behavior. Typical hemangiomas are commonly incidentally found and asymptomatic, characterized by the presence of fat and typical "spotted," "polka-dot" or coarse vertical trabeculae on CT. On MRI, the presence of fat and a striate pattern is typically seen, with less fat and more edema and postcontrast enhancement on atypical lesions. Features of aggressiveness include extension beyond the vertebral body, collapse, destruction of the cortex, and invasion of the epidural and paravertebral spaces.

Differential Diagnosis: Differential diagnoses for typical VHs include focal fat replacement, Modic type II changes, and postradiation changes.

Aggressive VHs may mimic plasmacytoma, metastases, chordoma, lymphoma, and epithelioid hemangioendothelioma. Typical features of VH may help, even though VH may coexist with another lesion. Angiography and biopsy may be necessary.

Treatment may be necessary for symptomatic or aggressive VHs, including vertebroplasty, transarterial embolization, ethanol injection, radiotherapy, surgery, or a combination of those.

Reference: Gaudino S, et al. A systematic approach to vertebral hemangioma. *Skeletal Radiol* 2015;44:25–36.

14 **Answer C.** Lymphoma with soft tissue component.

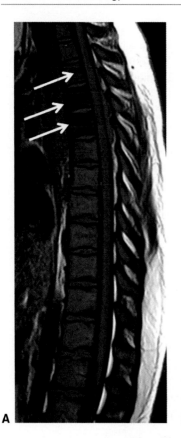
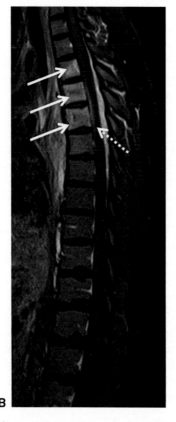
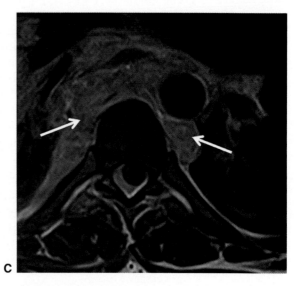

Imaging Findings: There is T1 hypointense marrow infiltration (A) with enhancement on postcontrast T1 sagittal image (B). Note sliver of ventral epidural soft tissue density (dotted arrow) on sagittal post contrast image (B) and paravertebral soft tissue on axial post contrast image (C).

Discussion: Vertebral column lymphoma of the vertebral column is a rare manifestation of lymphoma; however, it is one of the three most common malignancies of the vertebral column (with the most common being metastasis, followed by multiple myeloma). It is commonly seen in older individuals, with a slight male preponderance. Clinically, this can present as severe back pain and pathologic compression fractures, which may be severe leading to vertebra plana and neurologic deficits because of spinal canal extension. Pathologically, most commonly, these are due to diffuse large B cell lymphoma.

On imaging, it is characterized by infiltrative T1 hypointense and T2 hyperintense enhancing marrow abnormality that may have associated soft tissue components. CT and radiograph can show permeative bone destruction or sclerosis. Similar to infection, lymphoma can also cross the disc space and have presence of a sequestrum. The solid enhancing soft tissue component in the perivertebral space as shown in this case is highly unlikely with infectious causes. Management primarily relies upon chemotherapy and radiation therapy. In severe spinal canal extension and cord compression, surgical decompression may be warranted.

Reference: Koeller KK, Shih RY. Extranodal lymphoma of the central nervous system and spine. *Radiol Clin North Am* 2016;54(4):649–671.

15a **Answer C.** Long-standing process with bone remodeling. Note smooth undulating osseous remodeling with prominent dural ectasia seen on T2w MRI.

15b **Answer B.** Dural ectasia. In this, there is prominent dural ectasia in this patient with neurofibromatosis type 1.

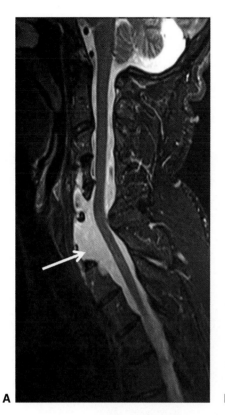
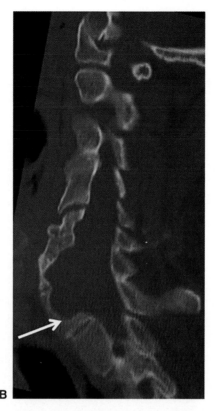
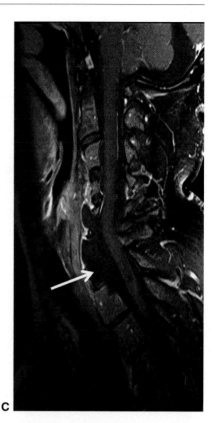

A　　　　　　　　　　B　　　　　　　　　　C

Imaging Findings: Sagittal STIR, sagittal reconstruction of CT in bone window, sagittal postcontrast fat-saturated T1 images are shown. There is enlargement of the CSF spaces along the midcervical spine with scalloping of the adjacent bone and enlargement of the neuroforamen with a left anterolateral meningocele (A, B). No bone destruction is seen. No abnormal postcontrast enhancement (C).

Discussion: Failure to confer resistance to the physiologic spinal CSF pulsation because of mesoderm dysplasia resulting in bone weakness and dural dysplasia (NF1) or connective tissue disorders (Marfan disease, Ehlers-Danlos) results in enlargement of the spinal CSF spaces, scalloping of the vertebral bodies, and widening of the foramina. There may be associated development of lateral meningocele, a dural diverticulum, extending through the widened foramen. As opposed to the meningocele, in dural ectasia, the dural enlargement is confined to the intraspinal compartment. The most common location is in the thoracolumbar spine, possibly because of contribution of relatively feeble muscles and negative pressure from the chest.

Posterior vertebral bone scalloping refers to the depth of the scalloping >3 mm in the thoracic and 4 mm in the lumbar segment. It can be associated with spinal instability and angular deformity.

Differential Diagnosis: The differential diagnosis for vertebral body scalloping includes spinal tumors, ankylosing spondylitis, achondroplasia, syringomyelia, mucopolysaccharidosis, Ehlers-Danlos, and Marfan syndrome.

References: Patel NB, Stacy GS. Musculoskeletal manifestations of neurofibromatosis type 1. *AJR Am J Roentgenol* 2012;199(1):W99–W106. doi: 10.2214/AJR.11.7811

Tortori-Donati P, Rossi A, Biancheri R, et al. Phakomatoses. In:Tortori-Donati P, Rossi A, eds. *Pediatric neuroradiology,* volume 1. Heidelberg, Germany: Springer, 2005:775–776.

16a **Answer B.** Dural AV fistula. Note the innumerable T2 flow voids seen primarily along the dorsal surface of the spinal cord. No nidus is visualized. The most likely diagnosis is a dural AV fistula.

16b **Answer C.** Myelopathy secondary to venous congestion. Also named "Foix-Alajouanine" syndrome, because of congestive ischemia in the cord resulting from venous hypertension arising from reflux into the perimedullary veins.

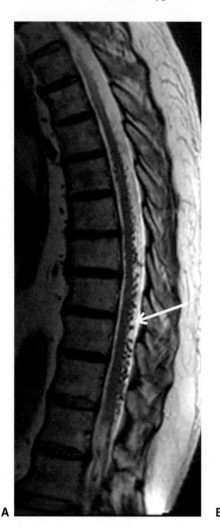
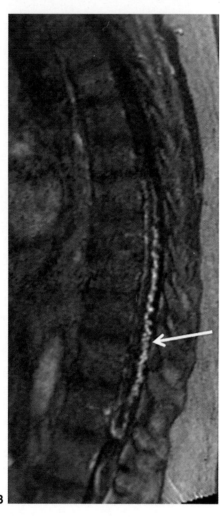
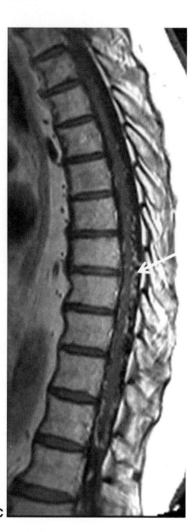

A B C

Imaging Findings: There are innumerable T2 flow voids along the surface of the cord (A) with flow-related enhancement seen on MRA and sagittal postcontrast T1w (B and C). These findings are most compatible with spinal dural AV fistula.

Discussion: Spinal dural AV fistula (DAVF) is an intradural abnormal AV shunt involving the radiculomeningeal arteries and radicular veins usually near the spinal nerve root. Also called a Type 1 malformation, it is the most common type of spinal vascular malformation, accounting for nearly 70% of cases.

The exact etiology is unclear, but it is commonly an acquired condition seen in 50 to 60 years age group, clinically presenting with nonspecific symptoms such as back pain or neurologic deficits associated with myelopathy. On imaging, these patients have numerous flow voids on T2 because of dilation of the perimedullary veins. MR angiogram with contrast can enhance the sensitivity of detection particularly in the low-flow shunts. There may be cord edema and ischemia from venous congestion because of reflux in the perimedullary veins.

Selective catheter angiogram may aid in detection of the site fistulous communication, which can be targeted for surgical removal or transarterial embolization.

Differential Diagnosis: Type 2 malformations, also known as glomus AVM are the most commonly seen intramedullary vascular malformations, accounting for 20% of all spinal vascular malformations. These lesions usually present in younger patients with acute neurologic deterioration secondary to hemorrhage usually in the cervicomedullary region. In contrast to Type 1, there is a nidus within the cord in Type 2 malformations.

References: Krings T, Geibprasert S. Spinal dural arteriovenous fistulas. *AJNR Am J Neuroradiol* 2009;30(4):639–648.

Saliou G, Krings T. Vascular diseases of the spine. *Handb Clin Neurol* 2016;136:707–716.

17   **Answer D.**   Subclavian steal syndrome. There is evidence of subclavian steal with occluded proximal left subclavian artery and flow in the postvertebral segment via a patent left vertebral artery. Note that this will result in retrograde flow in the ipsilateral vertebral artery on US. The vertebral artery itself is patent without evidence of dissection or severe stenosis.

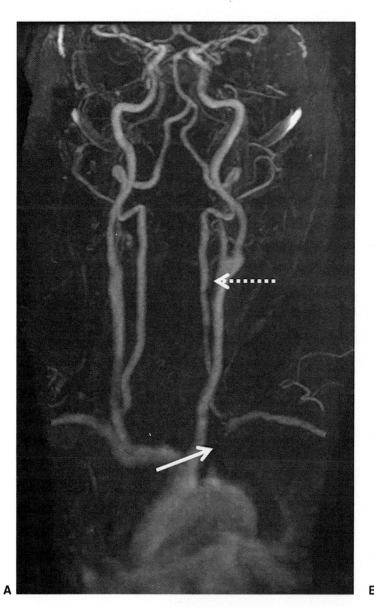

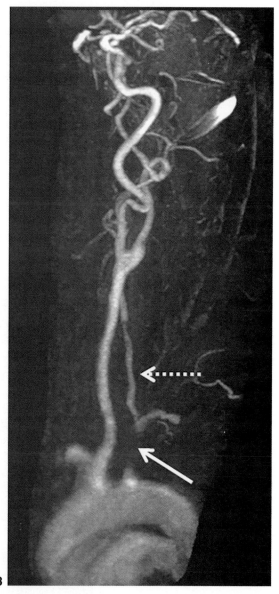

A

B

Imaging Findings: There is absence of flow-related signal in the proximal left subclavian artery (solid arrow A and B) with flow in the left vertebral artery (dotted arrow A and B) and subsequent reconstitution of the postvertebral subclavian artery.

Discussion: Subclavian steal syndrome is a hemodynamic abnormality resulting from retrograde flow from the vertebral artery to the subclavian artery in the setting of ipsilateral prevertebral subclavian or innominate stenosis or occlusion. This leads to diversion of blood from the posterior circulation resulting in symptoms of vertebrobasilar insufficiency such as syncope, ataxia, and vertigo and may be exacerbated by exertion, transient ischemic attack, or stroke. These patients often have concomitant upper extremity claudication, because the retrograde flow may not be sufficient for adequate tissue perfusion.

The occlusion or stenosis of subclavian/innominate may be due to underlying atherosclerotic disease, extrinsic compression, giant cell or Takayasu arteritis, etc. On imaging, US shows reversal of flow in the ipsilateral vertebral artery and CTA/MRA define the site of proximal occlusion or stenosis along with confirming patency of the vertebral artery. Management of the underlying stenosis is required to address the reversal of flow in the vertebral artery.

References: Kargiotis O, Siahos S, Safouris A, et al. Subclavian steal syndrome with or without arterial stenosis: a review. *J Neuroimaging* 2016;26(5):473–480.

Saha T, Naqvi SY, Ayah OA, et al. Subclavian artery disease: diagnosis and therapy. *Am J Med* 2017;130(4):409–416.

18a **Answer A.**   Central cord infarction because of severe hypotension. Note there is central cord involvement typically seen with severe hypotension that may occur in the intraoperative or immediate postoperative course. Toxicity from nitrous oxide (anesthetic gas) can result in myelopathy; however, typically, dorsal column involvement is seen. The distribution is unusual for anterior spinal artery infarction that supplies the anterior 2/3rd of the spinal cord.

18b **Answer C.**   Posterior cord infarction. The images show loss of ADC (C) in the posterior cord most compatible with posterior cord infarction in the current clinical setting of acute-onset myelopathy. Contrast can be used to definitively evaluate this finding, because inflammatory, neoplastic, infectious, or demyelinating conditions typically enhance, particularly in the acute phase for the nonneoplastic conditions.

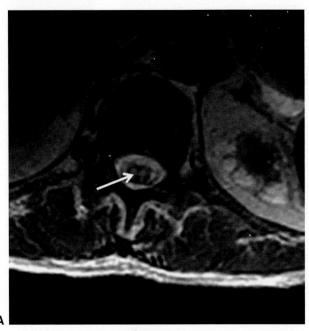

A

Figure 1

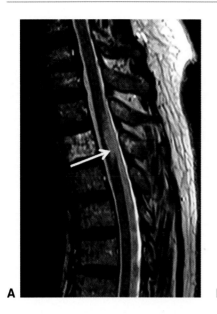 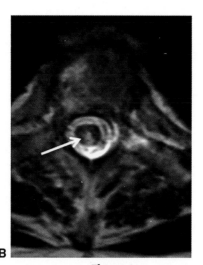 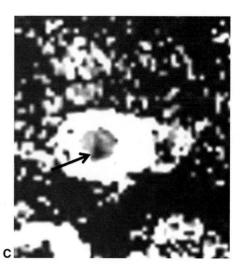

A · B · C

Figure 2

Imaging Findings: Figure 1. There is intrinsic T2 hyperintensity in the central cord predominantly affecting the gray matter. Although on imaging along in the absence of DWI, this is a highly nonspecific finding. In the clinical setting of acute onset, in the perioperative course, central cord infarct is the most likely diagnosis.

Figure 2. There is intrinsic T2 hyperintensity in the dorsal cord (A and B) with corresponding loss of signal on ADC map (C), compatible with cord acute infarction.

Discussion: Spinal cord infarction is a rare condition; however, it is associated with significant morbidity and mortality. Clinically, these patients present acutely with symptoms depending on the site of infarction ranging from autonomic dysfunction to paraplegia to minor weakness. Etiologic factors are diverse such as trauma, atherosclerosis, dissection, emboli, severe hypotension, underlying spinal vascular malformations, etc.

Most commonly seen is anterior spinal artery infarct, which supplies the anterior 2/3rd of the spinal cord, characterized by loss of motor function, pain and temperature sensation, and sparing of dorsal column function of vibration and proprioception. This is a single artery formed by fusion of vessels arising from the V4 segment of vertebral arteries with multiple contributions from other arteries, such as vertebral, intercostal, lumbar, inferior thyroid, and lateral sacral arteries and iliolumbar arteries and artery of Adamkiewicz. Artery of Adamkiewicz or arteria radicularis anterior magna is critical, given it supplies the lower 2/3rd of the spinal cord/conus. It has a variable origin from lumbar or intercostal arteries, typically on the left between T8 and L1, with a characteristic hairpin loop to anastomose with the anterior spinal artery.

Posterior spinal artery infarction is typically unilateral because this is a paired artery arising from the PICA. This leads to posterior roots, dorsal horn, and dorsal column involvement with loss of vibration and proprioception.

Rarely, central cord infarction can occur in the setting of severe hypotension resulting in spinothalamic sensory deficits.

MRI is the modality of choice for imaging cord infarction. On MRI, cord infarction can present with T2 hyperintensity, T1 hypointensity, and restricted diffusion on DWI. In the acute phase, enhancement is absent differentiating it from other inflammatory or neoplastic entities that tend to enhance in the acute phase.

References: Vargas MI, Gariani J, Sztajzel R, et al. Spinal cord ischemia: practical imaging tips, pearls, and pitfalls. *AJNR Am J Neuroradiol* 2015;36(5):825–830.

White ML, El-Khoury GY. Neurovascular injuries of the spinal cord. *Eur J Radiol* 2002;42(2):117–126.

12

Congenital and Developmental Abnormalities of the Spine

GAURAV JINDAL • PAMELA H. NGUYEN • RAFEEQUE BHADELIA

QUESTIONS

1   Patient A presents with cough-induced headaches. Patient B presents with upper extremity sensory deficits. MRI was performed for further assessment. Key images are shown below.

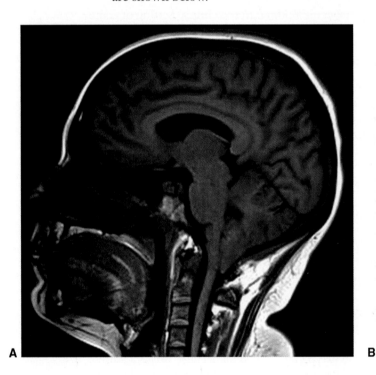

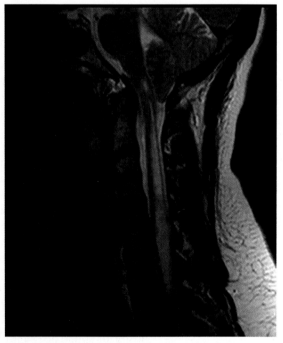

A

B

1a Which of the following is the most accurate diagnoses based on the images shown?

   A. Both patients have Chiari 1 malformation.
   B. Only patient A has Chiari 1.
   C. Only patient B has Chiari 1.
   D. Patient A has Chiari 1 and patient B has Chiari 2 malformation.

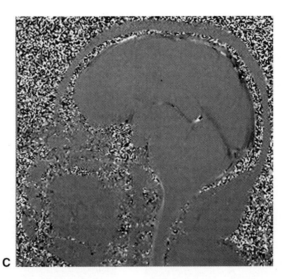

C

1b Additional advanced imaging was performed to understand the CSF flow dynamics, and the image is shown. Which of the following MR imaging sequences was used to obtain the image?

   A. 3D steady-state gradient echo sequence such as CISS/FIESTA
   B. Subtraction MR myelogram
   C. Phase-contrast sequence CSF flow
   D. 3D volumetric fast spin echo T1w

2 History withheld.

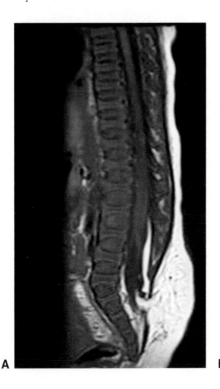

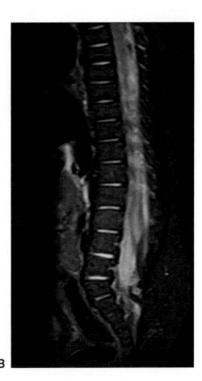

A   B

2a Which of the following is the most appropriate diagnosis?

    A. Lipoma of filum terminale
    B. Lipomyelocele
    C. Myelomeningocele
    D. Lipomyelomeningocele

2b Which of the following is true about this entity?

    A. Neural placode lipoma interface lies within the spinal canal.
    B. Neural placode lipoma interface projects beyond the spinal canal.
    C. Skin overlying the spinal dysraphic defect is disrupted.
    D. Normally positioned conus medullaris

3 Below are shown two contrasting developmental abnormalities in patients A and B. Key images from MRI are provided below.

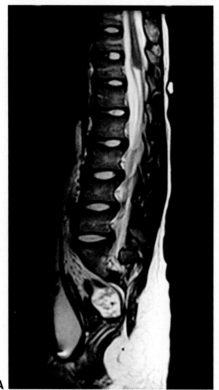
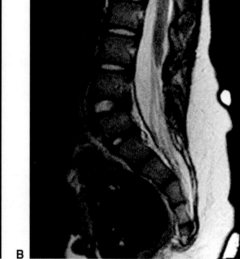

Patient A   Patient B

3a Which of the following is the most likely diagnosis in patient A?

    A. Type 1 caudal regression syndrome
    B. Type 2 caudal regression syndrome
    C. Tethered cord
    D. Myelomeningocele

3b Which of the following is the most likely diagnosis in patient B?

    A. Type 1 caudal regression syndrome

    B. Type 2 caudal regression syndrome

    C. Tethered cord

    D. Myelomeningocele

4 Incidental finding on an MRI lumbar spine performed for low back pain in an otherwise healthy patient. Key images from an MRI are provided below.

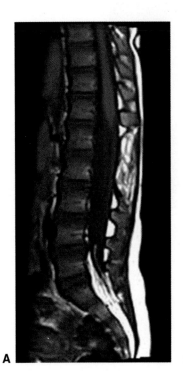
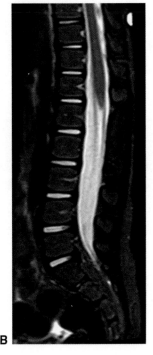
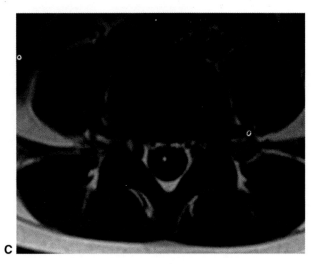

A   B   C

4a Which of the following is the most likely diagnosis?

    A. Fibrolipoma

    B. Dermoid

    C. Tethered cord

    D. Lipomyelocele

4b Which of the following associations are seen with this entity?

    A. Conus medullaris terminates at a normal position.

    B. Associated with spinal dysraphism

    C. Patients often have neurologic symptoms.

    D. Vertebral segmentation anomalies

5   Chronic low back pain without radiculopathy or neurologic symptoms. An MRI was performed for further assessment. Key images are shown below.

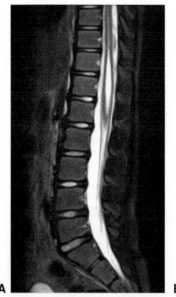

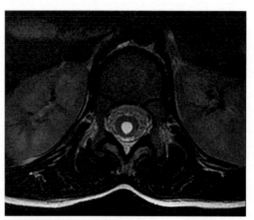

A   B

Images courtesy of Dr. Mai Lan Ho

Based on the above images, what is the most likely diagnosis?

A. Syringomyelia
B. Terminal ventricle
C. Myxopapillary ependymoma
D. Tethered cord

6   What is the most likely diagnosis?

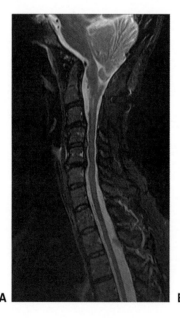

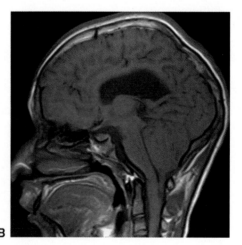

A   B

A. Chiari 1 malformation
B. Chiari 2 malformation
C. Low lying cerebellar tonsils
D. Dandy walker malformation

7   A 16-year-old female presents with back pain. Lateral radiographs of the lumbar spine demonstrate L5 pars defect with minimal anterior translation of L5 on S1.

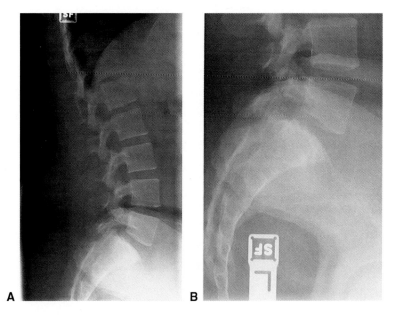

Which of the following is the likely etiology for the imaging findings above?

A. Acute traumatic injury
B. Congenital
C. Neoplastic
D. Repetitive stress injury

8   A young child with scoliosis presented for further evaluation. Key images from an MRI are shown below.

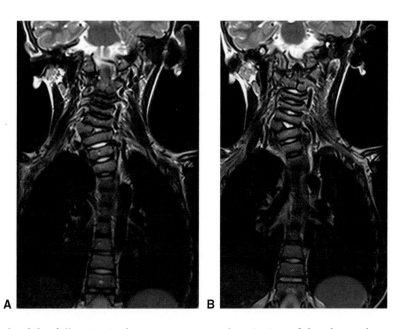

Which of the following is the most accurate description of the above abnormality?

A. Vertebral segmentation anomaly
B. Spinal dysraphism
C. Chiari 1 malformation
D. Aberrant left subclavian artery

9 Key image for a developmental abnormality is shown below.

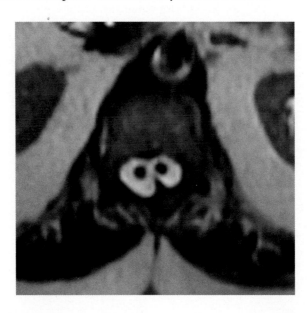

What is the diagnosis?

A. Congenital block vertebrae
B. Spinal dysraphism
C. Diastematomyelia
D. Dural ectasia

ANSWERS AND EXPLANATIONS

1a **Answer A.** Both patients have Chiari I malformation. Both patients have tonsillar ectopia with downward positioning of the cerebellar tonsils measuring at least 5 mm beyond the foramen magnum. There is an associated syrinx with patient B. These findings are compatible with Chiari 1 malformation.

1b **Answer C.** Phase-contrast sequence CSF flow. The image shown below (C) is a sagittal plane phase-contrast CSF flow sequence. The arrow points to the lack of flow-related signal in the dorsal subarachnoid CSF space at the cervicomedullary junction.

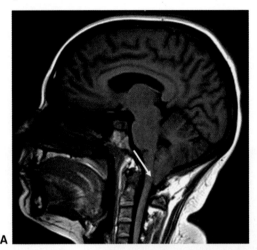 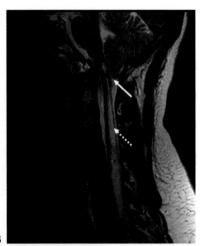

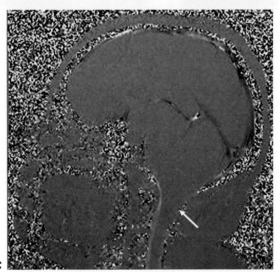

Imaging Findings: Sagittal T1w image in patient A and sagittal T2w image in patient B showing tonsillar ectopia (solid arrow A and B) with a syrinx seen in the upper cord in patient B (dotted arrow, B). Note lack of flow-related signal in the dorsal subarachnoid CSF space in phase-contrast CSF flow study in image C (solid arrow, C).

Discussion: Chiari 1 malformation.

Chiari 1 malformation is defined as inferior displacement of the cerebellar tonsils below the foramen magnum typically by at least 5 mm. It may be idiopathic or could be secondary to posterior fossa or craniovertebral junction anomalies. Caudally displaced tonsils are typically pointed or peg-like.

The most common complications of Chiari 1 result from altered CSF flow dynamics and include syringohydromyelia and hydrocephalus.

Chiari 1.5 is a more recently described entity, which combines features of Chiari 1 with inferior descent of the brainstem, typically the inferior margin of 4th ventricle (obex) lying below the foramen magnum.

Phase-contrast CSF flow imaging can be useful in evaluating CSF flow at the foramen magnum. Treatment in symptomatic patients most often consists of suboccipital craniectomy, and often also resection of the posterior arch of C1, with the goal to restore normal CSF flow.

References: Barkovich AJ. Congenital anomalies of the spine. In: Barkovich AJ, Raybaud C. (eds). *Pediatric neuroimaging*, 5th ed. Philadelphia, PA: Lippincott Williams & Wilkins, 2011.

Tubbs RS, Iskandar BJ, Bartolucci AA, et al. A critical analysis of the Chiari 1.5 malformation. *J Neurosurg* 2004;101(2 Suppl):179–183.

2a **Answer B.** Lipomyelocele. Sagittal T1 and STIR images show fat signal compatible with a lipoma, which is located between the neural placode ventrally and a spinal dysraphic defect dorsally. There is intact skin overlying the defect making the lesion most compatible with a lipomyelocele.

2b **Answer A.** Neural placode lipoma interface lies within the spinal canal. Because of the above explained relationship of the structures involved, the interface lies within the spinal canal.

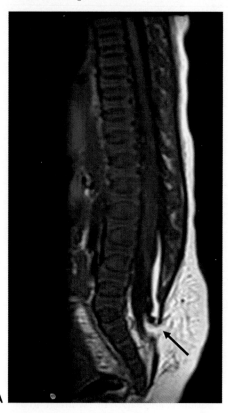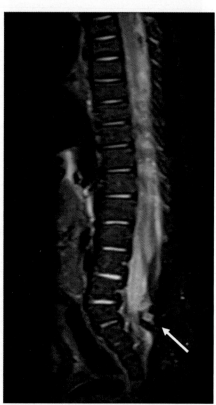

A   B

Imaging Findings: Sagittal T1w (A) and STIR (B) images show a tethered cord with a terminal syringomyelia. There is expansion of the lumbar spinal canal. There is fat containing signal compatible with a lipoma (black arrow) located between the neural placode ventrally and a sacral dysraphic defect dorsally with intact overlying skin (white arrow).

Discussion: Lipomyelocele.

Lipomyelocele refers to a skin-covered spinal dysraphism characterized by an intraspinal lipoma in contiguity with the subcutaneous fat via the dysraphic defect in the posterior elements. The neural placode is located within the spinal canal. If the neural placode projects through the dysraphic defect into the subcutaneous tissues, it is referred to as a lipomyelomeningocele. Location of the spinal lipoma may be intra- or extradural.

The cord is low lying and tethered to the intraspinal lipoma. There is typically mild expansion of the spinal canal and distention of the subarachnoid space at the level of lipomyelocele.

Differential Diagnosis: Imaging differentials include an intradural lipoma, which is characterized by an intact overlying dura and absence of communication with the subcutaneous fat. The spinal canal is not expanded although a tethered cord is often associated.

The other important differential is a myelomeningocele, which is an open spinal dysraphism where the neural placode projects outside the spinal canal and is not covered by the skin remaining exposed as a result to amniotic fluid in utero and air after birth.

References: Barkovich AJ. Congenital anomalies of the spine. In: Barkovich AJ, Raybaud C. (eds). *Pediatric neuroimaging*, 5th ed. Philadelphia, PA: Lippincott Williams & Wilkins, 2011.

Rufener SL, Ibrahim M, Raybaud CA, et al. Congenital spine and spinal cord malformations—pictorial review. *AJR Am J Roentgenol* 2010;194(3 Suppl):S26–S37.

3a   **Answer A.**   Type 1 caudal regression syndrome. Sagittal T2-weighted image demonstrates sacral agenesis beyond S1. The conus medullaris terminates at T11–T12 and appears blunted.

3b   **Answer B.**   Type 2 caudal regression syndrome. Sagittal T2-weighted images demonstrate low-lying conus terminating at inferior border of L3. There is agenesis of the coccyx.

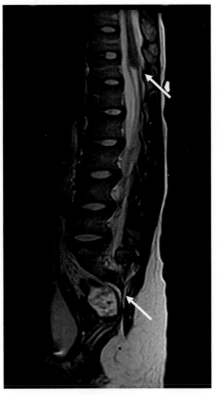

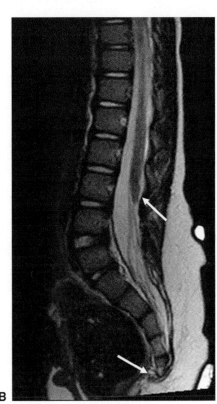

A

Patient A

B

Patient B

Discussion: Caudal regression syndrome.

Caudal regression syndrome is a complex congenital malformation characterized by varying degrees of lumbosacral agenesis/dysgenesis, along with malformations of the cord. Depending on the position of the conus, it is divided into two types:

Type 1: Abnormal high termination (above L1) of the conus, which is blunted or wedge shaped typically associated with sacral anomalies above S1.

Type 2: Low-lying tethered cord with less severe sacral agenesis, typically below S2.

Attention to the diagnosis is often directed initially during evaluation of associated genitourinary or gastrointestinal malformations. Most common GU malformations include renal agenesis and hydronephrosis, whereas associated GI anomalies are typically anal atresia and imperforate anus. Other than lumbosacral agenesis, patients may also have associated vertebral segmentation anomalies and the entire spine should be screened for complete evaluation. There is an association with diabetic embryopathy, especially in diabetic pregnant women on insulin.

Ultrasound screening in the first trimester may demonstrate a shortened crown–rump length, whereas second trimester fetal survey can better demonstrate the sacral agenesis as well as associated genitourinary malformations.

References: Barkovich AJ. Congenital anomalies of the spine. In: Barkovich AJ, Raybaud C. (eds). *Pediatric neuroimaging*, 5th ed. Philadelphia, PA: Lippincott Williams & Wilkins, 2011.

Stroustrup Smith A, Grable I, Levine D. Case 66: caudal regression syndrome in the fetus of a diabetic mother. *Radiology* 2004;230(1):229–233.

4a Answer A.   Fibrolipoma.

4b Answer A.   Conus medullaris terminates at normal position.

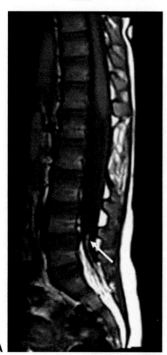
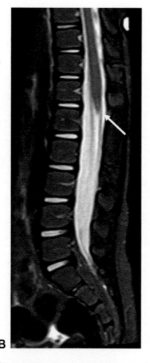
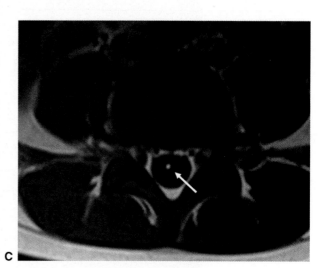

A   B   C

Imaging Findings: Sagittal T1w image demonstrates high signal within the filum at L4–S1 level, (arrow A) which is suppressed on the STIR images. Note normal position of the conus (arrow B). The distal fatty filum shows an abnormal dorsal location and appears tethered to the distal thecal sac. Axial T1 images with fat signal within the distal filum, which in this case, is not abnormally thickened. Findings compatible with a fatty filum or fibrolipoma.

Discussion: Fibrolipoma of filum terminale or fatty filum. Fatty filum refers to detection of fat in an otherwise normal size filum (transverse diameter <2 mm) in an asymptomatic patient. It is most commonly an incidental finding, which does not warrant further investigation.

Differential Diagnosis: It is important to differentiate from other fat-containing lesions such as intraspinal lipoma (larger in size), dermoid/epidermoid (more complex appearing) lipomyelocele (associated with posterior spinal fusion anomalies), and tethered cord (low-lying conus). MRI classically depicts high T1 signal within the filum, which is suppressed on fat-saturated sequences.

References: Barkovich AJ. Congenital anomalies of the spine. In: Barkovich AJ, Raybaud C. (eds). *Pediatric neuroimaging*, 5th ed. Philadelphia, PA: Lippincott Williams & Wilkins, 2011.

Bulsara KR, Zomorodi AR, Enterline DS, et al. The value of magnetic resonance imaging in the evaluation of fatty filum terminale. *Neurosurgery* 2004;54(2):375–379; discussion 379–380.

5 **Answer B.**   Terminal ventricle.

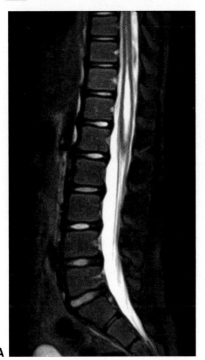
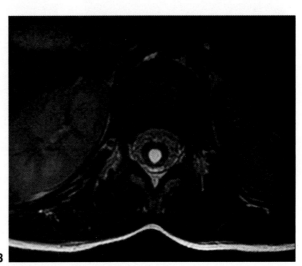

Images courtesy of Dr. Mai Lan Ho

Imaging Findings: Sagittal and axial T2w images demonstrate dilation of the central canal in the distal spinal cord. Note lack of complexity within the canal or associated signal changes in adjacent cord/conus.

Discussion: Terminal ventricle. Mild dilation of the central canal of the spinal cord in or around the conus medullaris is an incidental finding that warrants no further investigation in an asymptomatic patient in the absence of any evidence of enhancement, septations, eccentric location, or cord tethering.

Also referred to as ventriculus terminalis or fifth ventricle, it is often seen incidentally especially in pediatric population. It may sometimes be detected in newborns undergoing spinal cord ultrasound screening.

Differential Diagnosis: It is important to differentiate this entity from syringomyelia (which is usually accompanied by other developmental abnormalities) as well as neoplasms especially if there is cystic dilation of the central canal. Contrast-enhanced MRI is instrumental in depicting lack of enhancement, nodularity, or septations in patients with suspected neoplasms of the conus.

References: Ciappetta P, et al. Cystic dilation of the ventriculus terminalis in adults. *J Neurosurg Spine* 2008;8:92–99.

Coleman LT, et al. Ventriculus terminalis of the conus medullaris: MR findings in children. *AJNR Am J Neuroradiol* 1995;16(7):1421–1426.

6 **Answer B.** Chiari 2 malformation.

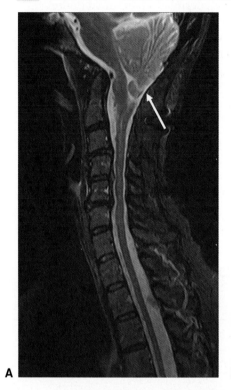
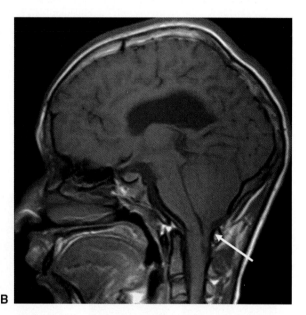

A   B

Imaging Findings: Sagittal STIR and Sag T1w images demonstrate a small posterior fossa with inferior displacement of the vermis (arrow, image A), cervicomedullary kinking (arrow image B), tectal beaking, and flattening of the 4th ventricle diagnostic of Chiari 2 malformation.

Discussion: Chiari 2 malformation.

Chiari 2 malformation is a congenital hindbrain malformation, which results from a developmentally small posterior fossa, which can no longer accommodate the normally growing brainstem and cerebellum. The cerebellum is displaced both superiorly through a widened tentorial incisura (with resulting mass effect on the tectum causing tectal beaking) as well as inferiorly into the upper cervical canal resulting in a flattening of 4th ventricle. It is important to recognize that unlike Chiari 1, it is the vermis that typically herniates inferiorly in Chiari 2 whereas Chiari 1 shows tonsillar herniation.

The cerebellum may also extend anterolaterally into the cerebellopontine angle cisterns ("wrapping around the brainstem") associated with concavity of the petrous bones.

Cervicomedullary kinking results from inferior displacement of the medulla into the cervical canal. Nearly all patients have a myelomeningocele, which requires closure immediately after birth. Supratentorial abnormalities are commonly present and include hydrocephalus, callosal dysgenesis, as well as gray matter abnormalities like heterotopias and polymicrogyria.

References: Barkovich AJ. Congenital anomalies of the spine. In: Barkovich AJ, Raybaud C. (eds). *Pediatric neuroimaging*, 5th ed. Philadelphia, PA: Lippincott Williams & Wilkins, 2011.

Geerdink N, van der Vliet T, Rotteveel JJ, et al. Essential features of Chiari II malformation in MR imaging: an interobserver reliability study—part 1. *Childs Nerv Syst* 2012;28(7):977–985. doi: 10.1007/s00381-012-1761-5

7 **Answer D.** Repetitive stress injury. The etiology is believed to be chronic stress-related injury resulting in a fracture of the pars interarticularis. It most often develops in the first decade of life and is not present at birth.

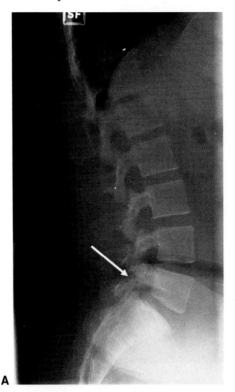 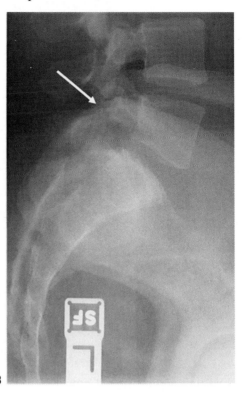

A   B

Imaging Findings: Lateral radiographs of the lumbar spine show an abnormal lucency in the pars interarticularis, the bony connection between the superior and inferior articular processes. This is a pars defect/spondylosis. It is most commonly seen at L5 followed by L4.

Discussion: Pars defect. Defects in the pars may result in varying degrees of anterolisthesis of the involved vertebra. The etiology is believed to be chronic stress-related injury resulting in a fracture of the pars interarticularis. It most often develops in the first decade of life and is not present at birth.

Radiographs and midline sagittal CT images can readily depict the bony defect with sclerotic edges as well as any associated anterior vertebral translation. On axial CT imaging, there is an elongation of the spinal canal with increased AP diameter. In addition to visualizing the pars defect, MRI can also depict reactive marrow changes. Other ancillary findings include horizontally oriented neural foramina and posterior wedging of the vertebral body.

Spondylolisthesis can also develop in the absence of pars defect in patients with degenerative facet arthropathy and acute fractures in the setting of trauma. Acute pars fractures, however, do not have sclerotic edges and there are often other associated fractures in the spine.

Treatment is mostly conservative with surgical fusion and/or posterior decompression reserved for cases with higher grades of anterolisthesis and neurologic deficits.

References: Jinkins JR, Matthes JC, Sener RN, et al. Spondylolysis, spondylolisthesis, and associated nerve root entrapment in the lumbosacral spine: MR evaluation. *AJR Am J Roentgenol* 1992;159(4):799–803.

Standaert CJ, Herring SA, Halpern B, et al. Spondylolysis. *Phys Med Rehabil Clin N Am* 2000;11:785.

8 **Answer A.** Vertebral segmentation anomaly.

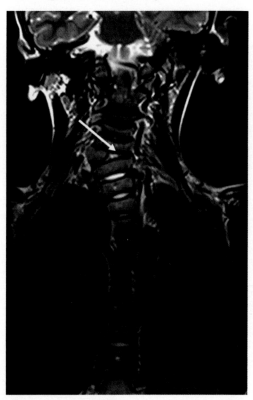

Imaging Findings: Coronal T2-weighted image shows a C6 hemivertebra (arrow).

Discussion: Vertebral segmentation anomaly.

Vertebral segmentation anomalies result from abnormal vertebral development during embryogenesis. These may be detected incidentally or during evaluation of patients with congenital scoliosis.

Segmentation anomalies include vertebral agenesis, hemivertebra, butterfly vertebra (sagittal cleft), coronal cleft, and block vertebra.

A lateral (right or left) hemivertebra results from lack of ossification of one-half of the vertebral body and present with congenital scoliosis. Ventral or dorsal hemivertebra results from lack of ossification in ventral or dorsal half of vertebral body. These may present with exaggerated kyphosis or lordosis.

Butterfly vertebra describes a sagittal cleft in the vertebral body and results from lack of fusion of lateral halves of the vertebral body. This is best seen on the coronal view.

Block vertebrae result from congenital fusion of the vertebral bodies, which can involve the anterior or posterior aspect of the vertebral bodies or both.

References: Barkovich AJ. Congenital anomalies of the spine. In: Barkovich AJ, Raybaud C. (eds). *Pediatric neuroimaging*, 5th ed. Philadelphia, PA: Lippincott Williams & Wilkins, 2011.

Kumar R, Guinto FC Jr, Madewell JE, et al. The vertebral body: radiographic configurations in various congenital and acquired disorders. *Radiographics* 1988;8(3):455–485.

9 Answer C. Diastematomyelia.

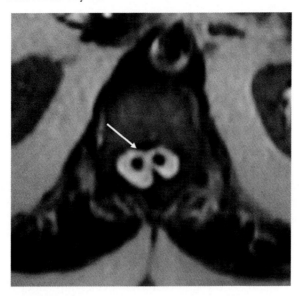

Imaging Findings: Axial T2w MR images reveal splitting of the spinal cord into two hemicords (arrow).

Discussion: Diastematomyelia/split cord malformation.

Diastematomyelia/split cord malformation refers to sagittal splitting of the spinal cord into two hemicords secondary to a bony or fibrocartilaginous septum. Each hemicord has an anterior and posterior horn with its associated nerve roots. The extent of cord involvement can be variable. It is most commonly seen in the thoracolumbar spine.

Split cord malformation is classically divided into two types:

Type 1: Two hemicords with individual dural sheaths
Type 2: Two hemicords within a common dural sheath

It is commonly associated with vertebral segmentation anomalies, intersegmental laminar fusion, and spinal dysraphism. Patients are most often diagnosed in childhood during evaluation of progressive scoliosis or presence of cutaneous stigmata such as hairy patch, which is seen in more than half the cases.

References: Huang SL, He XJ, Xiang L, et al. CT and MRI features of patients with diastematomyelia. *Spinal Cord* 2014;52:689–692. doi: 10.1038/sc.2014.68

Rufener SL, Ibrahim M, Raybaud CA, et al. Congenital spine and spinal cord malformations—pictorial review. *AJR Am J Roentgenol* 2010;194(3 Suppl):S26–S37.

13 Soft Tissue Neck

SYED ADIL AFTAB • DANIEL THOMAS GINAT

QUESTIONS

1 Identify the nodal level of the abnormal right neck lymph node shown on the following image:

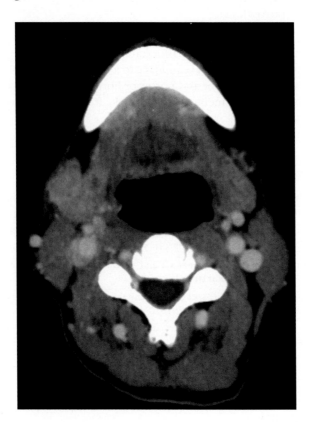

A. Level IA
B. Level IB
C. Level IIA
D. Level IIB

2   Identify the nodal level of the enlarged necrotic right neck lymph node shown on the following image:

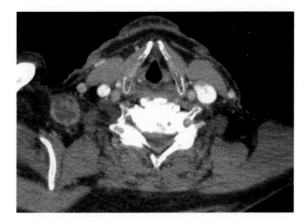

A. Level III
B. Level IV
C. Level VA
D. Level VB

3   The abnormality in the following image is attributable to a defect in which cranial nerve?

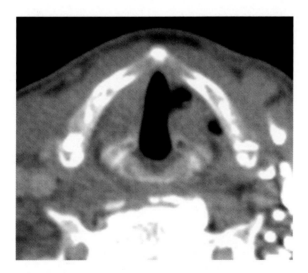

A. Glossopharyngeal nerve
B. Vagus nerve
C. Spinal accessory nerve
D. Hypoglossal nerve

4 In which space is the lesion on the following image located?

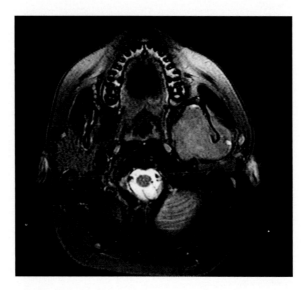

    A. Masticator space
    B. Parapharyngeal space
    C. Carotid space
    D. Parotid space

5 Which of the following statements is true in general about the condition depicted in the image below?

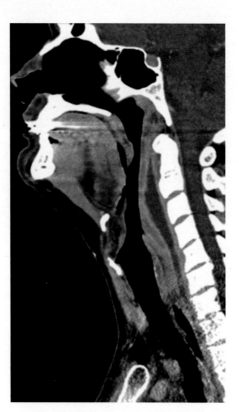

    A. The abnormality can potentially extend into the mediastinum via the danger space.
    B. The abnormality is more common in adults than in children.
    C. The abnormality most commonly arises from penetrating trauma.
    D. The presence of an enhancing wall does not differentiate this from an effusion.

6 The patient presented with neck pain for several weeks. The following CT of the neck without contrast was obtained. What is the most appropriate next step?

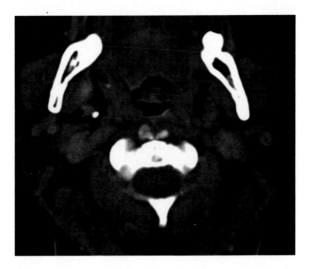

A. Surgery
B. Treatment with antibiotics
C. MRI of the neck
D. Treatment with NSAIDs

7 The patient presented with persistent sore throat for several days and new-onset chest pain. Physical examination reveals an inflamed erythematous mucosa with purulent exudate in the tonsils. The following CT of the neck with contrast was obtained. Which of the following is the most appropriate next step?

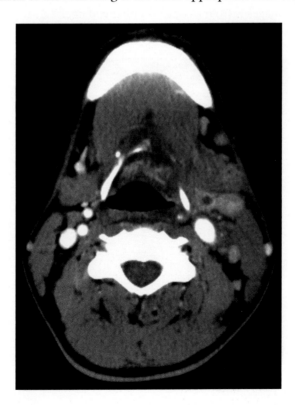

A. Incision and drainage
B. MRI of the neck
C. CT of the chest
D. Treatment with oral antibiotics

8   Which of the following is the most likely diagnosis based on the image below?

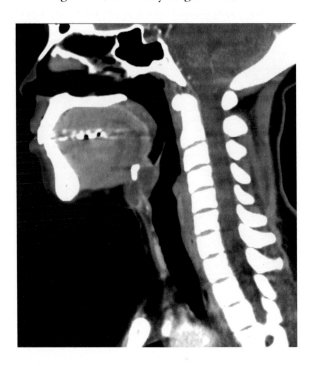

A. Ranula
B. Branchial cleft cyst
C. Thyroglossal duct cyst
D. Laryngocele

9   The following images is from a contrast-enhanced neck CT. Which of the following
is the most likely diagnosis?

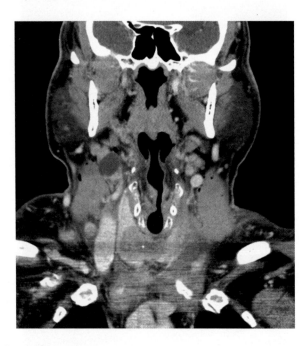

A. Lymphatic malformation
B. Mycobacterial lymphadenitis
C. Papillary thyroid cancer
D. Lymphoma

10 Which is the most likely tumor of origin based on the following image?

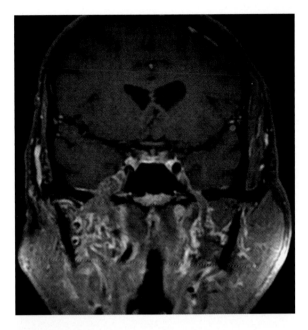

  A. Mucoepidermoid carcinoma
  B. Adenoid cystic carcinoma
  C. Warthin tumor
  D. Pleomorphic adenoma

11 The patient presented with dry eyes and dry mouth and underwent the following MRI. Which of the following is true regarding this condition?

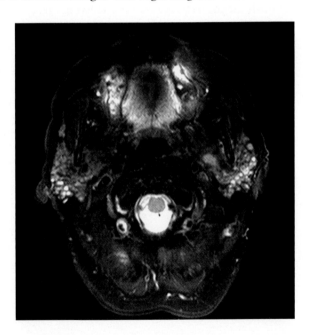

  A. It is more common in males than in females.
  B. There is an increased risk for developing lymphoma.
  C. The affected gland typically enlarges in late stage.
  D. It is rarely associated with interstitial lung disease.

12   Which best describes the location of the lesion shown on the following image?

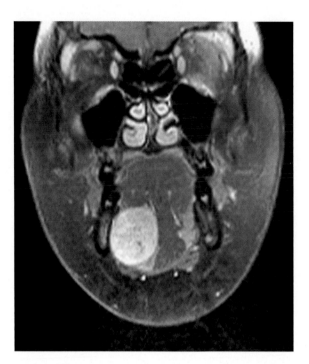

    A. Oral tongue
    B. Buccal mucosa
    C. Floor of the mouth
    D. Retromolar trigone

13   What is the most likely diagnosis based on the following images?

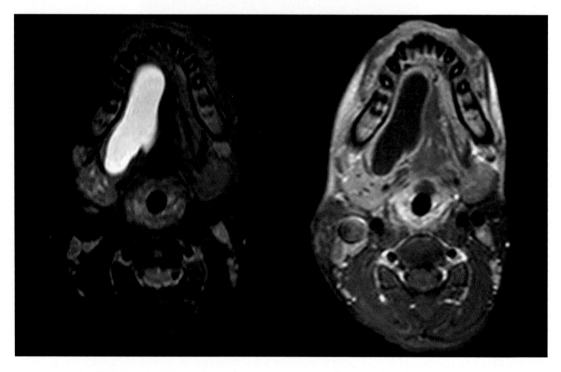

    A. Thyroglossal duct cyst
    B. Dentigerous cyst
    C. Adenoid cystic carcinoma
    D. Ranula

14 What is the most likely diagnosis for the cystic lesion shown in the following image?

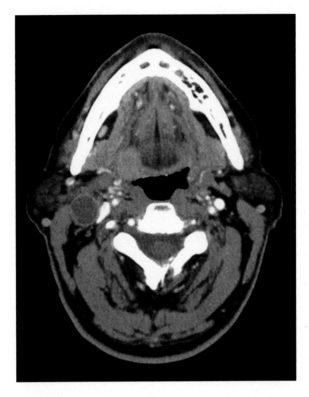

A. Branchial cleft cyst
B. Thyroid cancer metastasis
C. Oropharyngeal cancer metastasis
D. Peripheral nerve sheath tumor

15 In what space is the lesion depicted in the following image located?

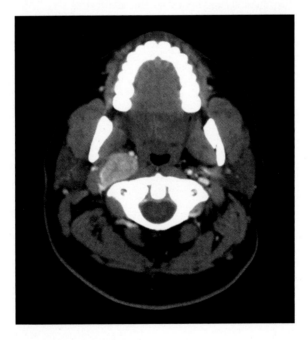

A. Pre-styloid parapharyngeal space
B. Post-styloid parapharyngeal space or carotid space
C. Parotid space
D. Pharyngeal mucosal space

16   Where is the lesion on the following image located?

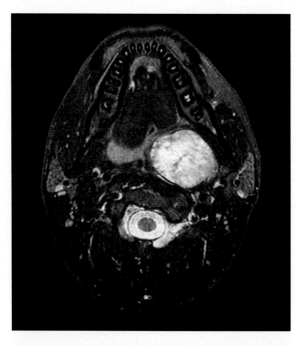

    A. Pre-styloid parapharyngeal space
    B. Post-styloid parapharyngeal space or carotid space
    C. Masticator space
    D. Pharyngeal mucosal space

17   Which of the following are true regarding pre styloid parapharyngeal space

    A. Pre-contrast T1-weighted images are the most accurate sequence to evaluate for the presence of fat surrounding the lesion
    B. Most common lesion is schwannoma
    C. Separated from post styloid space by the alar fascia
    D. Contains branches of the vagus nerve

ANSWERS AND EXPLANATIONS

1   **Answer B.**   Level IB.

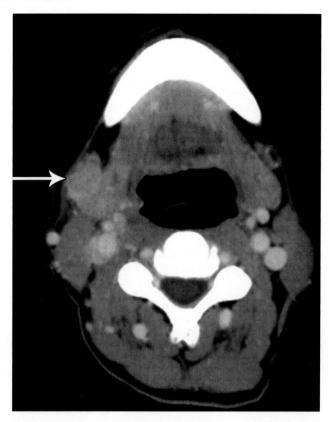

Imaging Findings: The axial CT image shows an abnormal lymph node anterolateral to the right submandibular gland (arrow).

2   **Answer C.**   Level VA.

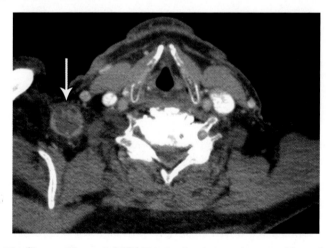

Imaging Findings: The axial CT image shows an abnormal lymph node located posterior to the posterior margin of the left sternocleidomastoid muscle (arrow), indicating that the node must be a level V lymph node. Although the cricoid cartilage is not visible on this image, the thyroid cartilage is evident, indicating that the node is above the level of the cricoid cartilage and therefore is a level VA lymph node.

Discussion: Level I lymph nodes include the submental (IA) and submandibular (IB) lymph node chains. Level IA nodes are between the anterior bellies of the digastric muscles. Level IB nodes are posterolateral to the anterior bellies of the digastric muscles. Level II lymph nodes constitute the internal jugular lymph node chain superior to the hyoid bone, which are anterior or immediately adjacent to the jugular vein (IIA) or posterior to the jugular vein deep to the sternocleidomastoid muscle (IIB). Level III lymph nodes involve the jugular chain between the hyoid and cricoid cartilage, and level IV lymph nodes involve the jugular chain below the cricoid cartilage. Level V is designated as all the lymph nodes of the posterior triangle of the neck (deep and posterior to the sternocleidomastoid muscle and above the clavicle). Level V nodes superior to the cricoid cartilage are designated as VA, whereas those inferior to the cricoid cartilage are designated VB. Level VI lymph nodes are in the space between the hyoid bone and manubrium anterior to the level III and IV nodal stations. Level VII nodes are in the superior mediastinum.

Reference: Forghani R, Yu E, Levental M, et al. Imaging evaluation of lymphadenopathy and patterns of lymph node spread in head and neck cancer. *Expert Rev Anticancer Ther* 2015;15(2):207–224.

3 **Answer B.** Vagus nerve.

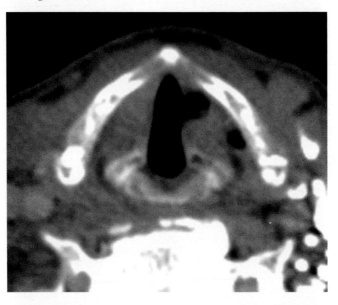

Imaging Findings: The axial CT image shows medialization of the posterior left vocal cord margin and dilation of the ipsilateral laryngeal ventricle.

Discussion: Vocal cord paralysis can result from impairment of the recurrent laryngeal branch of the vagus nerve. The nerve loops around the aortic arch on the left side and around the subclavian artery on the right side and courses through the tracheoesophageal grooves bilaterally. Although vocal cord paralysis can be observed on imaging, manifesting as dilation of the piriform sinus and ventricle, as well as medial rotation of the arytenoid, aryepiglottic fold, and posterior vocal cord, the role of imaging is mainly to identify a potential cause of the paralysis, such as tumors, and the field of view should extend from the brainstem to the upper mediastinum.

The glossopharyngeal nerve supplies the stylopharyngeus muscle.

The spinal accessory nerve supplies the sternocleidomastoid muscle and the trapezius muscle.

The hypoglossal nerve supplied the intrinsic tongue muscles.

Reference: Kwong Y, Boddu S, Shah J. Radiology of vocal cord palsy. *Clin Radiol* 2012;67(11):1108–1114.

4   **Answer A.**   Masticator space.

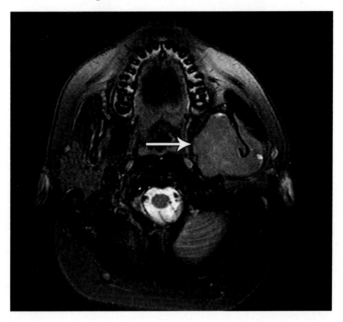

Imaging Findings: The axial fat-suppressed T2-weighted MRI shows a mass arising from the left mandible (arrow), which proved to be Ewing sarcoma.

Discussion: The suprahyoid head and neck spaces are subdivided by layers of the deep cervical fascia into the pharyngeal mucosal, parapharyngeal, carotid, parotid, masticator, retropharyngeal, and perivertebral spaces.

The masticator space contains the masseter, lateral pterygoid, medial pterygoid, and temporalis muscles, posterior portion of the mandible and inferior alveolar nerve, and internal maxillary artery. Tumors arising from the masticator space tend to displace the parapharyngeal fat pad medially.

Differential Diagnosis: Differential diagnosis or lesions in this location include inflammatory lesions from odontogenic source, vascular lesions like hemangioma and neoplasms arising from the mandible, trigeminal nerve branches or the muscles of mastication.

Reference: Gamss C, Gupta A, Chazen JL, et al. Imaging evaluation of the suprahyoid neck. *Radiol Clin North Am* 2015;53(1):133–144.

Fernandes T, Lobo JC, Castro R, Oliveira MI, and Som PM. Anatomy and pathology of the masticator space. *Insights Imaging* 2013;4(5):605–616.

5   **Answer A.**   The abnormality can potentially extend into the mediastinum via the danger space.

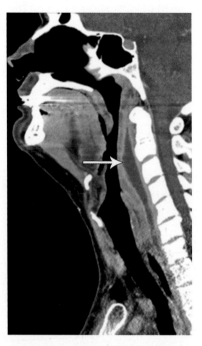

Imaging Findings: The sagittal contrast-enhanced CT of the neck demonstrates a rim-enhancing fluid collection posterior to the pharynx (arrow), consistent with a retropharyngeal abscess.

Discussion: The retropharyngeal space is located posterior to the pharynx and esophagus and constitutes the true retropharyngeal space, which extends inferiorly to the level of T1 to T6, and the "danger space," which extends into the mediastinum, down to the level of the diaphragm, allowing abscess in this space to spread inferiorly. Other complications of retropharyngeal abscess include airway and vascular compromise. Retropharyngeal abscesses most commonly arise from rupture of suppurative retropharyngeal lymph nodes and less often from spread of infection from contiguous spaces or penetrating trauma. Because retropharyngeal lymph nodes are more prominent in children, retropharyngeal abscesses are more common in this age group than in adults. On imaging, retropharyngeal abscesses typically appear as convex rim-enhancing fluid collections, as opposed to effusions, which have a bow-tie configuration in cross section and no rim enhancement.

Reference: Hoang JK, Branstetter BF, Eastwood JD, et al. Multiplanar CT and MRI of collections in the retropharyngeal space: is it an abscess? *AJR Am J Roentgenol* 2011;196(4):W426–W432.

6   **Answer D.**   Treatment with NSAIDs.

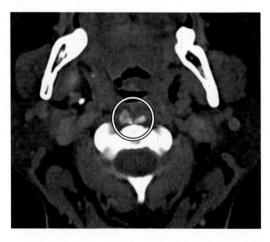

Imaging Findings: The axial CT depicts calcifications in the prevertebral space (encircled), along the bilateral longus colli tendons, related to calcific tendinitis.

Discussion: Calcific tendinitis of the longus colli muscle is an inflammatory reaction to deposition of calcium hydroxyapatite in the tendons of the longus colli muscle. Symptoms develop acutely and include neck pain, fever, dysphagia, odynophagia, and reduced neck range of movement. Inflammatory markers such as erythrocyte sedimentation rate can be elevated. The diagnosis is best made via CT depiction of calcification in the upper prevertebral space, but the degree of symptoms may be unrelated to the amount of calcification. MRI may demonstrate elevated T2 signal in the surrounding soft tissue due to edema. Antibiotics are not indicated for the treatment of calcific tendinitis of the longus colli muscle. Rather, this condition often responds well to conservative management with NSAIDs.

Reference: Eastwood JD, Hudgins PA, Malone D. Retropharyngeal effusion in acute calcific prevertebral tendinitis: diagnosis with CT and MR imaging. *AJNR Am J Neuroradiol* 1999;19(9):1789–1792.

7 **Answer C.**   CT of the chest.

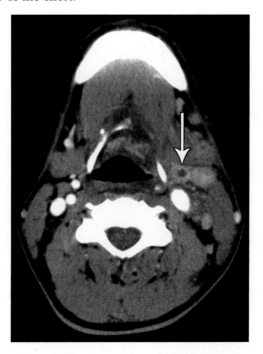

Imaging Findings: The CT of the neck demonstrates thrombus within the left internal jugular vein (arrow) and left oropharyngeal mucosal space edema. A chest CT also showed multiple septic emboli:

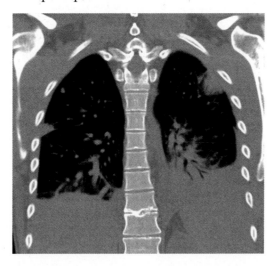

Discussion: Lemierre syndrome consists of an oropharyngeal infection associated with thrombophlebitis of the adjacent internal jugular vein. Bacteremia and distal septic thromboembolism, most often involving the lung, is a common complication of the syndrome. An oropharyngeal abscess may or may not be present. Classically, *Fusobacterium necrophorum* is considered to be the most common causative organism, although various other organisms can be responsible. The patient in this scenario presented with chest pain, which should raise the suspicion for pulmonary emboli, prompting further evaluation with a CT of the chest. A neck MRI does not add more information once the findings in the neck have been made on the neck and chest CTs. The infection related to Lemierre syndrome typically requires prolonged therapy with parenteral antibiotics as opposed to oral antibiotics. Incision and drainage are not necessary if there is no neck abscess.

Reference: Nguyen-Dinh KV, Marsot-Dupuch K, Portier F, et al. Lemierre syndrome: usefulness of CT in detection of extensive occult thrombophlebitis. *J Neuroradiol* 2002;29(2):132–135.

8 **Answer C.** Thyroglossal duct cyst.

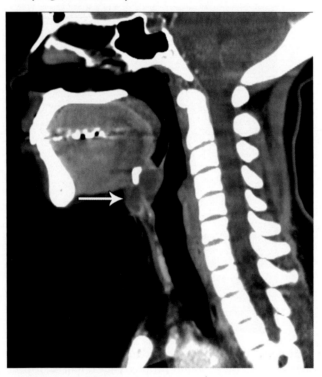

Imaging Findings: The sagittal CT image shows a midline lobulated cystic lesion (arrow) that extends from the tongue base to the anterior neck soft tissues inferior to the hyoid bone.

Discussion: Thyroglossal duct cysts are congenital anomalies that represent segments of the thyroglossal duct that do not regress. They are the most common congenital neck cyst. The lesions can be found in the midline or near the midline from the base of the tongue to the suprasternal region, but occur most commonly just below the level of the hyoid bone. Most lesions are in midline with off midline locations seen more inferiorly.

Reference: Miller MB, Rao VM, Tom BM. Cystic masses of the head and neck: pitfalls in CT and MR interpretation. *AJR Am J Roentgenol* 1992;159(3):601–607.

9 Answer C.   Papillary thyroid cancer.

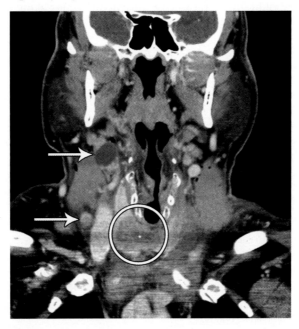

Imaging Findings: The coronal CT images shows cystic and solid left cervical lymph nodes (arrows) and a mass in the right lobe of the thyroid gland with calcification (encircled).

Discussion: Lymph node metastases from papillary thyroid carcinoma may be the initial manifestation of the cancer and are often cystic with walls that range from thin/imperceptible to thick enhancing nodular. The lesions may be hypervascular, contain septations and calcify. Imaging findings may mimic second branchial cleft cyst.

Reference: Wunderbaldinger P, Harisinghani MG, Hahn PF, et al. Cystic lymph node metastases in papillary thyroid carcinoma. *AJR Am J Roentgenol* 2002;178(3):693–697.

10 Answer B.   Adenoid cystic carcinoma.

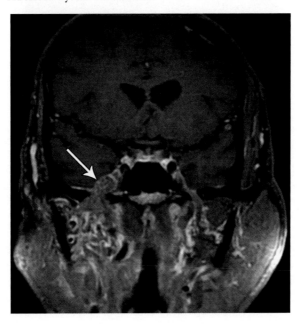

Imaging Findings: The fat-suppressed postcontrast MR image demonstrates widening of the right foramen ovale by enhancing tumor along the trigeminal nerve (arrow).

Discussion: Adenoid cystic carcinoma is the second most common malignancy involving the parotid gland and the most common malignancy involving the other salivary glands. Furthermore, adenoid cystic carcinoma has a particular propensity for perineural tumor spread, which appears as thickening and abnormal enhancement of the affected nerves.

Mucoepidermoid carcinoma is less likely than adenoid cystic carcinoma to undergo perineural spread and can be low grade with well-defined margins or high grade with infiltration and bone erosions.

Warthin tumors are benign salivary gland tumors that are most commonly located in the parotid gland tail and associated with smoking. They are bilateral or multifocal in up to 20% of cases and are the most common neoplastic cause of multiple solid parotid masses. The tumors can be hypermetabolic on FDG-PET and consist of solid and/or cystic components.

Pleomorphic adenomas, or benign mixed tumors, are the most common salivary gland tumors and most often appear as well-circumscribed, mildly lobulated, enhancing, predominantly T2 hyperintense masses:

Reference: Badger D, Aygun N. Imaging of perineural spread in head and neck cancer. *Radiol Clin North Am* 2017;55(1):139–149.

11 Answer B.   There is an increased risk for developing lymphoma.

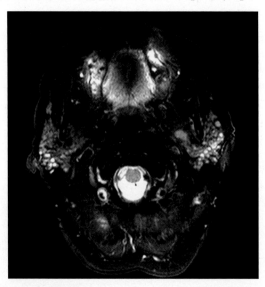

Imaging Findings: The axial MRI depicts variable-sized cystic lesions in bilateral slightly enlarged parotid glands.

Discussion: In the setting of xerophthalmia and xerostomia, this finding of cystic foci in the parotid glands should raise suspicion of Sjogren syndrome, which is an autoimmune disorder involving mainly the salivary and lacrimal glands and is associated with hyperactivity of the B lymphocytes and with autoantibody production. It most commonly affects females and is usually seen in the fourth or fifth decade of life. There is a known significant risk of interstitial lung disease in patients with Sjogren syndrome, although the reported frequency ranges from 9% to 75%. Of note, parotid gland lymphoepithelial cysts seen in the setting of HIV can have a similar appearance although symptoms of xerophthalmia and xerostomia as shown in the presented case are more typical of Sjogren syndrome.

Reference: Yousem DM, Kraut MA, Chalian AA. Major salivary gland imaging. *Radiology* 2000; 216(1):19–29.

12 **Answer C.** Floor of the mouth.

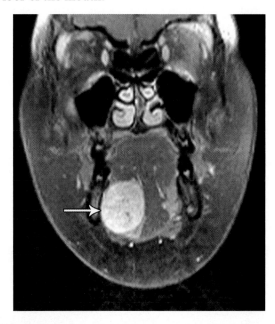

Imaging Findings: The coronal fat-suppressed postcontrast coronal T1-weighted MRI shows a mass (arrow) in the right sublingual space (a part of the floor of mouth) that displaces the sublingual gland inferiorly. The mass proved to be a schwannoma.

Discussion: The subdivisions of the oral cavity include the lips, floor of the mouth, oral tongue, buccal mucosa, gingiva, hard palate, and retromolar trigone. The floor of the mouth is situated between the oral tongue and mylohyoid, lateral to the root of the tongue, and medial to the mandible. The floor of the mouth contains the sublingual glands, the deep portion of the submandibular glands, submandibular ducts, lingual artery and vein, lingual nerve, and hypoglossal and glossopharyngeal nerves. Lesions in the floor of mouth include ranulas, epidermoid or dermoid cysts, lymphatic malformation, lipoma, schwannomas and malignancies (predominantly squamous cell carcinoma).

Reference: La'porte SJ, Juttla JK, Lingam RK. Imaging the floor of the mouth and the sublingual space. *Radiographics* 2011;31(5):1215–1230.

13 **Answer D.** Ranula.

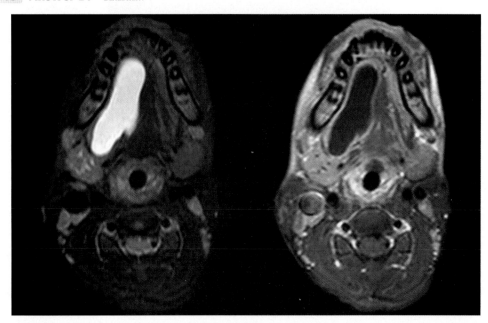

Imaging Findings: Axial fat-suppressed T2-weighted (A) and fat-suppressed post-contrast T1-weighted (B MR images show a large cystic mass in the right sublingual space with diffuse peripheral enhancement and signs of sialadenitis in the adjacent right submandibular gland.

Discussion: Ranulas are sublingual gland mucoceles. These can be confined to the sublingual space or extend into the submandibular space as plunging ranulas. Ranulas may display high or low T1 signal on MRI, depending on protein content, but typically demonstrate high T2 signal. Plunging ranulas feature a tapering connection with the sublingual space, which is often referred to as the "tail sign". When infected, ranulas can display mural enhancement and inflammation of the surrounding soft tissues. Differential considerations for ranulas on imaging include lymphatic malformations, inclusion cysts, and abscesses.

Reference: Kurabayashi T, Ida M, Yasumoto M, et al. MRI of ranulas. *Neuroradiology* 2000;42:917–22.

14 **Answer C.** Oropharyngeal cancer metastasis.

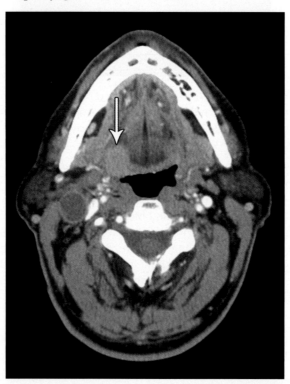

Imaging Findings: Axial CT image shows a cystic right level 2 lymph node and a right tongue base tumor (arrow) compatible with squamous cell carcinoma.

Discussion: Smoking, alcohol, and HPV are risk factors for the development of oropharymgeal squamous cell carcinoma. The imaging findings for HPV-positive versus HPV-negative oropharyngeal squamous cell carcinomas tend to differ. HPV-positive oropharyngeal squamous cell carcinomas tend to appear as tumors with well-defined borders and cystic lymph node metastases, while HPV-negative squamous cell carcinoma primary tumors tend to be poorly defined and the metastatic lymph nodes tend to solid or partly necrotic. The cystic lymph nodes associated with HPV-positive squamous cell carcinomas can resemble branchial cleft cysts, but the presence of an underlying malignancy should be excluded on head and neck imaging, endoscopy, and/or FNA/biopsy in adults.

Reference: Cantrell SC, Peck BW, Li G, et al. Differences in imaging characteristics of HPV-positive and HPV-Negative oropharyngeal cancers: a blinded matched-pair analysis. *AJNR Am J Neuroradiol* 2013;34(10):2005–2009.

15 **Answer B.** Post-styloid parapharyngeal space or carotid space.

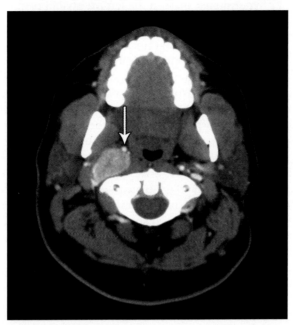

Imaging Findings: Axial CT image shows and avidly enhancing right suprahyoid mass that anteriorly displaces the internal carotid artery (arrow) and represents a paraganglioma.

Discussion: The post-styloid parapharyngeal space is almost synonymous with the carotid space and contains the carotid artery, internal jugular vein, lymph nodes, and IX-XII, cervical sympathetic chain, and glomus bodies. The main differential diagnosis for post-styloid parapharyangeal space tumors includes nerve sheath tumors, paragangliomas, nodes and pseudoaneurysms. Tumors in this space tend to displace the parapharyngeal fat pad and carotid artery anteriorly.

Reference: Fruin ME, Smoker WR, Harnsberger HR. The carotid space in the suprahyoid neck. *Semin Ultrasound CT MR* 1990;11(6):504–519.

16 **Answer A.** Pre-styloid parapharyngeal space.

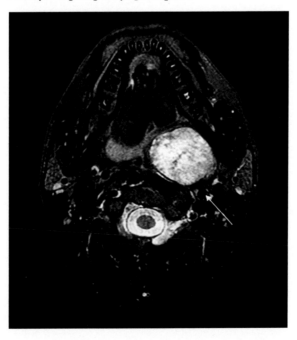

Imaging Findings: Axial STIR image shows a mildly lobulated, but well-defined predominantly T2 hyperintense mass in the left pre-styloid parapharyngeal space. The carotid is diplaced posteriorly by the mass (arrow)

Discussion: The pre-styloid parapharyngeal space contains minor or ectopic salivary gland tissue, branches of the mandibular division of the trigeminal nerve, internal maxillary artery, ascending pharyngeal artery, and pharyngeal venous plexus. This space is separated from the post-styloid parapharyngeal space by the tensor-vascular-styloid fascia, which extends from the tensor velipalatini muscle with styloid process. Pleomorphic adenoma is the most common neoplasm of pre-styloid parapharyngeal space. These benign tumors typically display nodular enhancement, high T2 signal, a T2 dark rim, and lobulated, but well-defined margins. Additional lesions that may arise within the pre-styloid parapharyngeal space include other salivary gland neoplasms, certain types of second branchial cleft cysts, and peripheral nerve sheath tumors. Otherwise, most abnormalities that involve the pre-styloid parapharyngeal space actually arise from adjacent spaces. The direction of the displacement of the parapharyngeal fat pat is a useful indicator as to the space of origin of lesions.

Reference: Gupta A, Chazen JL, Phillips CD. Imaging evaluation of the parapharyngeal space. *Otolaryngol Clin North Am* 2012;45(6):1223–1232.

17 **Answer A.**   Pre-contrast T1-weighted images are the most accurate sequence to evaluate for the presence of fat surrounding the lesion.

Discussion: Please refer to Answer 16.

14 Nose and Paranasal Sinuses

DANIEL THOMAS GINAT • DANIEL CHOW

QUESTIONS

1 Which label corresponds to the uncinate process?

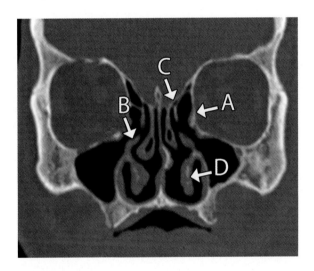

2 Where does the nasolacrimal duct drain?
   A. Frontoethmoid recess
   B. Sphenoethmoid recess
   C. Middle meatus
   D. Inferior meatus

3 Which of the following variants is correctly paired with the potential complication from endoscopic sinus surgery?
   A. Lamina papyracea dehiscence: olfactory bulb injury
   B. Sphenoid sinus dehiscence: internal carotid artery injury
   C. Cribriform plate asymmetry: optic nerve injury
   D. Retained Haller cell: persistently obstructed frontal sinus drainage

4 Which is the most likely diagnosis based on the image below?

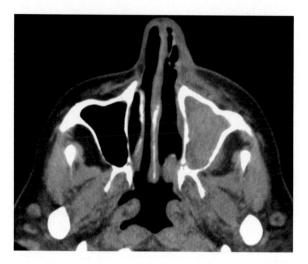

A. Acute invasive fungal rhinosinusitis
B. Allergic fungal sinusitis
C. Pott puffy tumor
D. Mycetoma

5 Which is the most likely diagnosis based on the image below?

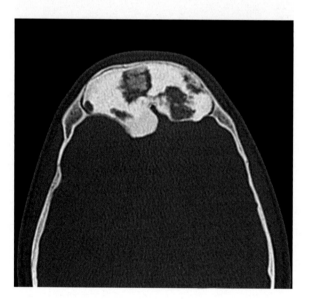

A. Osteoma
B. Mucocele
C. Paget disease
D. Fibrous dysplasia

6 What is the most likely diagnosis in a male teenager with epistaxis?

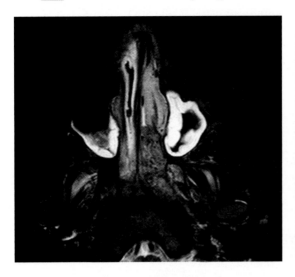 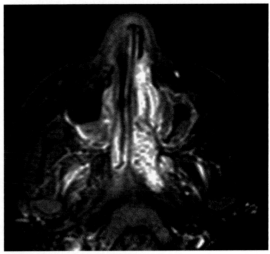

A. Rhabdomyosarcoma
B. Encephalocele
C. Juvenile nasal angiofibroma
D. Chondrosarcoma

7 Which of the following is true regarding juvenile nasal angiofibroma?

A. It is a malignant neoplasm.
B. It is avascular.
C. It arises from foramen rotundum.
D. It can erode bone.

8 Which is the most likely diagnosis based on the image below?

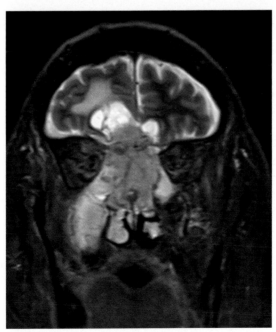

Image courtesy of Dr. Jason Johnson.

A. Nasopharyngeal carcinoma
B. Nasal polyposis
C. Esthesioneuroblastoma
D. Inverted papilloma

9   Which of the following statements is true regarding sinonasal masses?

   A. Esthesioneuroblastoma is the most common sinonasal malignancy.
   B. Cysts on MRI along the intracranial margin of a sinonasal mass are highly suggestive of esthesioneuroblastoma.
   C. CT is better than MRI for differentiating between trapped secretions and tumor.
   D. Esthesioneuroblastoma arises from the sinonasal respiratory epithelium.

10   Which of the following is true regarding nasal glial heterotopia (nasal gliomas)?

   A. Most demonstrate diffuse enhancement.
   B. They represent neoplasms.
   C. They generally do not have an intracranial connection.
   D. They commonly present with epistaxis.

11   Which is the most likely diagnosis based on the images below?

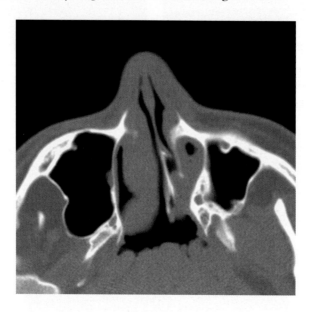

   A. Choanal atresia
   B. Dermoid
   C. Pyriform aperture stenosis
   D. Foreign body

12   Which of the following is true regarding choanal atresia?

   A. It is most commonly only membranous.
   B. It is less common than is pyriform aperture stenosis.
   C. It is always symptomatic at birth.
   D. It can be associated with CHARGE syndrome.

13 What is the most likely diagnosis in a 45-year-old male with painless growing mass.

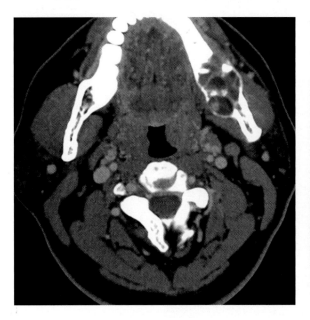 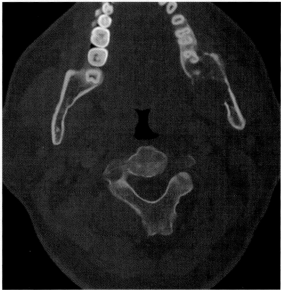

A. Ameloblastoma
B. Aneurysmal bone cyst
C. Dentigerous cyst
D. Keratocystic odontogenic cyst

14 Which of the following statements is true regarding ameloblastoma?

A. More commonly presents in children
B. Is painless
C. Malignant transformation is common.
D. Over half arise from dentigerous cysts.

15 A 15-year-old male presents with jaw mass. What is the diagnosis?

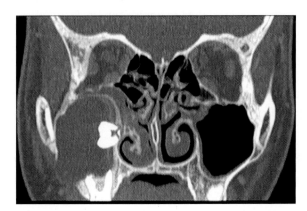

A. Ameloblastic carcinoma
B. Dentigerous cyst
C. Keratocystic odontogenic tumor
D. Periapical cyst

ANSWERS AND EXPLANATIONS

1 **Answer B.**

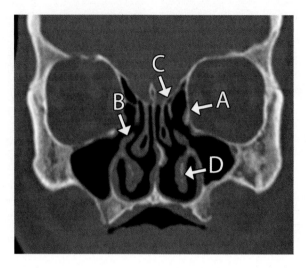

Discussion:
A: The lamina papyracea is the medial orbital wall.

B: The uncinate process is a bony projection alongside the infundibulum.

C: The cribriform plate is the roof of the nasal cavity, through which the olfactory nerves are transmitted. The cribriform plate is composed of a medial and lateral lamella on each side.

D: The inferior turbinate is the largest of the nasal turbinates and is covered by scroll-shaped mucosa that can vary in thickness.

Reference: Vaid S, Vaid N. Normal anatomy and anatomic variants of the paranasal sinuses on computed tomography. *Neuroimaging Clin N Am* 2015;25(4):527–548.

2 **Answer D.** Inferior meatus.

Discussion: The nasolacrimal duct extends from the lacrimal sac to the inferolateral nasal cavity. In particular, tears drain into the inferior meatus, which is located lateral to the inferior turbinate. The frontal, anterior ethmoid, and maxillary sinuses drain into the middle meatus. The frontal sinuses drain into the frontoethmoid recess, while the sphenoid sinuses drain into the sphenoethmoid recess. The sphenoid and posterior ethmoid sinuses then collectively drain into the superior meatus.

Reference: Vaid S, Vaid N. Normal anatomy and anatomic variants of the paranasal sinuses on computed tomography. *Neuroimaging Clin N Am* 2015;25(4):527–548.

3 **Answer B.** Sphenoid sinus dehiscence: internal carotid artery injury.

Discussion: There are several important anatomical variants and acquired abnormalities that can compromise the success of endoscopic sinus surgery. Dehiscence of the lamina papyracea can be congenital or acquired through trauma and can predispose to intraorbital injury during surgery, particularly the medial rectus muscle. Depending on the location of a sphenoid sinus dehiscence, the internal carotid artery, optic nerve, and trigeminal nerve are potentially at risk of injury during surgery. An asymmetric, particularly a low-lying, cribriform plate can lead to an increased risk of injury of the olfactory apparatus or adjacent brain parenchyma or branches of the anterior cerebral artery. Haller cells are anterior ethmoid air cells that extend along the floor of the orbits, lateral to the sagittal plane of the lamina papyracea, and can contribute to obstruction of the infundibulum.

Reference: Hoang JK, Eastwood JD, Tebbit CL, et al. Multiplanar sinus CT: a systematic approach to imaging before functional endoscopic sinus surgery. *AJR Am J Roentgenol* 2010;194(6):W527–W536.

4 **Answer A.** Acute invasive fungal rhinosinusitis.

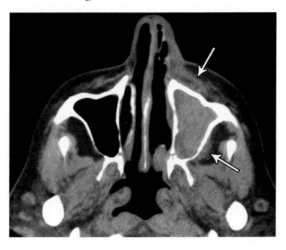

Imaging Findings: The axial CT image shows hyperattenuating material within the left maxillary sinus, as well as periantral fat infiltration (arrows).

Discussion: Acute invasive fungal rhinosinusitis is an aggressive infection often caused by *Aspergillus* species and *Mucor* species in diabetic and/or immunocompromised individuals. The presence of periantral fat infiltration, bone dehiscence, orbital invasion, septal ulceration, pterygopalatine fossa, nasolacrimal duct, and lacrimal sac involvement are potential signs of acute invasive fungal rhinosinusitis on imaging. On the other hand, allergic fungal sinusitis is a relatively common and indolent type I IgE-mediated allergic response to inhaled fungal spores and manifests as hyperattenuating allergic mucin with the sinuses.

Pott puffy tumor represents a subperiosteal abscess and/or epidural abscess associated with frontal osteomyelitis and sinusitis.

A mycetoma is a fungus ball, which characteristically contains calcifications that can be visible on CT.

Reference: Middlebrooks EH, Frost CJ, De Jesus RO, et al. Acute invasive fungal rhinosinusitis: a comprehensive update of CT findings and design of an effective diagnostic imaging model. *AJNR Am J Neuroradiol* 2015;36(8):1529–1535.

5 **Answer A.** Osteoma.

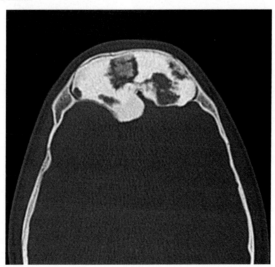

Imaging Findings: The axial CT image shows a mass with very high attenuation bone and areas of lower attenuation in the expanded frontal sinuses.

Discussion: Osteomas are benign tumors that characteristically display very dense bone formation, but may also contain lower attenuation fibrous areas. These lesions most commonly occur in the frontal and ethmoid sinuses. Giant osteomas can expand the sinuses and can be complicated by pneumocephalus and meningitis.

Mucoceles can also expand the paranasal sinuses, but do not display bone attenuation.

Paget disease can contain areas of dense bone, producing a "cotton wool" appearance, but arises from the skull itself rather than from within the sinus and tends to be a more diffuse process.

Fibrous dysplasia can be expansile and contain ground-glass components, but does not contain such dense bone as in osteomas.

Reference: Earwaker J. Paranasal sinus osteomas: a review of 46 cases. *Skeletal Radiol* 1993;22(6):417–423.

6 Answer C. Juvenile nasal angiofibroma.

7 Answer D. It can erode bone.

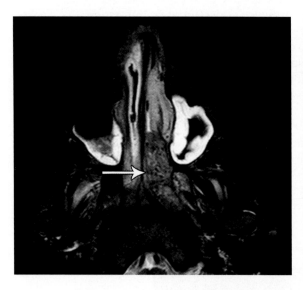 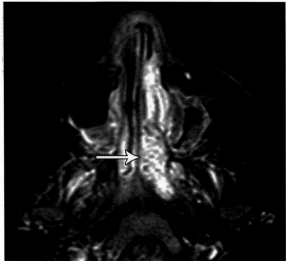

Discussion: Please refer to answer 6.

Imaging Findings: Axial fat-suppressed T2-weighted and postcontrast T1-weighted MR images shows an avidly enhancing mass with prominent flow voids in the left nasal cavity and nasopharynx, centered at the sphenopalatine foramen (arrows).

Discussion: Juvenile nasal angiofibromas are benign, vascular tumors that classically occur in young males presenting with epistaxis. The tumors arise from the sphenopalatine foramen and extend into the posterior nasal cavity and pterygopalatine fossa. Furthermore, juvenile nasal angiofibromas often erode bone of the medial pterygoid plate, which can be depicted on CT. On MRI, flow voids and intense contrast enhancement are typical. The lesions can be amenable to embolization prior to surgery.

Rhabdomyosarcomas are among the most common pediatric head and neck malignancies and can appear as destructive soft tissue tumors.

Encephaloceles are herniations of brain tissue along with variable amounts of cerebrospinal fluid. MRI is useful for depicting the intracranial connections.

Chondrosarcomas are unusual in the sinonasal region and appear as soft tissue tumors with calcified matrix and may erode or remodel the sinus walls.

Reference: Lloyd G, Howard D, Lund VJ, et al. Imaging for juvenile angiofibroma. *J Laryngol Otol* 2000;114(9):727–730.

8 **Answer C.** Esthesioneuroblastoma.

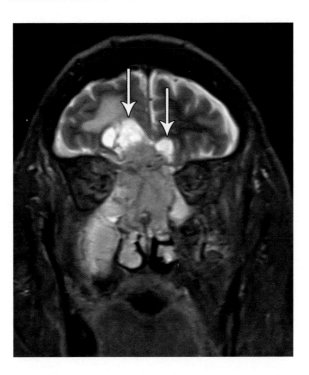

Imaging Findings: Coronal T2-weighted MRI shows a bulky sinonasal tumor with intracranial extension and associated cysts along the intracranial margin (arrows).

Discussion: Esthesioneuroblastoma (ENB), is a malignant tumor of neural crest origin, and arises from the olfactory epithelium of the superior nasal cavity. It has a bimodal age of presentation in the second and sixth decades. On CT, it presents as soft tissue mass in the nasal vault, often with bony destruction. MRI is superior to define the extent of tumor intracranially and to differentiate tumor from entrapped secretions. The presence of cysts along the intracranial margin of a sinonasal mass is highly suggestive of esthesioneuroblastoma.

Nasal polyposis is associated with allergic rhinitis and can appear as multiple mass lesions with peripheral enhancement due to inflamed mucosa.

Nasopharyngeal carcinoma is often associated with EBV infection, more commonly occurs in adults, and typically arises from the fossa of Rosenmuller.

Inverted papillomas are most commonly located in the maxillary sinus or nasal cavity and classically display a "cerebriform" pattern of enhancement.

Reference: Som PM, Lidov M, Brandwein M, et al. Sinonasal esthesioneuroblastoma with intracranial extension: marginal tumor cysts as a diagnostic MR finding. *AJNR Am J Neuroradiol* 1994;15(7):1259–1262.

9 **Answer B.** Cysts on MRI along the intracranial margin of a sinonasal mass are highly suggestive of esthesioneuroblastoma.

Discussion: Please refer to answer 8.

10 **Answer C.** They generally do not have an intracranial connection.

Discussion: Nasal glial heterotopias are congenital anomalies consisting of ectopic cerebrospinal fluid and/or dysplastic brain tissue and therefore do not have a visible intracranial connection. The antiquated term nasal glioma is a misnomer, because these lesions are not neoplastic. They may be external, internal, or a combination of the two with respect to the nasal cavity and can cause nasal obstruction. The imaging features of nasal glial heterotopia vary based on the types of contents, but the contents typically do not enhance much at all.

Reference: Ginat DT, Robson CD. Diagnostic imaging features of congenital nose and nasal cavity lesions. *Clin Neuroradiol* 2015;25:3–11.

11 **Answer A.** Choanal atresia.

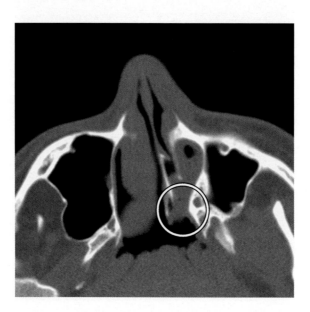

Imaging Findings: The axial CT image shows both membranous and bony occlusion of the left posterior choana (encircled).

Discussion: Choanal atresia results from the failure of resorption of the buccopharyngeal membrane and may present with nasal obstruction early in life or rhinosinusitis later in life. There is always a bony component, which can be complete or partial along with a membranous component. There is characteristic bowing of the nasal septum and nasoantral wall toward the atresia. Choanal atresia is associated with other congenital anomalies up to 50%, most commonly CHARGE syndrome, which is a genetic disorder that consists of ocular coloboma, heart defects, choanal atresia, retarded growth, genital anomalies, and ear anomalies.

Pyriform aperture stenosis is also a congenital malformation defined by a pyriform aperture width of <4 mm in a newborn. This condition is often associated with other midline anomalies, such as a solitary mega incisor and syntelencephaly. Low-dose CT is useful for delineating the narrow airway.

Reference: Ginat DT, Robson CD. Diagnostic imaging features of congenital nose and nasal cavity lesions. *Clin Neuroradiol* 2015;25:3–11.

12 **Answer D.** It can be associated with CHARGE syndrome.

Discussion: Please refer to answer 11.

13 **Answer A.** Ameloblastoma.

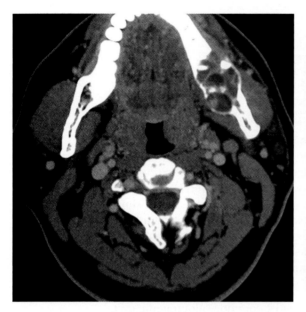 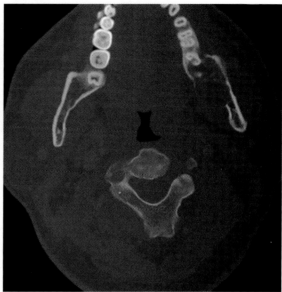

Imaging findings: Contrast-enhanced CT with bone and soft tissue windows demonstrates a multiloculated cystic expansile mass within the left mandible. Bone window demonstrates a thinned cortex with multiple coarse septations giving a bubbly appearance. Soft tissue windows demonstrate a central hyperdense and mildly enhancing mural nodule. The lesion itself is located along the course of the left inferior alveolar nerve.

Discussion: Ameloblastomas represent 1% of all lesions of the mandible and maxilla but are the second most common odontogenic tumor, representing 35%. These are benign epithelial odontogenic tumors, with 20% reportedly arising from dentigerous cysts. Clinically, these commonly present as painless masses in adulthood. Less than 1% may develop malignant transformation to an ameloblastic carcinoma.

On imaging, these appear as multilocular, mixed cystic and solid masses. The mandible is more commonly involved than is the maxilla and most commonly in the mandibular ramus region. Differential may include dentigerous cysts, keratocystic odontogenic cysts, odontogenic myxomas, and aneurysmal bone cysts. With regard to the dentigerous and keratocystic odontogenic cysts, the absence of nodular enhancement is useful in differentiating them from ameloblastomas.

References: Bharatha A, Pharoah MJ, Lee L, et al. Pictorial essay: cysts and cyst-like lesions of the jaws. *Can Assoc Radiol J* 2010;61(3):133–143.

Diagnostic imaging: head and neck. Elsevier. ISBN: 9780323443012. https://www.elsevier.com/books/diagnostic-imaging-head-and-neck/koch/978-0-323-44301-2

Dunfee BL, Sakai O, Pistey R, et al. Radiologic and pathologic characteristics of benign and malignant lesions of the mandible. *Radiographics* 2006;26(6):1751–1768.

14 **Answer B.** Is painless.

Discussion: Please refer to answer 13.

15 Answer B.   Dentigerous cyst.

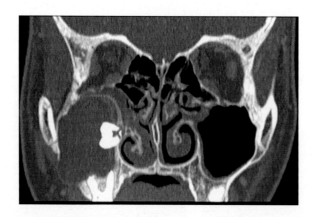

Imaging findings: Noncontrast CT of the face demonstrates a well-circumscribed, unilocular expansile cyst surrounding the crown of an unerupted tooth, compatible with a dentigerous cyst. A odontogenic keratocyst may have a similar unilocular cystic mass; however, it would typically surround the entire unerupted tooth. An ameloblastic carcinoma would be expected to have a more multilocular appearance with enhancing soft tissue nodules. Lastly, a periapical cyst would be expected to be associated with the root of a tooth and demonstrate associated periodontal disease.

Discussion: Dentigerous cysts are the second most common odontogenic cyst, preceded by periapical cysts. These represent benign developmental cysts, felt to form because of the hydrostatic force due to accumulation of fluid between enamel epithelium and the surface of the crown of the unerupted tooth. Like ameloblastomas, these are typically painless at presentation.

The third mandibular molar is the most common location. On imaging, CT demonstrates a thin-walled and well-circumscribed cystic structure surrounding the crown of an unerupted tooth. Note, these may be indistinguishable from unilocular ameloblastomas, which is the primary differential consideration.

References: Bharatha A, Pharoah MJ, Lee L, et al. Pictorial essay: cysts and cyst-like lesions of the jaws. *Can Assoc Radiol J* 2010;61(3):133–143.

Diagnostic imaging: head and neck. Elsevier. ISBN: 9780323443012. https://www.elsevier.com/books/diagnostic-imaging-head-and-neck/koch/978-0-323-44301-2

Dunfee BL, Sakai O, Pistey R, et al. Radiologic and pathologic characteristics of benign and malignant lesions of the mandible. *Radiographics* 2006;26(6):1751–1768.

15 Orbit

DANIEL THOMAS GINAT

QUESTIONS

1   What nerve supplies the structure denoted in the following image?

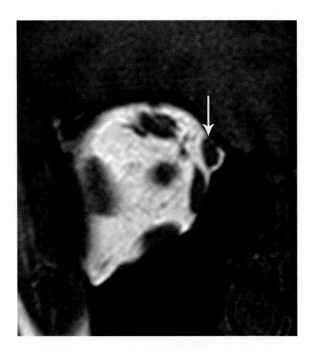

A. Cranial nerve 3
B. Cranial nerve 4
C. Cranial nerve 6
D. Cranial nerve 7

2 With which syndrome is the abnormality shown on the following image most closely associated?

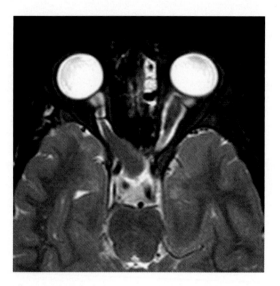

A. Neurofibromatosis type 1
B. Neurofibromatosis type 2
C. Tuberous sclerosis complex
D. von Hippel-Lindau syndrome

3 Which of the following is true regarding optic nerve gliomas?

A. The presence of cystic components is less common with sporadic optic nerve gliomas than those in patients with neurofibromatosis type 1.
B. Sporadic tumors are less likely to progress than are those associated with neurofibromatosis type 1.
C. The tumors tend to be smaller and maintain the original shape of the optic pathways in patients with neurofibromatosis type 1.
D. Extension beyond the optic pathway at diagnosis is less common in patients with neurofibromatosis than those without.

4 Which of the following is the most likely diagnosis based on the following image?

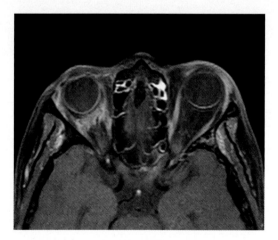

A. Melanoma metastasis
B. Neuroblastoma metastasis
C. Lung cancer metastasis
D. Breast cancer metastasis

5   What is the most likely diagnosis based on the following imaging obtained in a
pediatric patient with a rapidly growing right orbital mass?

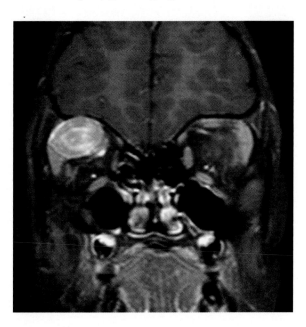

A. Rhabdomyosarcoma
B. Retinoblastoma
C. Meningioma
D. Lymphangioma

6   Which of the statements is true regarding the abnormalities shown in the following
image?

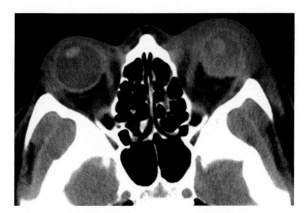

A. The left globe contour is deformed by retrobulbar hemorrhage.
B. There is left intraocular air.
C. Ultrasound is contraindicated for evaluating the left globe.
D. There is complete left lens dislocation.

7   What is the most likely diagnosis based on the following image?

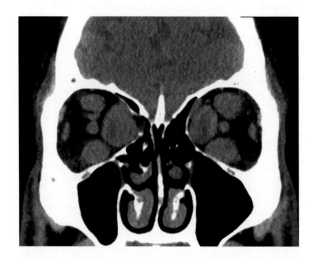

A. Sarcoidosis
B. Orbital inflammatory syndrome
C. Thyroid eye disease
D. Lymphoma

8   Which muscle is most commonly involved in thyroid eye disease?

A. Medial rectus
B. Inferior rectus
C. Lateral rectus
D. Superior rectus

9   Which statement is correct regarding the following image in a patient with fever and proptosis?

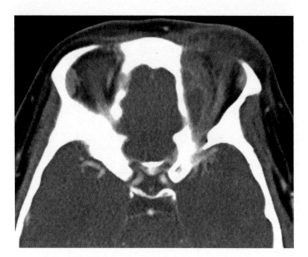

A. Oral antibiotics are sufficient treatment.
B. CT is more sensitive than is MRI for detecting intracranial complications.
C. Bone erosions must be present for the spread to infection.
D. Acute bacterial rhinosinusitis is the most common cause.

10 What is the most likely diagnosis in this infant based on the following image?

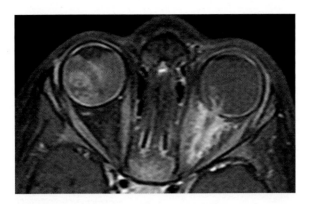

A. Rhadomyosarcoma
B. Retinoblastoma
C. Persistent hyperplastic primary vitreous
D. Infantile fibromatosis

11 Which of the following is true regarding the complication related to treatment of retinoblastoma shown in the following image?

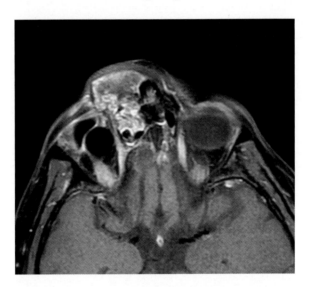

A. Chondrosarcoma is the most common histological type.
B. The majority of cases occur within 2 years following treatment.
C. CT is superior to MRI for depicting matrix mineralization.
D. This is a manifestation of trilateral retinoblastoma.

12 Which of the following most likely coincides with the findings on the following image?

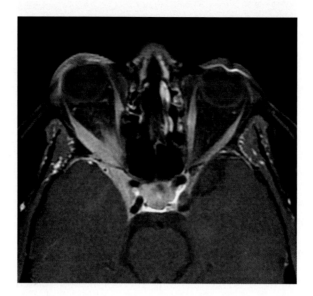

    A. Tolosa-Hunt syndrome
    B. Duane syndrome
    C. Brown syndrome
    D. One-and-a-half syndrome

13 What is the most likely diagnosis based on the following image?

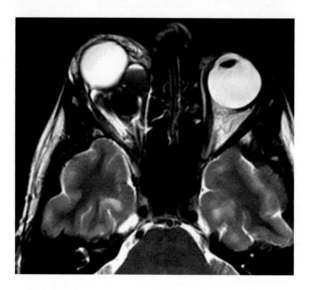

    A. Lymphatic malformation
    B. Venous malformation
    C. Arteriovenous malformation
    D. Cavernous hemangioma

14 What is the most likely diagnosis for the abnormality shown on the following image?

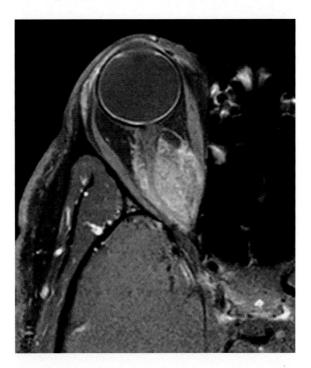

A. Choroidal melanoma
B. Optic nerve glioma
C. Schwannoma
D. Optic nerve sheath meningioma

ANSWERS AND EXPLANATIONS

1 **Answer B.** Cranial nerve 4.

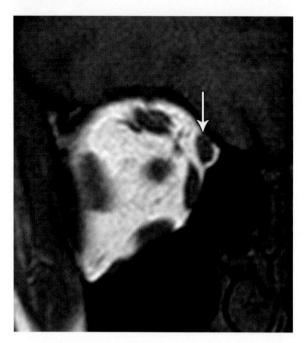

Imaging Findings: The arrow in the coronal T1-weighted MR image points to the superior oblique muscle.

Discussion: The superior oblique muscle internally rotates and abducts the globe. It is the only structure supplied by cranial nerve 4, or the trochlear nerve. The superior rectus, medial rectus, inferior rectus, levator palpebrae superioris, and inferior oblique muscles are supplied by cranial nerve 3, or the oculomotor nerve. The lateral rectus muscle is supplied by cranial nerve 6, or the abducens nerve. The orbicularis oculi muscle is supplied by cranial nerve 7, or the facial nerve.

Reference: Braffman BH, Naidich TP, Chaneles M. Imaging anatomy of the normal orbit. *Semin Ultrasound CT MR* 1997;18(6):403–412.

2 **Answer A.** Neurofibromatosis type 1.

3 **Answer D.** Extension beyond the optic pathway at diagnosis is less common in patients with neurofibromatosis than those without.

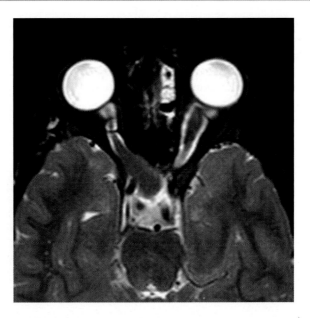

Imaging Findings: The axial T2-weighted MRI shows expansion of the bilateral optic nerve gliomas with dilation of the optic nerve sheaths in a patient with neurofibromatosis type 1.

Discussion: Up to 70% of patients with optic nerve gliomas have neurofibromatosis type 1. The orbital portions of the optic nerves are most commonly involved in patients with neurofibromatosis type 1, whereas the optic chiasm is the most common site of involvement in patients without neurofibromatosis type 1. The tumors tend to be smaller and maintain the original shape of the optic pathways in patients with neurofibromatosis type 1. Conversely, extension beyond the optic pathway at diagnosis is less common in patients with neurofibromatosis than those without. The presence of cystic components is more common with sporadic optic nerve gliomas than those in patients with neurofibromatosis type 1. Sporadic tumors are more likely to progress than are those associated with neurofibromatosis type 1.

Reference: Kornreich L, Blaser S, Schwarz M, et al. Optic pathway glioma: correlation of imaging findings with the presence of neurofibromatosis. *AJNR Am J Neuroradiol* 2001;22(10):1963–1969.

4 **Answer D.** Breast cancer metastasis.

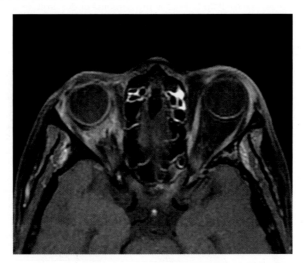

Imaging Findings: The axial fat-suppressed postcontrast T1-weighted MRI shows an infiltrative, enhancing retro-orbital lesion and associated enophthalmos.

Discussion: Metastases represent the most common orbital malignancy overall. Common primary tumors for orbital metastases include melanomas and breast and lung cancers in adults and neuroblastoma in children. Although most orbital metastases typically present with proptosis, scirrhous breast carcinoma metastases can present with enophthalmos due to soft tissue contraction.

Reference: Purohit BS, Vargas MI, Ailianou A, et al. Orbital tumours and tumour-like lesions: exploring the armamentarium of multiparametric imaging. *Insights Imaging* 2016;7(1):43–68.

5 **Answer A.** Rhabdomyosarcoma.

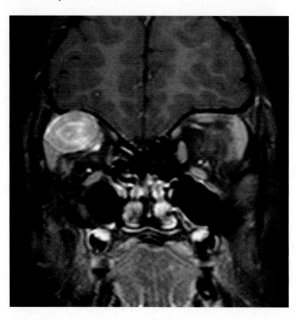

Imaging Findings: The coronal fat-suppressed postcontrast T1-weighted MRI shows an enhancing extraconal mass in the right superotemporal orbit.

Discussion: Rhabdomyosarcoma is the most common primary orbital malignancy in the pediatric population. It can present as an aggressive, rapidly growing mass or an indolent mass that can mimic a benign tumor. The tumors are usually in the extraconal space and enhance. There may be associated bone erosions and intracranial or paranasal sinus extension.

Reference: Mafee MF, Pai E, Philip B. Rhabdomyosarcoma of the orbit. Evaluation with MR imaging and CT. *Radiol Clin North Am* 1998;36(6):1215–1227, xii.

6 **Answer C.** Ultrasound is contraindicated for evaluating the left globe.

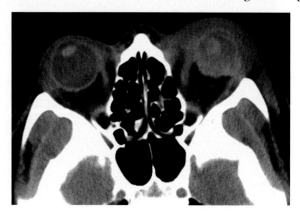

Imaging Findings: The axial CT image shows a deformed and shrunken left globe with partial posterior lens dislocation, intraocular hemorrhage, and extensive periorbital edema.

Discussion: Open-globe injuries are a contraindication for ultrasound because of compromised intraocular pressure. Rather, CT is appropriate for evaluating such cases. The characteristic findings associated with globe rupture include abnormal size and contours of the globe, or "flat tire" sign. There may also be associated intraocular hemorrhage, retinal detachment, and lens dislocation, which results from zonular fiber disruption. With partial detachment, the lens remains in the anterior portion of the globe, whereas with complete dislocation, the lens tends to fall to the posterior part of the globe. Anterior dislocation is less common.

Reference: Sung EK, Nadgir RN, Fujita A, et al. Injuries of the globe: what can the radiologist offer? *Radiographics* 2014;34(3):764–776.

7   **Answer C.**   Thyroid eye disease.

8   **Answer B.**   Inferior rectus.

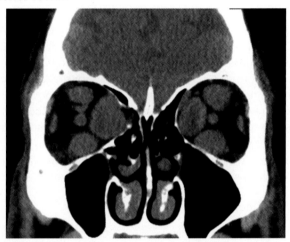

Imaging Findings: The coronal CT image shows enlargement of the bilateral inferior, medial, and superior rectus muscles with areas of hypoattenuation in the medial rectus muscles.

Discussion: Thyroid eye disease, or dysthyroid orbitopathy or Graves ophthalmopathy, is the most common cause of exophthalmos in adults. It is an autoimmune disease that involves the inferior, medial, superior, and lateral rectus muscles and oblique muscles in descending order of frequency, with the corresponding mnemonic "IMSLO." Additional imaging findings include increased orbital fat, lacrimal gland enlargement, eyelid edema, stretching of the optic nerve, tenting of the posterior globe, and intramuscular fat deposition. Involvement is usually bilateral and symmetric, but can be unilateral.

Reference: LeBedis CA, Sakai O. Nontraumatic orbital conditions: diagnosis with CT and MR imaging in the emergent setting. *Radiographics* 2008;28(6):1741-1753.

9 **Answer D.** Acute bacterial rhinosinusitis is the most common cause.

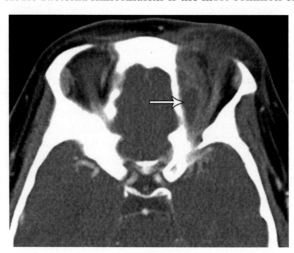

Imaging Findings: The axial postcontrast CT image shows a left medial orbit rim-enhancing subperiosteal fluid collection (arrow).

Discussion: Orbital subperiosteal abscesses appear as lenticular rim-enhancing fluid collections. These most result from acute bacterial sinusitis, which can spread through into the orbit through the ophthalmic venous system. Thus, bone erosions are often not visible on CT. Management of subperiosteal orbital abscesses may require surgical decompression in addition to intravenous antibiotics. Intracranial complications associated with the orbital infection include cavernous sinus thrombosis, abscess, and meningitis. MRI is generally more sensitive than is CT for detecting such complications.

Reference: Dankbaar JW, van Bemmel AJ, Pameijer FA. Imaging findings of the orbital and intracranial complications of acute bacterial rhinosinusitis. *Insights Imaging* 2015;6(5):509–518.

10 **Answer B.** Retinoblastoma.

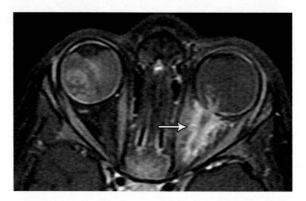

Imaging Findings: Axial fat-suppressed post-contrast T1-weighted MRI shows bilateral intraoacular tumors, as well as intraconal extension on the left (arrow).

11 **Answer C.** CT is superior to MRI for depicting matrix mineralization.

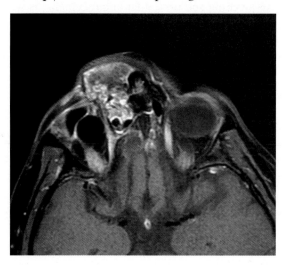

Imaging Findings: Axial fat-suppressed post-contrast T1-weighted MRI shows a heterogeneous right periorbital mass, adjacent to the right orbital implant and prosthesis related to prior enucleation for retinoblastoma.

Discussion: Retinoblastoma is the most common intraocular childhood malignancy and can be sporadic or hereditary, particularly in association with p53 mutations. High-resolution MRI is useful for evaluating the presence of extraocular tumor extension and the possibility of trilateral retinoblastoma involving the pineal gland. CT often demonstrates calcifications within retinoblastomas. In the past, radiation therapy was used considerably to treat retinoblastoma, but more recently there has been a trend towards emphasize on other treatment options.

Osteosarcoma is the most common second malignant neoplasm in survivors of retinoblastoma treated with radiation. Osteosarcoma after radiation typically develops after a latency period of 5–10 years. CT is superior for depicting matrix mineralization, periosteal reaction, and cortical destruction, whereas MRI is better for delineating soft-tissue and marrow infiltration and differentiating tumor from sinus secretions. Matrix mineralization and periosteal new bone formation favors a diagnosis of osteosarcoma over other neoplasms and a destructive mass is generally not associated with radiation osteitis.

Reference: Rauschecker AM, Patel CV, Yeom KW, et al. High-resolution MR imaging of the orbit in patients with retinoblastoma. *RadioGraphics* 2012;32(5):1307–1326.

12 **Answer A.** Tolosa-Hunt syndrome.

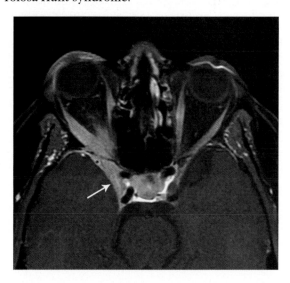

Imaging Findings: Axial fat-suppressed post-contrast T1-weighted MRI shows right lateral rectus swelling and orbital fat enhancement, as well as enhancing soft tissue in the right cavernous sinus (arrow).

Tolosa-Hunt syndrome is a clinical entity that is often attributable to inflammatory pseudotumor or idiopathic orbital inflammation. The diagnostic criteria for Tolosa-Hunt syndrome include the following:

- Unilateral orbital pain persisting for weeks if untreated.
- Paralysis of the third, fourth and/or sixth cranial nerves and/or cavernous sinus abnormality by MRI or biopsy.
- Paralysis coincides with the onset of pain or follows it within 2 weeks.
- Pain and paralysis resolve within 72 hours when treated adequately with corticosteroids.

MRI is useful for assessing patients with Tolosa-Hunt syndrome. MRI can demonstrateabnormal signal, enhancement, and enlargement of the cavernous sinuses, as well as contiguous involvement of the orbital apex contents and subtemporal region. Differential diagnoses based on imaging include meningioma, lymphoma, and sarcoidosis.

Reference: Yousem DM, Atlas SW, Grossman RI, et al. MR imaging of Tolosa-Hunt syndrome. *AJNR Am J Neuroradiol* 1989;10(6):1181–1184.

13 **Answer A.** Lymphatic malformation.

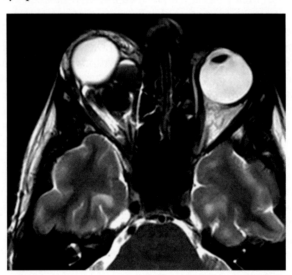

Imaging Findings: Axial T2-weighted MRI shows a multicystic mass in the right orbit with fluid-fluid levels, proptosis, and infiltration of the right eyelid.

Discussion: Lymphatic malformations are low-flow vascular malformations and can be macrocystic and/or microcystic. MRI is useful for delineating lymphatic malformations, which classically exhibit fluid-fluid levels in the cystic components and infiltrate across multiple tissue planes. Patients often experience multiple recurrences. Macrocystic lymphatic malformations are amenable to treatment usingsclerosing agents. However, lymphatic malformations are difficult lesions to treat because they do not respect tissue planes.

Reference: Lally SE. Update on orbital lymphatic malformations. *Curr Opin Ophthalmol* 2016;27(5):413–415.

14 **Answer D.** Optic nerve sheath meningioma.

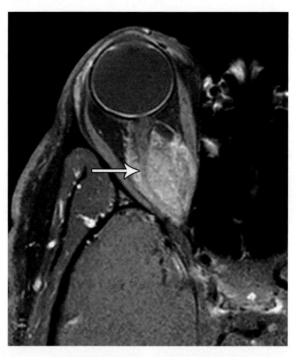

Imaging Findings: Axial fat-suppressed post-contrast T1-weighted MRI shows an enhancing mass surrounding the orbital portion of the right optic nerve (arrow), which represents an optic nerve sheath meningioma.

Discussion: Optic nerve sheath meningiomas typically present with painless, slowly gradual vision loss due to optic nerve atrophy. Tumor surrounding the optic nerve classically has a "tram-track" configuration on axial image, but can be eccentric. MRI is the optimal modality for delineating optic nerve sheath meningiomas, which display diffuse enhancement. However, intratumoralcalcifications, which are present in up to half of cases, are most conspicuous on CT.

Reference: Tailor TD, Gupta D, Dalley RW, et al. Orbital neoplasms in adults: clinical, radiologic, and pathologic review. *RadioGraphics* 2013;33(6):1739–1758.

16 Sella, Suprasellar, and Parasellar Lesions

ERNST GARCON • GUL MOONIS

QUESTIONS

1   A 41-year-old female presents with galactorrhea. An initial MRI was performed, top row (A and B). The patient was subsequently started on oral cabergoline; images C and D in the bottom row are from 5-month follow-up MRI.

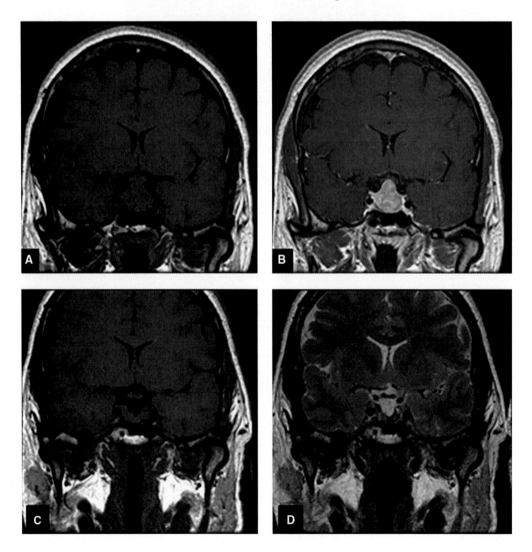

1a Based on the clinical picture and complete response to medical therapy, which of the following is the most likely diagnosis?

    A. Nonfunctioning macroadenoma

    B. Prolactinoma

    C. Rathke cleft cyst

    D. Lymphocytic hypophysitis

1b What other symptoms may be anticipated in this case based on the lesion size and location?

    A. Facial numbness

    B. Right-sided upper and lower extremity weakness

    C. Visual abnormalities

    D. Speech abnormalities

2 A 45-year-old female presents with headache and an abnormal MRI. There are no associated endocrine abnormalities or visual field defects.

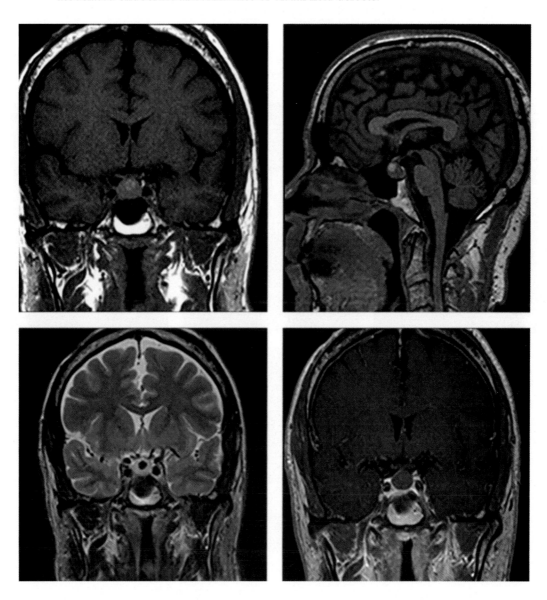

2a What is the most likely diagnosis?

    A. Cystic craniopharyngioma
    B. Cystic pituitary adenoma
    C. Rathke cleft cyst
    D. Intrasellar dermoid cyst
    E. Arachnoid cyst

2b Patient declined surgical intervention, and therefore, this lesion was managed conservatively. On a subsequent 6-month follow-up visit, an ophthalmologic examination was performed and bitemporal hemianopsia was noted. There was no loss in visual acuity. No new symptoms or associated endocrine abnormalities.

In the above clinical setting, what are the expected changes on follow-up MRI?

    A. Extrinsic compression of the prechiasmatic optic nerves
    B. Extrinsic compression of the optic chiasm
    C. Infiltration of cavernous sinus with cranial nerve involvement
    D. Extrinsic compression of bilateral cavernous ICAs

3 A 5-year-old girl presented with acute onset of abrupt staring and brief giggle or laughter, followed by right upward gaze deviation. Brain MRI without and with gadolinium was performed, and selected images are submitted for review.

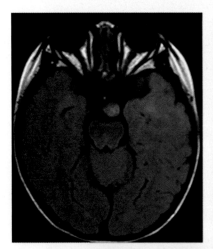
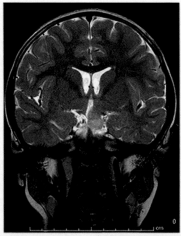
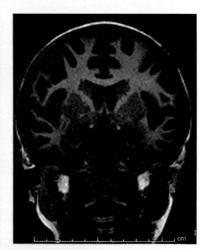

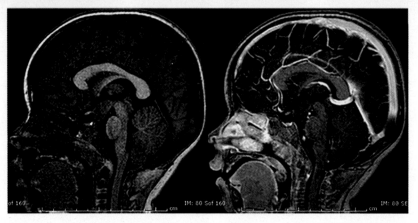

3a The most likely diagnosis is:

    A. Optic nerve glioma
    B. Hypothalamic hamartoma
    C. Pituitary microadenoma
    D. Germinoma

3b   Which of the following is true about this entity?

   A. Responds to medical treatment
   B. Patients have cortisol deficiency
   C. Follows gray matter on all sequences without enhancement
   D. Precocious puberty is seen with intrahypothalamic location of the lesion

4   A 45-year-old woman with diplopia on lateral gaze.

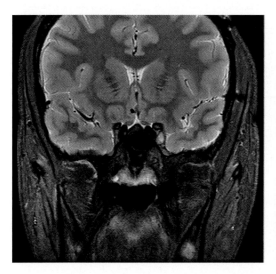 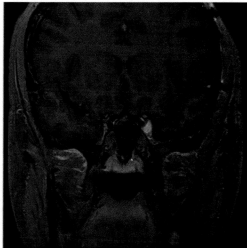

4a   In which anatomic space is the lesion located?

   A. Sella turcica
   B. Cavernous sinus
   C. Hippocampus
   D. Frontal lobe

An additional postgadolinium image is submitted below:

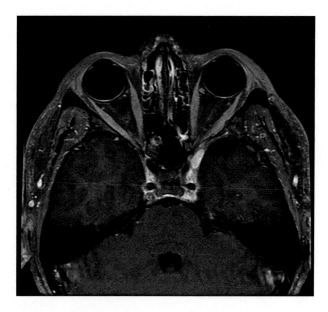

4b   What is the most likely diagnosis?

   A. Meningioma
   B. Aneurysm
   C. Schwannoma
   D. Pituitary adenoma

5 A 19-year-old male presents with polyuria and lethargy. Brain MRI was done without and with gadolinium.

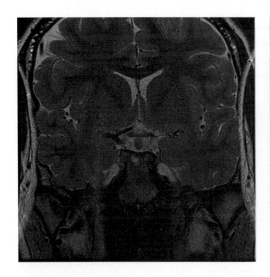 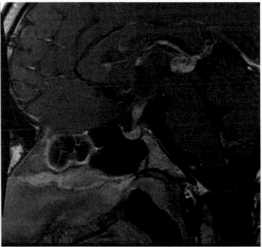

5a The patient's clinical symptoms are best explained by a lesion in the following locations:

A. Hypothalamus
B. Thalamus
C. Hippocampus
D. Tectal plate

5b The most likely diagnosis is:

A. Pineocytoma
B. Germinoma
C. Hypothalamic hamartoma
D. Pilocytic astrocytoma

6 A 35-year-old female presented with decreased frequency of menstrual periods. Brain MRI without and with gadolinium was done, and selected images are submitted for review.

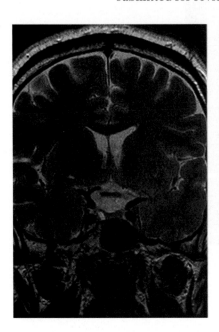 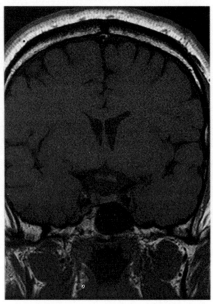 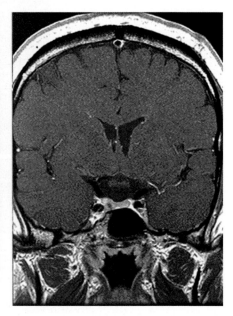

The most likely diagnosis is:

A. Pituitary microadenoma
B. Hypothalamic hamartoma
C. Cavernous sinus thrombosis
D. Neurocysticercosis

7 A 25-year-old with upward gaze palsy, nonreactive pupils to light stimuli and nystagmus. Brain MRI with gadolinium was performed, and selected postgadolinium images are submitted for review.

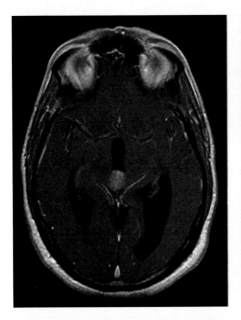 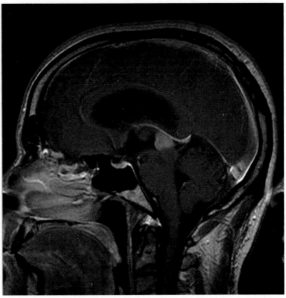

7a The patient clinical presentation is best explained by:

A. Compression of the superior colliculi
B. Obstructive hydrocephalus
C. Mass effect upon the optic chiasm
D. Tumor infiltration of CN VI

7b What is the most likely diagnosis?

A. Vein of Galen malformation
B. Epidermoid
C. Pineocytoma
D. Meningioma

8   A 25-year-old with fever and headaches. CT images of the brain and paranasal sinuses were acquired with IV contrast.

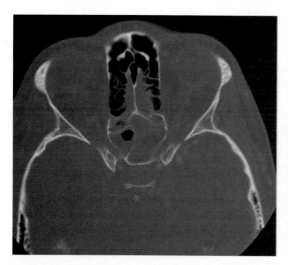 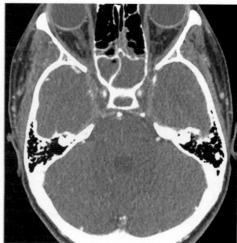

8a   The most critical finding is in which structure?

    A. Cavernous sinuses
    B. Cerebellum
    C. Orbits
    D. Pons

Brain MRI was performed without gadolinium, and selected images are submitted for review.

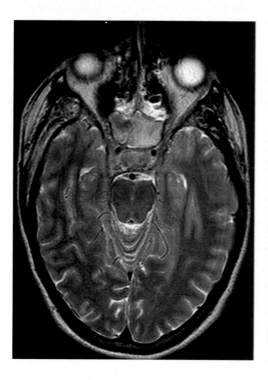 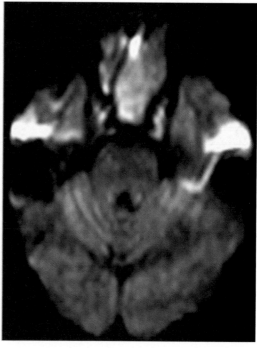

8b   What is the next best step in imaging evaluation?

   A. MRA of the COW without IV contrast
   B. MRA of the neck without IV contrast
   C. Postgadolinium T1-weighted images of the brain
   D. Refer to neurointerventional suite for clot retraction

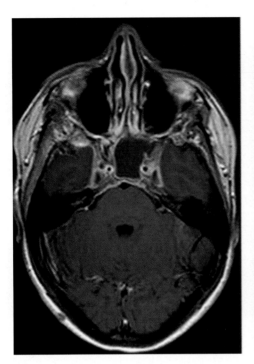
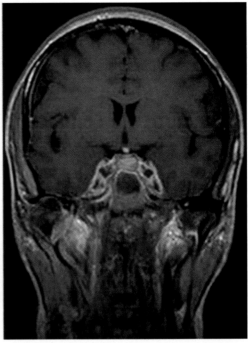

8c   What is the most likely diagnosis based on the post gadolinium images above?

   A. Acute meningitis
   B. Chronic sphenoid sinusitis
   C. Tolosa-Hunt syndrome
   D. Cavernous sinus thrombosis

9   A 15-year-old woman with bitemporal hemianopia has the following MRI:

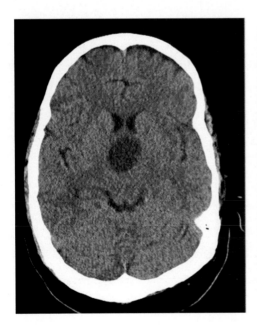
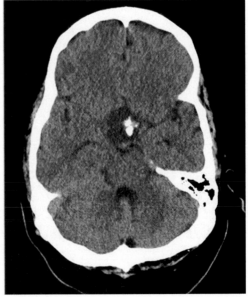

9a   What is the next best step?

   A. CT scan of the brain with IV contrast
   B. MRA
   C. Recommend transsphenoidal surgery
   D. MRI of the pituitary with gadolinium

Additional images are submitted below.

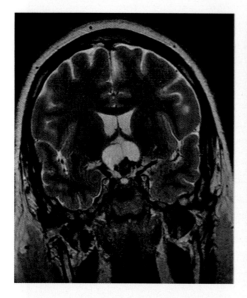
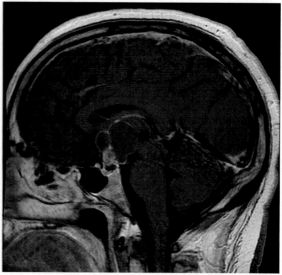

9b   What is the most likely diagnosis?

   A. Craniopharyngioma
   B. Pituitary macroadenoma
   C. Arachnoid cyst
   D. Rathke cleft cyst

10   A recently postpartum woman presents with headache, nausea, and vomiting and is found to have hypopituitarism on lab evaluation.

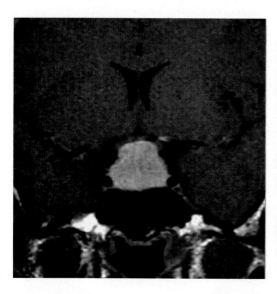
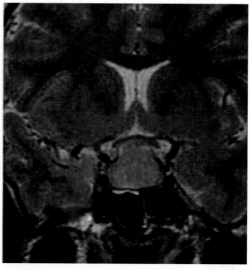

10a What is the most likely diagnosis?

    A. Pituitary hemorrhage
    B. Pituitary adenoma
    C. Lymphocytic hypophysitis
    D. Metastatic disease

10b Which of the following is true about Lymphocytic Hypophysitis?

    A. Easily distinguised from pituitary adenoma on imaging
    B. Can be related to medications
    C. Calcification is common
    D. A normal but compressed pituitary gland can be identified in most cases

ANSWERS AND EXPLANATIONS

1a **Answer B.** Prolactinoma. This sellar/suprasellar enhancing mass in the current clinical setting and complete response to cabergoline (a dopamine receptor agonist) is compatible with a prolactinoma.

1b **Answer C.** Visual abnormalities. Sellar/suprasellar adenomas can result in visual symptoms because of extrinsic compression of the optic chiasm. The superior edge of this lesion is contacting and upward displacing the optic chiasm (A and B); therefore, the patient is at risk for visual symptoms.

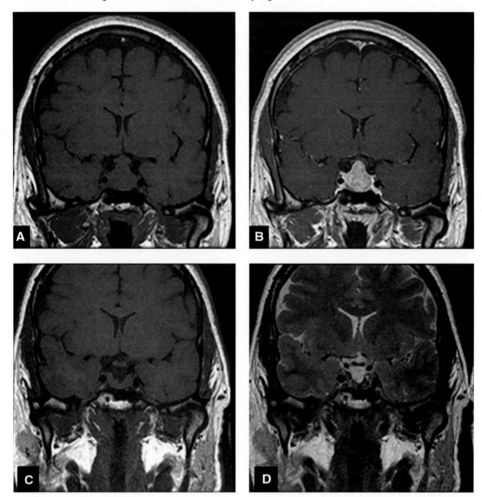

Imaging Findings: A sellar/suprasellar mass is shown. It is T1W hypointense (A) and homogenously enhancing on postcontrast images (B) with the superior edge of the lesion contacting and upward displacing the optic chiasm. Based on these images, there is no cavernous sinus invasion or ICA occlusion. This lesion is completely resolved on the posttreatment follow-up images (C and D).

Discussion: Pituitary adenomas, in this case prolactinoma, are commonly benign intracranial neoplasms. Prolactinomas, accounting for 40% to 60% of all pituitary adenomas are typically treated with dopamine agonists as a first-line treatment. Refractory lesions with neuro-ophthalmic implications can be managed with surgery/radiotherapy. These lesions are mostly benign and noninvasive in nature. Commonly, these are noted as incidental findings on MRI or autopsy. Occasionally, more aggressive atypical variants may also be seen.

    Rarely, these may present acutely as pituitary apoplexy, as a result of intratumoral hemorrhage or ischemia, with visual symptoms, headache, and ophthalmoplegia. These are typically lesions confined to the pituitary gland; lesions <10 mm in size are referred to as microadenomas; the lesions larger than 10 mm are referred to as macroadenomas.

On imaging, these are typically iso- to hypointense to the pituitary gland on T1W sequences and enhance slower than the native pituitary gland. For this reason, they are most conspicuous as hypoenhancing lesions on early postcontrast images; this is particularly true for microadenomas because of their small size. Subsequently on delayed phases, these lesions may "wash-in," whereas native pituitary "washes-out" making them isoenhancing to surrounding tissue. Dynamic contrast-enhanced pituitary MRI can therefore help in identifying microadenomas. Secondary signs of microadenoma may be infundibular deviation and superior border convexity. However, both of these signs are nonspecific in isolation and may be seen with normal variants. Macroadenoma may have locally invasive features, erosion of sellar floor, invasion into the cavernous sinus, and encasement of the cavernous ICA. These larger lesions are also prone to hemorrhage, ischemia, and necrosis.

References: Go JL, Rajamohan AG. Imaging of the sella and parasellar region. *Radiol Clin North Am* 2017;55(1):83–101.

Johnsen DE, Woodruff WW, Allen IS, et al. MR imaging of the sellar and juxtasellar regions. *Radiographics* 1991;11(5):727–758.

2a **Answer C.** Rathke cleft cyst.

2b **Answer B.** Extrinsic compression of the optic chiasm.

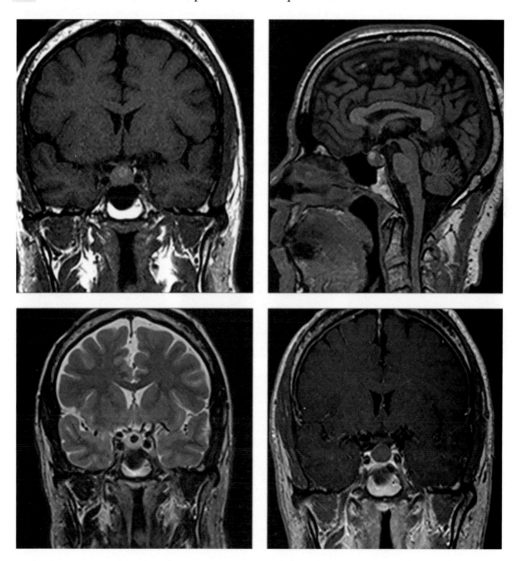

Imaging Findings: An intrasellar cystic lesion that is hyperintense on precontrast T1-weighted sequence (A) and hyperintense on T2-weighted sequence (B). On postcontrast sequences, the lesion is isointense to the enhancing pituitary gland and does not displace the pituitary infundibulum (C). The above features are most consistent with Rathke cleft cyst.

Discussion: Rathke cleft cyst is a congenital nonneoplastic lesion derived from the embryonic Rathke pouch. The Rathke pouch is interposed between the anterior pituitary gland that migrates rostrally from the primitive oral cavity and the posterior pituitary gland that migrates inferiorly from the diencephalon. The anterior wall of the Rathke pouch proliferates to form the anterior lobe of the pituitary gland and pars tuberalis, and the posterior wall contributes to the posterior lobe. The intervening cleft subsequently involutes in early gestational life. Lack of regression of this cleft may lead to the formation of a Rathke cleft cyst.

Majority of these lesions are incidental and remain asymptomatic.

On MRI RCC can be T1 hyperintense (due to protien content) or hypointense and T2 hyperintense (majority) or T2 iso/hypointense without enhancement.

A T2 hypointense intracystic nodule is characteristic as in this case. Lesions can be purely sellar or sellar/suprasellar.

Differential Diagnosis: Differential diagnosis of this lesion is either a cystic craniopharyngioma or a cystic pituitary adenoma, which can often be indistinguishable on imaging. The lack of calcifications and septations, cyst wall enhancement, and presence of T2 hypointense intracystic nodule support the diagnosis of RCC.

Reference: Byun WM, et al. MR imaging findings of Rathke's cleft cysts: significance of intracystic nodules. *AJNR Am J Neuroradiol* 2000;21:485–488.

3a **Answer B.** Hypothalamic hamartoma. The clinical presentation and imaging findings are consistent with hypothalamic hamartoma.

3b **Answer C.** Follows gray matter on all sequences without enhancement.

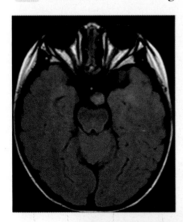
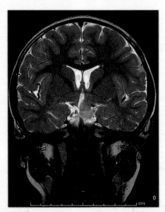
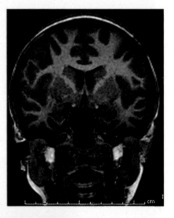

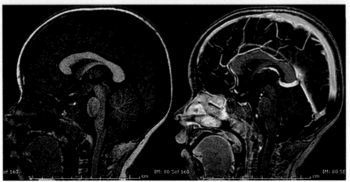

Imaging Findings: Axial FLAIR-weighted and coronal T2- and T1-weighted images show a sausage-shaped mass in the hypothalamus contiguous with the left mammillary body. The mass is isointense to gray matter on all sequences without a cystic component. Pre- and postgadolinium sagittal T1-weighted images show no enhancement. There is no sellar extension. The optic chiasm is intact.

Discussion: Hypothalamic hamartomas are benign malformations mainly found in the first two decades of life with a male predominance. Histologic examination shows a mixture of mature neuronal and glial cells and an overall resemblance to normal hypothalamic gray matter. They are classified as parahypothalamic or intrahypothalamic hamartomas. Parahypothalamic hamartomas are pedunculated masses that are attached to the floor of the hypothalamus by a narrow base and more likely to be associated with precocious puberty rather than with gelastic seizures. Intrahypothalamic hamartomas are sessile masses with a broad attachment to the hypothalamus. They appear to lie within the substance of the hypothalamus itself and associated more often with gelastic seizures than with precocious puberty.

MRI is the imaging modality of choice to make the diagnosis. The lesion can be sessile or pedunculated and closely follows gray matter signal on all imaging without enhancement after intravenous administration of gadolinium.

Most cases are refractory to medical treatment, and a surgical resection is needed to control the clinical symptoms.

Differential diagnosis: The main differential diagnoses are optic nerve glioma and germinoma. Both lesions do not follow gray matter signal and strongly enhance after intravenous gadolinium.

References: Freeman JL. The anatomy and embryology of the hypothalamus in relation to hypothalamic hamartomas. *Epileptic Disord* 2003;5(4):177–186.

Freeman JL, Coleman LT, Wellard RM, et al. MR imaging and spectroscopic study of epileptogenic hypothalamic hamartomas: analysis of 72 cases. *AJNR Am J Neuroradiol* 2004:25(3):450–462.

4a **Answer B.** Cavernous sinus. The abnormality is located inside the cavernous sinus lateral to the sella turcica (choice A), medial to the temporal lobe and hippocampus (choice C), and inferior to the frontal lobe (choice D).

4b **Answer C.** Schwannoma. The most likely diagnosis is a cavernous sinus schwannoma.

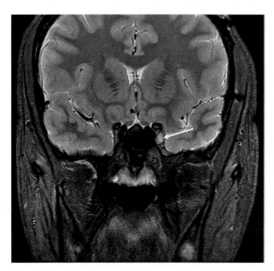
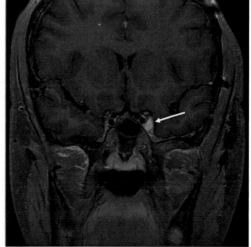

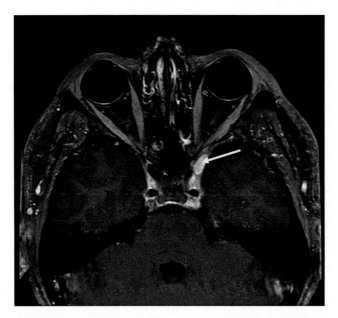

Imaging Findings: Coronal fat-suppressed T2-weighted image demonstrate a focus of hyperintense T2-weighted signal in the prominent left cavernous sinus compared to the contralateral side (*arrows*). Contrast-enhanced coronal and axial T1-weighted images with fat suppression demonstrate a homogenously enhancing nodule within the left cavernous sinus that corresponds to the T2 signal abnormality.

Discussion: Cavernous sinus schwannoma is a slow-growing benign tumor that originates from the cranial nerves that travel into the cavernous sinus. It is most commonly found in middle-aged and elderly women. Although the clinical presentation may vary based on the size of the lesion, deficits of the parent cranial nerves are usually the initial complain.

The cavernous sinus is a pair of dural venous sinus with a unique anatomic arrangement in the skull base. The cranial nerves III, IV, V1, and V2 travel along the lateral wall of the sinus. The internal carotid artery and the cranial nerve VI run inside the dural venous sinus.

MRI is the imaging modality of choice in the imaging evaluation of a patient with clinical suspicion of cavernous sinus schwannoma. Schwannomas are typically hyperintense on T2 with prominent postgadolinium enhancement. The T1-weighted signal is usually iso- to hypointense. Large lesion can have a cystic component or demonstrate low GRE signal. Lesions tend to be in the lateral wall of the cavernous sinus (as in this case) because they arise from cranial nerves traveling along the lateral wall.

Differential diagnosis: The main differential diagnosis considerations are meningioma, cavernous carotid aneurysm, or pituitary adenoma. A meningioma will demonstrate avid postgadolinium enhancement with narrowing of the cavernous ICA and associated dural tail or thickening. A cavernous sinus aneurysm shows a flow void on T2-weighted images. Pituitary adenoma is primarily a sellar mass with cavernous sinus invasion and lateral displacement of the cavernous ICA.

Reference: Skolnik AD, Loevner LA, Sampathu DM, et al. Cranial nerve schwannomas: diagnostic imaging approach. *Radiographics* 2016;36(5):1463–1477.

5a **Answer A.** Hypothalamus. The patient presents with symptoms consistent with central diabetes insipidus (CDI). which is seen with lesions of the hypothalamus and infundibulum.

5b **Answer B.**   Germinoma. This is the most likely diagnosis in a young adult with CDI and enhancing lesions in the pineal gland and pituitary stalk.

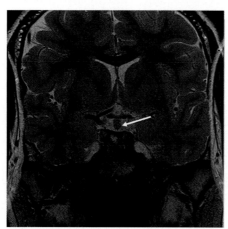 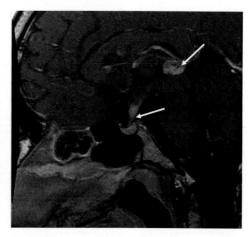

Imaging Findings: Coronal T2-weighted image of the brain demonstrates a thick pituitary stalk in midline position, isointense to the adjacent brain parenchyma. Midline postgadolinium T1-weighted image shows enhancing masses in the pineal region and suprasellar cistern in the infundibular recess. There is mild compression of the tectal plate without complete obstruction.

Discussion: Germ cell tumors are the most common pineal region tumor and can be categorized as germinomatous (germinoma) or nongerminomatous (teratoma, choriocarcinoma, yolk sac tumor, etc.). Germinomas are pure germ cell tumors of the central nervous system and are almost exclusively found in patients under 20, with a marked male predominance. They arise from entrapped totipotent germ cells, usually in the midline. The most common locations are pineal region or suprasellar cistern. Synchronous intracranial germinoma is rare and represent only 5% to 10% of all intracranial germinomas. Only 5% to 10% of all germ cell tumors are found as synchronous lesion in pineal and suprasellar region.

The clinical presentation depends on the anatomic location of the lesions. A patient with pineal germinoma may present with signs of increased intracranial pressure, hydrocephalus, or Parinaud syndrome. Suprasellar lesions in the supraoptic recess may compress the optic chiasm to cause visual field defects or infiltrate the infundibular recess to cause central diabetes insipidus. Laboratory testing for serum and csf levels of relevant oncoproteins including beta HCG and AFP should be performed in the preoperative workup of these patients.

On CT scan, the pineal lesions are dense, engulf the calcified pineal gland, and demonstrate homogenous enhancement. On MRI, these lesions are iso- or hyperintense to the adjacent brain tissue on T1- and T2-weighted images; may contain calcifications, cysts, or hemorrhages; and demonstrate strong postgadolinium enhancement.

The treatment depends on specific location, size, and extension of the disease. Radiotherapy is the mainstay of treatment. The entire neural axis should be images to exclude leptomeningeal disease after surgery. Radiation combined with chemotherapy offers an excellent prognosis with a 5-year survival rate around 90%.

Differential diagnosis: In the pineal region, pineoblastoma and pineocytoma are the main considerations. In the suprasellar cistern, pilocytic astrocytoma is the primary consideration in children.

References: Liang L, Korogi Y, Sugahara T, et al. MRI of intracranial germ cell tumors. *Neuroradiology* 2002;44(5):382–388.

Parker JP, Waziri A. Preoperative evaluation of pineal tumors. *Neurosurg Clin N Am* 2011;22(3):353–358.

Wang L, Yamaguchi S, Burstein MD, et al. Novel somatic and germline mutations in intracranial germ cell tumours. *Nature* 2014;511(7508):241–245.

6   Answer A.   Pituitary microadenoma.

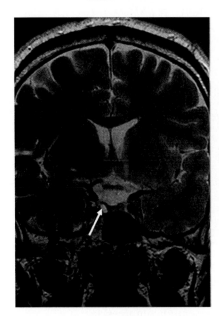
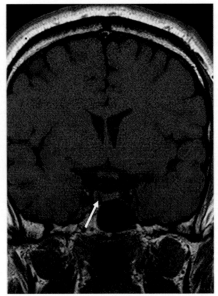
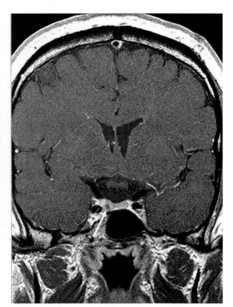

Imaging Findings: Coronal T2w, pre and post contrast T1w images through the sella show a T2 hyperintense, hypoenhancing focus suggesting a microadenoma.

Discussion: Pituitary microadenomas are adenomas of the pituitary gland that are <10 mm in size. They are benign, slow-growing tumors with a higher incidence in young African American females.

The clinical presentation depends on its functional status and the type of releasing hormones. Prolactin-secreting tumors are the most common tumors, followed by gonadotropic (FSH-LH) and somatotropic (GH)-secreting adenomas. The excess hormonal production may result in galactorrhea, decrease in menstrual frequency, acromegaly, or gigantism.

MRI of the brain with a pituitary protocol using high-resolution precontrast coronal T2-weighted, sagittal and coronal T1-weighted, and postgadolinium dynamic T1-weighted images is the imaging modality of choice. Microadenomas may be iso- to hypointense on T1WI and iso- to hyperintense on T2WI, often with a lack of enhancement compared to the rest of the gland on early postgadolinium images. Dynamic sequences demonstrate a rounded region of delayed enhancement compared to the rest of the gland. Symptomatic patients with repeatedly normal MRI may benefit from an inferior petrosal sinus sampling in the neurointerventional suite to confirm the presence of an occult MRI lesion.

Medical treatment designed to control the effect of the secreting hormone is preferred over surgical resection.

Differential diagnosis: The differential diagnosis includes Rathke cleft cysts that follow simple fluid signal on MRI and craniopharyngiomas that are larger with calcification and cystic components.

Reference: Bartynski WS, Lin L. Dynamic and conventional spin-echo MR of pituitary microlesions. *AJNR Am J Neuroradiol* 1997;18(5):965–972.

7a **Answer A.** Compression of the superior colliculi. The patient presents with clinical findings consistent with Parinaud syndrome (PS) indicating compression of the superior colliculi by a solid enhancing mass in the pineal region, as noted on the MRI.

7b **Answer C.** Pineocytoma. The most likely diagnosis of an enhancing solid pineal mass in a young adult is a pineocytoma among the choices provided.

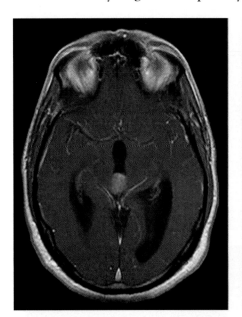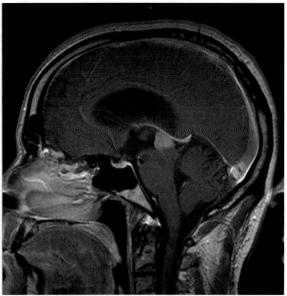

Imaging Findings: Axial postgadolinium T1-weighted images demonstrate a mild enlargement of the lateral and third ventricles, with a homogenously enhancing mass in the posterior third of the third ventricle. Sagittal T1-weighted postgadolinium images reveal that the mass is located in the pineal region with mass effect upon the tectal plate and obstruction of the aqueduct of Sylvius causing a noncommunicating hydrocephalus.

Discussion: Pineocytomas are benign parenchymal neoplasms of the pineal gland that can be seen at any age but more commonly seen in the second decade of life. They are slow-growing tumor that may be asymptomatic for a long time until they cause mass effect upon the tectum with secondary obstruction of the aqueduct.

   The clinical manifestations include signs and symptoms related to the compression of the superior colliculi or obstructive hydrocephalus. Compression of the superior colliculi will result in PS characterized by the classic triad of upward gaze palsy, light-near pupillary reflex dissociation, and convergence–retraction nystagmus. Aqueductal obstruction cause increased intracranial pressure with headaches and papilledema.

   CT scan shows a pineal region mass isodense to the brain tissue, often with peripheral calcification in a useful pattern that helps to differentiate it from other pineal region masses like germinoma that engulfs the calcifications. On MRI, the lesion is solid (occasionally with cystic degeneration), iso- to hypointense on T1-weighted images, and iso- to hyperintense on T2-weighted images with brisk postgadolinium enhancement.

   The treatment is surgical resection with a very good prognosis.

Differential diagnosis: The differential diagnosis includes other pineal parenchymal lesion like pineoblastoma, germinoma, astrocytoma, or metastatic diseases to the pineal gland.

Reference: Reis F, et al. Neuroimaging of pineal tumors. *J Neuroimaging* 2006;16(1):52–58.

8a **Answer A.**   Cavernous sinuses. Note low attenuation within the cavernous sinuses on CT with contrast.

8b **Answer C.**   Postgadolinium T1-weighted images of the brain.

8c **Answer D.**   Cavernous sinus thrombosis.

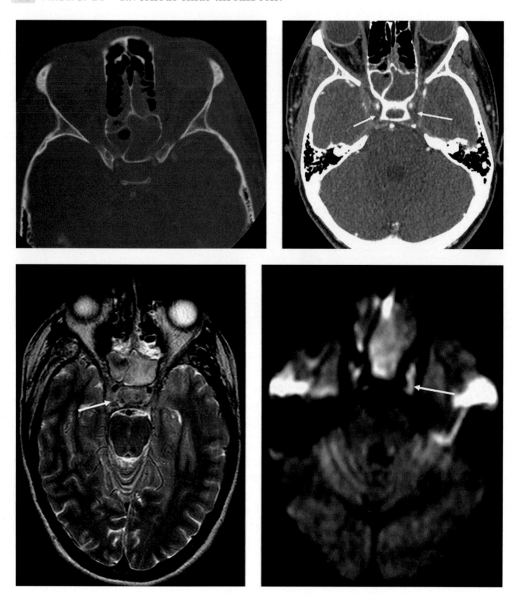

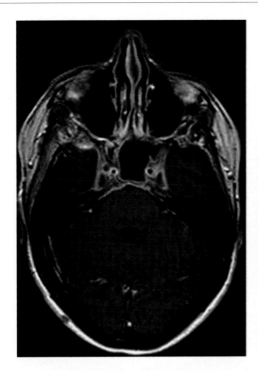
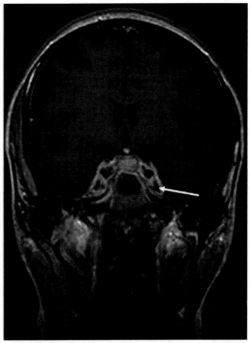

Imaging Findings: Axial CT images show sinus inflammatory changes and low attenuation within cavernous sinuses on post contrast image.

There are corresponding T2 hyperintensity, restricted diffusion and rim enhancing filling defects compatible with cavernous sinus thrombosis (or septic thrombophlebitis).

Discussion: Cavernous sinus thrombosis or septic thrombophlebitis is a rare condition, most commonly infectious in nature, with a high mortality and morbidity rate. The diagnosis on imaging requires a high index of suspicion if there is associated infection of the paranasal sinus or dental infection and cavernous sinus abnormalities. *Staphylococcus aureus* is the most common organism.

The most common clinical symptom is headaches. Focal neurologic symptoms and/or seizures may also occur. Isolated CN III palsy is thought to be an early manifestation. Orbital signs including chemosis, periorbital swelling, and exophthalmos may be present.

Imaging mainstay of diagnosis is CT or MRI with contrast and thin sections through the cavernous sinus. Postcontrast CT and MRI show enhancement defects within the cavernous sinuses.

Differential diagnosis: Bilateral cavernous carotid fistula that may present with prominent bilateral cavernous sinus and intraluminal flow voids rather than thrombi. The superior ophthalmic veins are usually very prominent.

References: Absoud M, Hikmet F, Dey P, et al. Bilateral cavernous sinus thrombosis complicating sinusitis. *J R Soc Med* 2006;99(9):474–476.

Razek AA, Castillo M. Imaging lesions of the cavernous sinus. *AJNR Am J Neuroradiol* 2009;30(3):444–452.

9a **Answer D.** MRI of the pituitary with gadolinium.

9b **Answer A.** Craniopharyngioma.

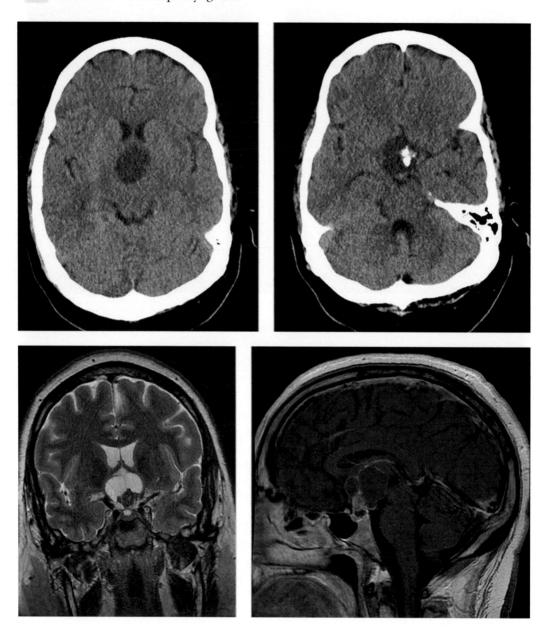

Imaging Findings: Noncontrast head CT demonstrates a partly calcified cystic mass.

Coronal T2-weighted image and sagittal T1-weighted postgadolinium image demonstrate a mixed cystic and solid mass with septation and enhancing solid component, most compatible with a craniopharyngioma.

Discussion: Craniopharyngiomas are benign tumors that arise from neoplastic transformation of ectopic embryonal remnants of the hypophyseal duct through which the Rathke pouch migrates to form the anterior pituitary gland. They are found in patients of all ages and sex with a bimodal distribution, the first peak around 10 to 15 years old and the second peak around 60 years old. Although they are histologically benign grade I lesions, their proximity to the pituitary stalk, hypothalamus, optic apparatus, and the circle of Willis and tendency to adhere to critical structures can create morbidity. They also have high rates of recurrence.

The clinical presentation includes visual changes, headaches, and behavioral changes. Short stature, decreased libido, amenorrhea, and diabetes insipidus are among the hormonal imbalances reported.

CT may demonstrate cyst, calcification, and soft tissue components. MRI with its multiplanar capability easily depicts size, extent, and consistency (solid and cystic). Imaging can help differentiate the adult papillary type from the childhood adamantinomatous type that is usually larger and contains calcification.

Surgical resection using a transsphenoidal or a craniotomy approach is the treatment of choice with adjunct radiotherapy for incomplete surgical resection.

Differential diagnosis: The differential diagnosis includes lesions with sellar and suprasellar component like a pituitary adenoma. Other considerations are Rathke cleft cyst that usually demonstrates no soft tissue component and teratoma that contain fat.

References: Cohen LE. Update on childhood craniopharyngiomas. *Curr Opin Endocrinol Diabetes Obes* 2016;23(4):339–344. doi:10.1097/MED.0000000000000264.

Lee IH, Zan E, Bell WR, et al. Craniopharyngiomas: radiological differentiation of two types. *J Korean Neurosurg Soc* 2016;59(5):466–470.

10a **Answer C.**   Lymphocytic hypophysitis.

10b **Answer B.**   Can be related to medications.

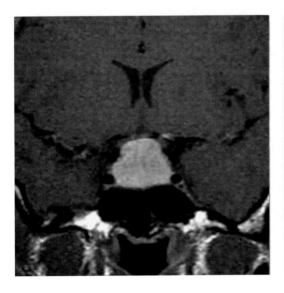
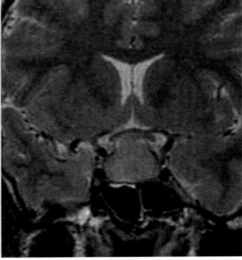

Imaging Findings: There is diffuse enlargement of the pituitary gland with mass effect on the optic chiasm. Normal pituitary gland is not visible.

Discussion: Lymphocytic hypophysitis is a disorder characterized by autoimmune inflammation of the pituitary gland resulting in pituitary dysfunction. Lymphocytic hypophysitis is most commonly diagnosed in women during pregnancy or in the postpartum period and can be associated with other types of autoimmune disease. Recently, hypophysitis has also been described in patients undergoing treatment with ipilimumab, an immunotherapy agent used in patients with melanoma and renal cell carcinoma. The clinical presentation varies depending on the pituitary segment that is affected. In lymphocytic adenohypophysis (LAH), which is more common, an early destruction of the ACTH-producing cells is characteristic. Lymphocytic infundibuloneurohypophysitis (LINH) affects the stalk and posterior pituitary and typically presents as acute-onset diabetes insipidus (DI). Lymphocytic Infudibulopanhypophysitis (LIPH) includes features of both anterior and posterior pituitary involvement. The diagnosis can be challenging in many cases, because distinction from pituitary adenomas and other sellar masses is difficult both clinically and on imaging. The histopathology consists of monoclonal lymphocytic infiltrate with variable fibrosis.

Imaging studies of patients with lymphocytic hypophysitis usually demonstrate diffuse homogeneous pituitary enlargement with or without enlargement of the pituitary stalk and a characteristic "pear-shaped" appearance. A normal pituitary gland is not identified, which helps distinguish it from a pituitary adenoma.

References: Hamnvik OP, Laury AR, Laws ER Jr, et al. Lymphocytic hypophysitis with diabetes insipidus in a young man. *Nat Rev Endocrinol* 2010;6(8):464–470. doi:10.1038/nrendo.2010.104.

Rivera JA. Lymphocytic hypophysitis: disease spectrum and approach to diagnosis and therapy [review]. *Pituitary* 2006;9(1):35–45.

17 Skull Base

DANIEL CHOW • DANIEL THOMAS GINAT • GUL MOONIS

QUESTIONS

Regarding the following image:

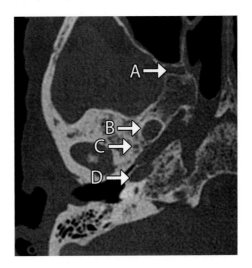

1 Which of the letter corresponds to foramen spinosum?

Regarding the following image:

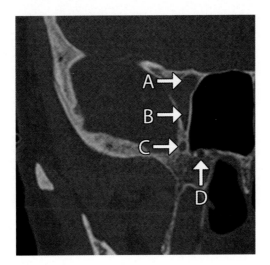

459

2   Which letter corresponds to foramen rotundum?

Regarding the following image:

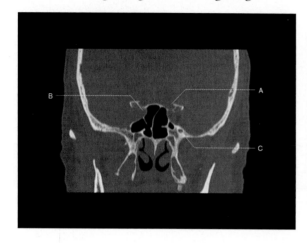
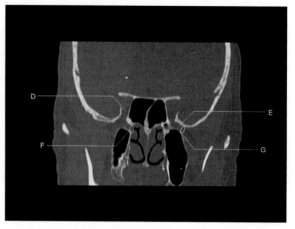

3   The superior ophthalmic vein passes through which structure?
   A.
   B.
   C.
   D.
   E.
   F.

4   Juvenile nasopharyngeal angiofibromas arise from which region?
   A.
   B.
   C.
   D.
   E.
   F.
   G.

Regarding the following image:

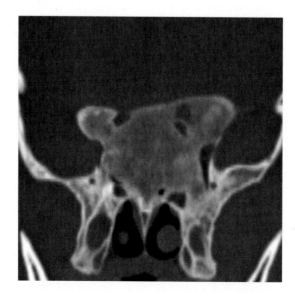

5 Which is the most likely diagnosis?

A. Metastatic disease
B. Osteomyelitis
C. Intraosseous lipoma
D. Fibrous dysplasia

6 Which of the following is associated with polyostotic fibrous dysplasia?

A. McCune-Albright syndrome
B. Ollier syndrome
C. Gardner syndrome
D. Cowden syndrome

7 Based on the image below, which is the next best test for further evaluation?

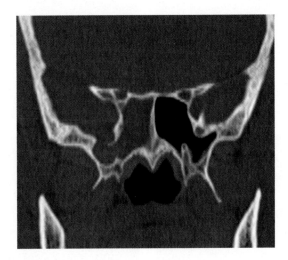

A. Cerebral angiography
B. Biopsy
C. Bone scan
D. MRI

8 Based on the following images, which of the following is the most likely diagnosis?

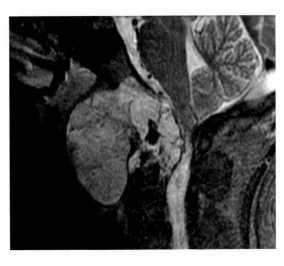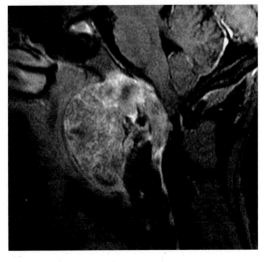

A. Chondrosarcoma
B. Aneurysmal bone cyst
C. Chordoma
D. Pituitary adenoma

9 A 74-year-old male with prior history of diabetes presented with pus drainage from the right ear with new right facial weakness. What is the most likely diagnosis?

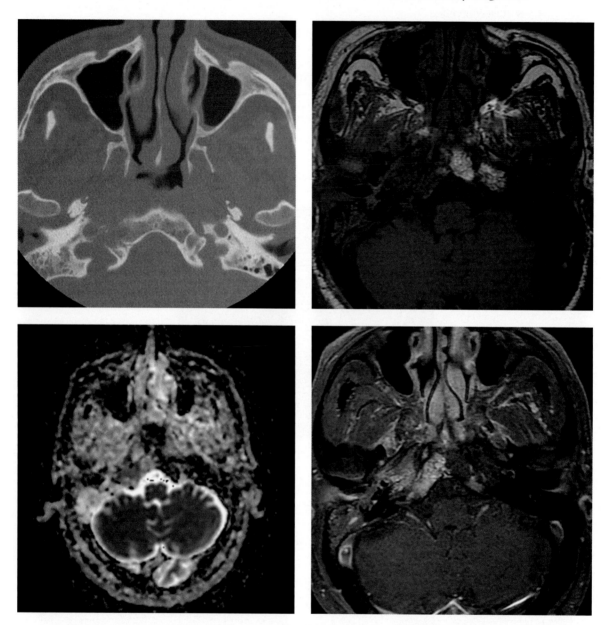

A. Lymphoma
B. Nasopharyngeal carcinoma
C. Metastasis
D. Skull base osteomyelitis

10 What is the most common pathogen responsible for typical skull base osteomyelitis?

A. *Aspergillus*
B. *Mucor*
C. *Pseudomonas*
D. *S. aureus*

11 A 68-year-old male presents with hearing loss over 3 years and some tinnitus.

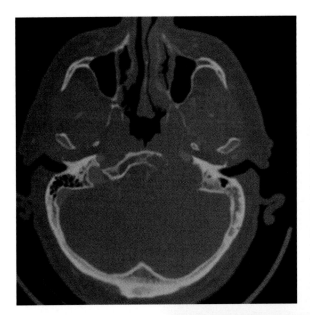

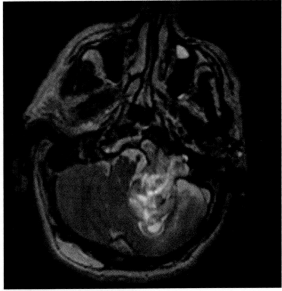

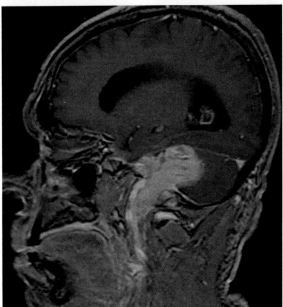

11a What is the location of the lesion?

    A. Petrous apex
    B. Internal auditory canal
    C. Jugular foramen
    D. Middle ear

11b What is the most likely diagnosis?

    A. Glomus jugulare paraganglioma
    B. Meningioma
    C. Metastasis
    D. Schwannoma

12   A 34-year-old female presents with headaches.

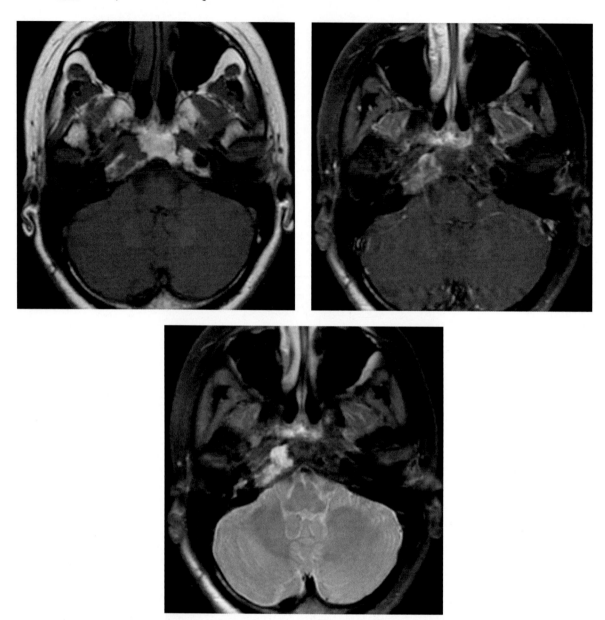

Based on the location and imaging features, what is the most likely diagnosis?

A. Chondrosarcoma
B. Chordoma
C. Ecchordosis physaliphora
D. Plasmacytoma

13   A 29-year-old male presents with headaches.

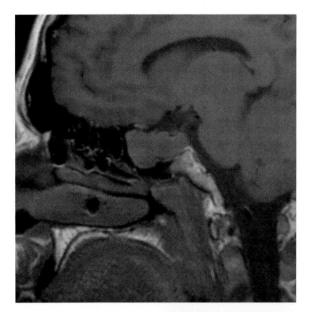 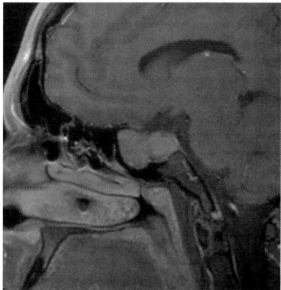

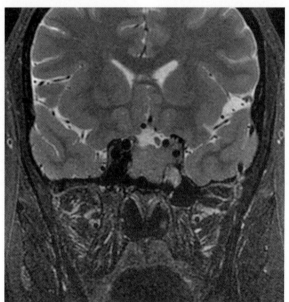

What is the most likely diagnosis?

A. Chondrosarcoma
B. Chordoma
C. Invasive pituitary macroadenoma
D. Plasmacytoma

14 A 55-year-old male presents with left preauricular swelling.

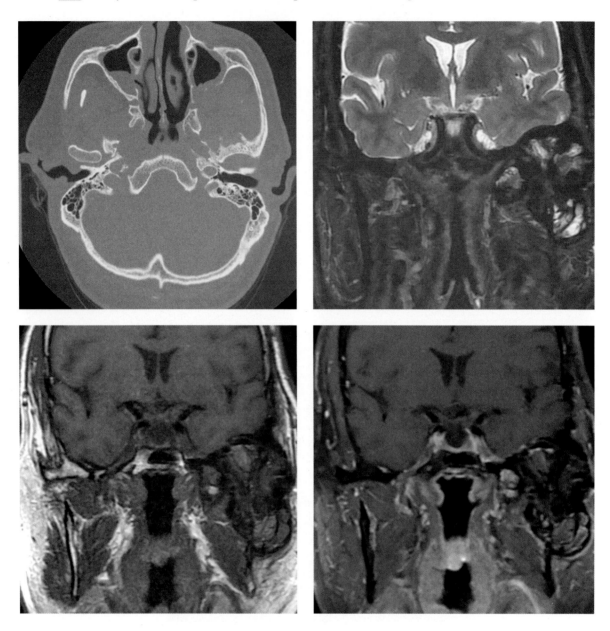

What is the diagnosis?

A. Calcium pyrophosphate dihydrate deposition
B. Chondrosarcoma
C. Pigmented villonodular synovitis
D. Synovial chondromatosis

15 A 40-year-old male being worked up for refractory headaches presents with recently worsening. Below are provided key images from nonenhanced head CT and contrast-enhanced MRI. Where is the lesion centered based on these images?

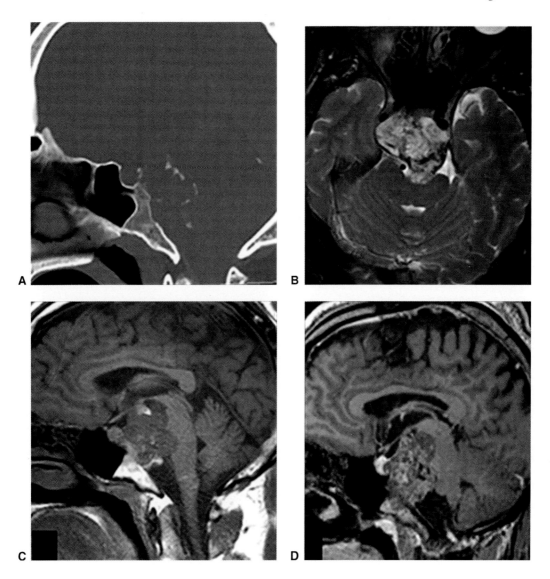

A. Sella/suprasellar
B. Prepontine/retroclival region
C. Hypothalamus
D. Floor of the third ventricle

16 Which of the following statements is most accurate about chordoma?

A. This is a locally aggressive lesion arising from a notochordal remnant.
B. This is a benign indolent lesion arising from a notochordal remnant.
C. This lesion does not arise from a notochordal remnant and is primarily a sellar mass.
D. This lesion does not arise from a notochordal remnant and is primarily a pontine mass.

17   Which of the following features have been shown to favor the diagnosis of chondrosarcoma compared to chordoma?

    A. Off-center location and relatively higher ADC measurements

    B. Midline location and relatively lower ADC

    C. Presence of calcifications or bone destruction on CT

    D. T2W hyperintensity and lobulated morphology

ANSWERS AND EXPLANATIONS

1 **Answer C.**

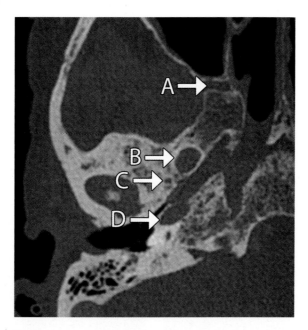

Imaging Findings: A: Pterygopalatine fossa; B: foramen ovale; C: foramen spinosum; D: carotid canal.

2 **Answer C.**

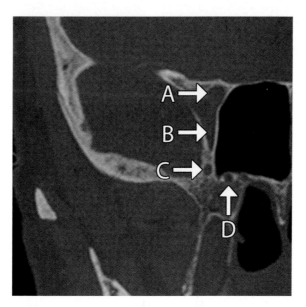

Imaging Findings: A: Optic canal; B: superior orbital fissure; C: foramen rotundum; D: vidian canal.

Discussion: The pterygopalatine fossa contains the pterygopalatine ganglion, descending palatine artery, maxillary division of trigeminal nerve, and nerve of the pterygoid canal. Foramen ovale is an opening in the greater wing of the sphenoid that transmits the mandibular nerve, accessory meningeal artery, lesser petrosal nerve, and emissary veins. Foramen spinosum is an opening in the greater wing of the sphenoid that transmits the middle meningeal artery. The carotid canal transmits the internal carotid artery and sympathetic plexus. The optic canal transmits the optic nerve. The superior orbital fissure transmits the ophthalmic (V1), oculomotor (III), trochlear (IV), and abducens (VI) nerves, as well as the superior and inferior ophthalmic veins.

Foramen rotundum transmits the maxillary (V2) division of the trigeminal nerve to the pterygopalatine fossa. The Vidian canal transmits the Vidian nerve (combination of the greater superficial petrosal nerve and the deep petrosal nerve) to the pterygopalatine fossa.

Reference: Policeni BA, Smoker WR. Imaging of the skull base: anatomy and pathology. *Radiol Clin North Am* 2015;53(1):1–14.

3 **Answer B.**   The superior ophthalmic vein passes through the superior orbital fissure, which is inferior to the anterior clinoid process, choice B.

4 **Answer F.**   Juvenile nasopharyngeal angiofibromas (JNAs) arise at the sphenopalatine foramen, choice F.

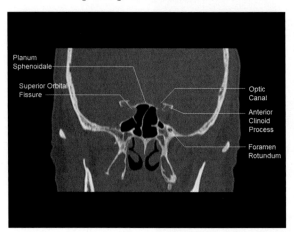
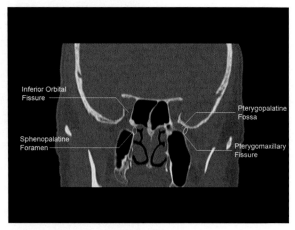

Imaging Findings: The various foramen and important bony landmarks of the central and anterior skull base are labeled.

Discussion: Depicted are images of the anterior and central skull base. The anterior clinoid process forms from the medial aspect of the lesser wing of the sphenoid bone. This is an important landmark as the optic canal is medial to this (choice A), and the superior orbital fissure (SOF) is immediately inferior to this (choice B). Inferior to this is the inferior orbital fissure (IOF) (choice D). Notice that the IOF communicates with the pterygopalatine fossa (PPF) (choice E). Medially, this fossa is connected to the nasal region through the sphenopalatine foramen (SPF) (choice F) and laterally to the infratemporal fossa through the pterygomaxillary fissure (PMF) (choice G). The PPF empties posteriorly into foramen rotundum (choice C). Thus, malignant tumors of the sinonasal region or cheek may use CNV2 as a perineural route for intracranial spread.
Important structures:

- Optic canal: CNII, ophthalmic artery
- SOF: CNIII, CNIV, CNV1, CNVI, and the superior ophthalmic vein
- IOF: Infraorbital artery, vein, and nerve
- Foramen rotundum: CNV2 and emissary veins

Reference: Policeni BA, Smoker WR. Imaging of the skull base: anatomy and pathology. *Radiol Clin North Am* 2015;53(1):1–14.

5 **Answer D.**   Fibrous dysplasia.

6 **Answer A.** McCune-Albright syndrome.

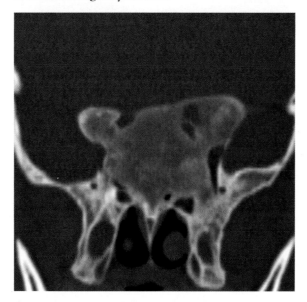

Imaging Findings: The coronal CT image shows an expansile lesion with ground-glass attenuation involving the sphenoid bone.

Discussion: Fibrous dysplasia is a benign condition characterized by abnormal proliferation of fibrous tissue in bone that most commonly affects the ethmoid and sphenoid bones when the skull base is involved. Skull base fibrous dysplasia typically has an expansile, "ground-glass" appearance on CT but may contain cystic components. Cranial nerves may be compressed, requiring debulking surgery. Polyostotic fibrous dysplasia can be a manifestation of McCune-Albright syndrome, along with endocrine dysfunction, abnormal pigmentation, and precocious puberty. Ollier syndrome is a nonhereditary disorder of multiple enchondromas. Gardner syndrome is an autosomal dominant disease and consists of gastrointestinal polyps, multiple osteomas, and desmoid tumors.

Cowden syndrome is autosomal dominant and consists of multiple hamartomas.

Reference: Lustig LR, Holliday MJ, McCarthy EF, et al. Fibrous dysplasia involving the skull base and temporal bone. *Arch Otolaryngol Head Neck Surg* 2001;127(10):1239–1247.

7 **Answer D.** MRI.

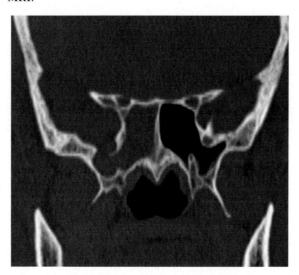

Imaging Findings: The coronal CT image shows a defect in the right lateral sphenoid wall and opacification of the right sphenoid sinus.

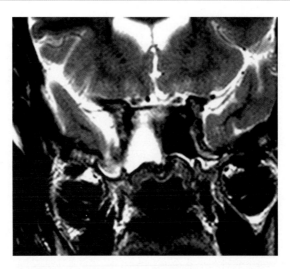

The corresponding coronal T2-weighted MRI shows herniation of a portion of the right temporal lobe through the sphenoid wall defect.

Discussion: Spontaneous lateral sphenoid cephaloceles arise from bony defects in the lateral sphenoid, in the absence of predisposing factors such as trauma, surgery, mass, or congenital skull base malformation. Sphenoid arachnoid pits and empty or partially empty sella are commonly associated findings, suggesting altered CSF dynamics as a causative factor. CT and MRI are complementary in evaluating these lesions, where CT can readily depict the bone defect and MRI can delineate the herniated contents.

Reference: Settecase F, Harnsberger HR, Michel MA, et al. Spontaneous lateral sphenoid cephaloceles: anatomic factors contributing to pathogenesis and proposed classification. *AJNR Am J Neuroradiol* 2014;35(4):784–789.

8 **Answer C.** Chordoma.

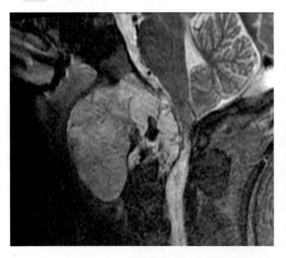 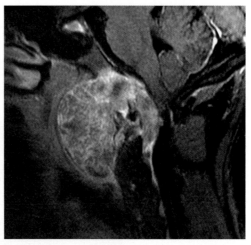

Imaging Findings: Sagittal T2-weighted and fat-suppressed postcontrast T1-weighted MRI shows an expansile mass arising from the midline basiclivus with erosion of the upper cervical spine and mass effect upon the cervicomedullary junction.

Discussion: Chordomas are malignant neoplasms derived from embryonic remnants of the primitive notochord and are typically located in the midline. The tumors display variable signal and enhancement on MRI and often abut critical anatomic structures, such as the carotid and basilar arteries, and the brainstem, which limits resection and delivery of high-dose radiation. Chondrosarcomas are also malignant neoplasms, but tend to be centered at the petroclival synchondrosis. Aneurysmal bone cysts are expansile bone lesions as well but classically display fluid levels and can occur in conjunction with other tumors. The tumor is not located near the sella and therefore is not a pituitary adenoma.

Reference: Erdem E, Angtuaco EC, Van Hemert R, et al. Comprehensive review of intracranial chordoma. *Radiographics* 2003;23(4):995–1009.

9 **Answer D.** Skull base osteomyelitis. Images depict extensive infection of the right skull base compatible with osteomyelitis (choice D). The other choices are in the differential but less likely. A soft tissue mass that locally invades the adjacent bony structures would be expected for non-Hodgkin lymphoma. Nasopharyngeal carcinoma is a good thought, but there are no provided images that demonstrate a dominant mass within the nasopharyngeal mucosal space. Metastasis generally occurs in the setting of known primary tumor with multiple lesions more frequently seen.

10 **Answer C.** *Pseudomonas.* The most common pathogen cultured in typical skull base osteomyelitis (SBO) is *Pseudomonas* (choice C), which is identified in 98% of cases. Pathogens encountered in atypical cases include gram-positive bacteria, *mucor*, and *Aspergillus*.

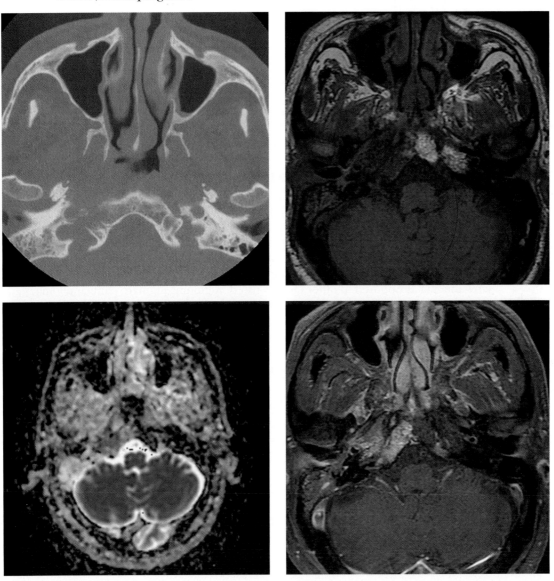

Imaging Findings: Axial bone window CT through the skull base demonstrates cortical destruction of the right hemiclivus and opacification of the mastoid air cells. Axial T1-weighted images demonstrate that the right hemiclivus has lost its normal marrow fat signal. Fat-saturated postgadolinium images demonstrate abnormal marrow enhancement with some abnormal enhancement within the subjacent nasopharyngeal soft tissues. ADC images demonstrate that the area of signal abnormality demonstrates reduced diffusion.

Discussion: Skull base osteomyelitis is relatively uncommon but potentially life-threatening condition. It is most commonly encountered in elderly diabetic patients with necrotizing otitis externa (also known as malignant otitis externa). Atypical SBO usually arises from invasive sinusitis rather than necrotizing otitis externa and may be seen in any age group. Risk factors for atypical SBO may include immunocompromised status (HIV and chronic steroid use) or chronic inflammatory sphenoid sinus disease.

Imaging features of SBO are similar to osteomyelitis encountered elsewhere in the skeletal system. CT findings include cortical destructive and erosive changes involving the central skull base, including the clivus and petrous apex. T1-weighted images demonstrate loss of normal marrow fat, which exhibits abnormal marrow enhancement on postcontrast images. T2 fat-saturated images typically demonstrate increased signal because of inflammation and edema. Diffusion-weighted images typically demonstrate reduced diffusion. However, the degree of diffusivity is typically not as low compared to lymphoma or nasopharyngeal carcinoma, which may be a potential problem-solving tool.

References: Chang PC, et al. Central skull base osteomyelitis in patients without otitis externa: imaging findings. *AJNR Am J Neuroradiol* 2003;24(7):1310–1316.

Diagnostic imaging: head and neck. Elsevier. ISBN: 9780323443012. https://www.elsevier.com/books/diagnostic-imaging-head-and-neck/koch/978-0-323-44301-2

Ozgen B, et al. Diffusion MR imaging features of skull base osteomyelitis compared with skull base malignancy. *AJNR Am J Neuroradiol* 2011;32(1):179–184.

11a **Answer C.** Jugular foramen. Images depict well-defined tubular mass expanding the jugular foramen with a large soft tissue component invaginating into the cerebellum. The margins of the contralateral jugular foramen are pristine.

11b **Answer D.** Schwannoma. Axial T2 images demonstrate a characteristic fusiform appearance with a waist within the jugular foramen. Bony margins are scalloped rather than permeative as would be expected with a paraganglioma. A meningioma would have hyperostosis and sclerotic bony pattern of involvement. Additionally, there are multiple intramural cysts, which is more characteristic of a schwannoma as opposed to other entities listed. A glomus jugulare paraganglioma and meningioma are in the differential but less likely based on imaging features. Specifically, a paraganglioma would be expected to demonstrate a "salt and pepper" appearance because of numerous foci of slow and high flow. There is no definite enhancing dural tail to suggest a meningioma. Additionally, the growth pattern of meningioma would be expected to be centrifugal.

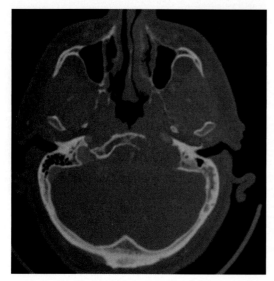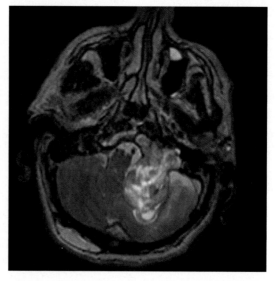

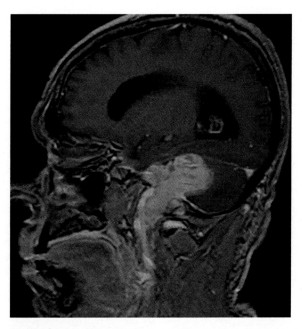

Imaging Findings: Contrast-enhanced axial bone window CT through the skull base demonstrates enlargement of jugular foramen. Axial T2 images demonstrate a fusiform mass with a waist at the jugular foramen. Multiple intramural cysts are also identified. Sagittal postcontrast images demonstrate that the mass follows a craniocaudal course, growing inferiorly along the expected course of the glossopharyngeal nerve (CNIX).

Discussion: Schwannomas are the second most common tumor at the jugular foramen with glomus jugulare paragangliomas being the most common and meningiomas the third most common. When encountered in this location, the glossopharyngeal nerve is the most common origin. Clinically, these patients present similarly to patients with vestibular schwannomas, including symptoms of sensorineural hearing loss. Patients may also exhibit pulsatile tinnitus related to dural sinus thrombosis and multiple other cranioneuropathies. The overwhelming majority of cases are sporadic with <10% associated with neurofibromatosis type 2.

Imaging features are similar to that of schwannomas in other locations. Specifically, the appearance of a tubular or dumbbell-shaped mass is relatively well circumscribed. These lesions do not demonstrate flow voids, which is useful in distinguishing them from paragangliomas. When small, these lesions demonstrate uniform enhancement but may demonstrate nonenhancing intramural cystic components when large, as in this case.

References: Eldevik OP, et al. Imaging findings in schwannomas of the jugular foramen. *AJNR Am J Neuroradiol* 2000;21(6):1139–1144.

Diagnostic imaging: head and neck. Elsevier. ISBN: 9780323443012. https://www.elsevier.com/books/diagnostic-imaging-head-and-neck/koch/978-0-323-44301-2

Wilson MA, et al. Jugular foramen schwannomas: diagnosis, management, and outcomes. *Laryngoscope* 2005;115(8):1486–1492.

12 **Answer A.**   Chondrosarcoma. Images depict a heterogeneously enhancing solitary soft tissue clival mass that is off midline with imaging features compatible with a chondrosarcoma.

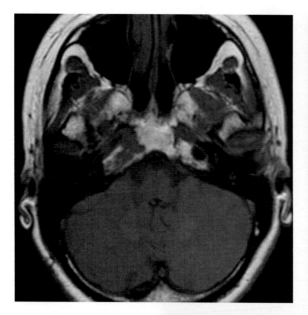
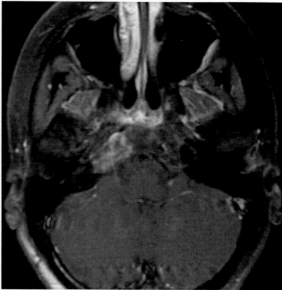
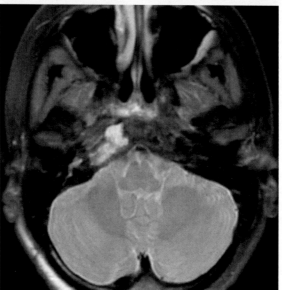

Imaging Findings: There is an enhancing T2 hyperintense mass at the right petroclival junction in a location characteristic for chondrosarcoma.

Discussion: Chondrosarcomas are malignant cartilaginous tumors. Although the majority occur at the long bones and pelvis, approximately 2% may be seen at the craniofacial regions. When these occur at the clivus, the primary differential consideration is a chordoma, which is a more common tumor and shares many imaging features. The most helpful feature in this case is location, as the majority of chondrosarcomas are off midline, whereas chordomas occur midline. Diffusion imaging may also be helpful with one series demonstrating significant higher ADC values with chondrosarcomas compared to chordomas.

Clinically, chondrosarcomas may present at any age group but, like chordomas, have a mean age of presentation around the fourth decade. Patients tend to present with headaches +/− other cranial nerve palsies.

Chondrosarcomas at the skull base appear similar to other locations. Specifically, CT images depict an expansile mass with chondroid matrix. T1-weighted images demonstrate low intensity because of fibrocartilaginous elements. T2 images demonstrate increased signal with areas of decreased intensity that reflect calcifications. When encountered in the skull base, the typical location is off midline, centered at the petro-occipital fissure.

Differential Diagnosis: As mentioned above, chordomas share many imaging features with chondrosarcomas but would be expected to demonstrate a midline location rather than lateral. Ecchordosis physaliphora is an ectopic notochordal remnant that manifests as a nonenhancing cystic mass. Skull base plasmacytoma demonstrates homogenous enhancement (rather than heterogenous) and is T2 isointense (rather than hyperintense) and would be expected to occur in an older patient.

References: *Diagnostic imaging: head and neck.* Elsevier. ISBN: 9780323443012. https://www.elsevier.com/books/diagnostic-imaging-head-and-neck/koch/978-0-323-44301-2

Murphey MD, et al. From the archives of the AFIP: imaging of primary chondrosarcoma: radiologic-pathologic correlation. *Radiographics* 2003;23(5):1245–1278.

Yeom KW, et al. Diffusion-weighted MRI: distinction of skull base chordoma from chondrosarcoma. *AJNR Am J Neuroradiol* 2013;34(5):1056–1061.

13 **Answer C.**   Invasive pituitary macroadenoma. Images depict a mass that invades the central skull base that is inseparable from a soft tissue mass within the sella and most suggestive of an invasive pituitary macroadenoma.

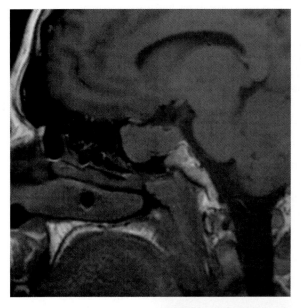
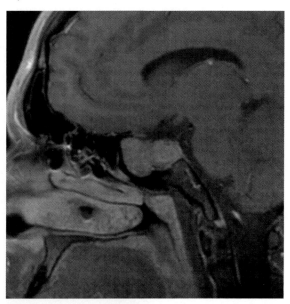
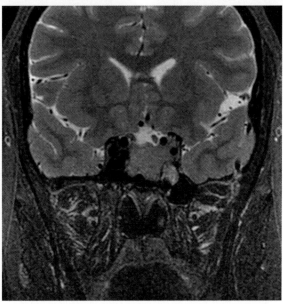

Imaging Findings: There is a homogenously enhancing, lobulated mass within an expanded sella. Sagittal images demonstrate that the mass invades the sphenoid sinus anteriorly as well as the posterior margins of the clivus. Coronal images demonstrate that the mass extends into the left cavernous sinus, where it encases the left cavernous internal carotid artery, which otherwise demonstrates a maintained flow void.

Discussion: Recognizing that the mass is inseparable and contagious with the sellar soft tissue mass is key for making this diagnosis. It is important to assess the cavernous sinus for invasion, which may be frequently encountered and may impact respectability. Assessment of cavernous sinus invasion may be challenging because of subjacent fat and venous plexus; however, >270 degree involvement is considered highly suggestive of invasion. Clinically, these patients may present with pituitary hormonal dysfunction and visual field defects because of compression upon the optic chiasm.

On imaging, CT demonstrates a soft tissue mass centered within the sella, with hemorrhage and calcifications infrequently encountered. On MR, pituitary macroadenomas are typically T1 isointense with homogenous enhancement. Note that enhancement may become heterogenous as the tumor enlarges. Imaging on T2 is typically isointense with larger lesions potentially demonstrating areas of internal cystic degradation.

References: *Diagnostic imaging: head and neck.* Elsevier. ISBN: 9780323443012. https://www.elsevier.com/books/diagnostic-imaging-head-and-neck/koch/978-0-323-44301-2

Knosp E, et al. Pituitary adenomas with invasion of the cavernous sinus space: a magnetic resonance imaging classification compared with surgical findings. *Neurosurgery* 1993;33(4):610–617.

Pisaneschi M, et al. Imaging the sella and parasellar region. *Neuroimaging Clin N Am* 2005;15(1):203–219.

14 **Answer C.** Pigmented villonodular synovitis. Pigmented villonodular synovitis (PVNS) of the temporomandibular joint. The other three choices are in the differential but less likely based on imaging.

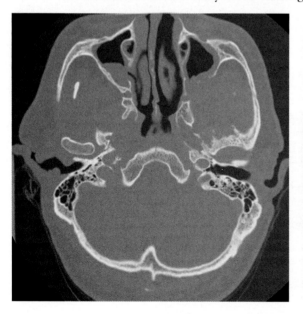
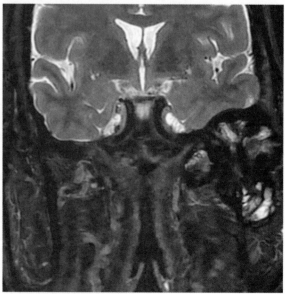

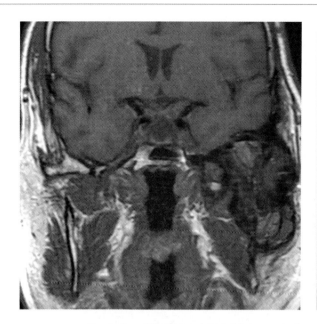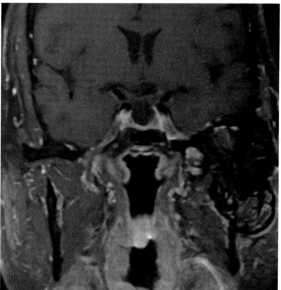

Imaging Findings: Axial bone window CT through the temporomandibular joint (TMJ) reveals left-sided rounded erosive lesions involving the zygomatic arch of the TMJ. Coronal T2-weighted MR demonstrates peripheral blooming surrounding a lobulated mass because of hemosiderin deposition. There are multiple areas of focal increased signal compatible with cystic change. Precontrast T1 images demonstrate a hypointense mass with peripheral decreased signal. Postcontrast images demonstrate minimal enhancement of the central portions.

Discussion: PVNS is a benign but locally aggressive disease of the synovial joints or tendons. It is most commonly encountered in the knee but may affect any synovial joint, including the TMJ. Clinically, this presents in middle-aged adults (between 2nd and 4th decades) and presents with trismus or preauricular pain. Treatment includes surgical resection with a relatively low recurrence rate.

    On imaging, CT may demonstrate erosive changes of the TMJ, including the mandibular condyle. The absence of calcified nodules and ground-glass calcifications distinguishes this entity from synovial chondromatosis and CPPD, respectively. MR findings demonstrate a synovial proliferation with surrounding hemosiderin deposition. The hemosiderin deposition results in a characteristic peripheral rim of susceptibility. Enhancement is variable but typically demonstrates less enhancement than chondrosarcomas and giant cell tumors.

Differential Diagnosis: Calcium pyrophosphate dihydrate deposition (CPPD) presents with diffusely ground-glass calcified nodules within the TMJ. Chondrosarcoma would typically present with more heterogenous enhancement than depicted in this case. Lastly, synovial chondromatosis would present with calcified nodules.

References: Bemporad JA, et al. Pigmented villonodular synovitis of the temporomandibular joint: diagnostic imaging and endovascular therapeutic embolization of a rare head and neck tumor. *AJNR Am J Neuroradiol* 1999;20(1):159–162.

Diagnostic imaging: head and neck. Elsevier. ISBN: 9780323443012. https://www.elsevier.com/books/diagnostic-imaging-head-and-neck/koch/978-0-323-44301-2

Le WJ, et al. Pigmented villonodular synovitis of the temporomandibular joint: CT imaging findings. *Clin Imaging* 2014;38(1):6–10.

15   **Answer B.**   Prepontine/retroclival region. Based on these images, the mass epicenter is most accurately located in the prepontine cistern or retroclival location. The sella is anterior and largely spared. The hypothalamic region/tuber cinereum and floor of third ventricle are along the superior edge of the lesion.

16   **Answer A.**   This is a locally aggressive lesion arising from a notochordal remnant. This lesion is most likely a chordoma. A benign notochordal remnant that may be seen in the same location but has no potential for local invasion or metastasis is ecchordosis physaliphora. Just based on the lesion location alone, sellar or pontine origin is unlikely.

17   **Answer A.**   Off-center location and relatively higher ADC measurements. Off-center location and relatively higher ADC measurements have been reported with chondrosarcoma, a differential diagnosis for this lesion.

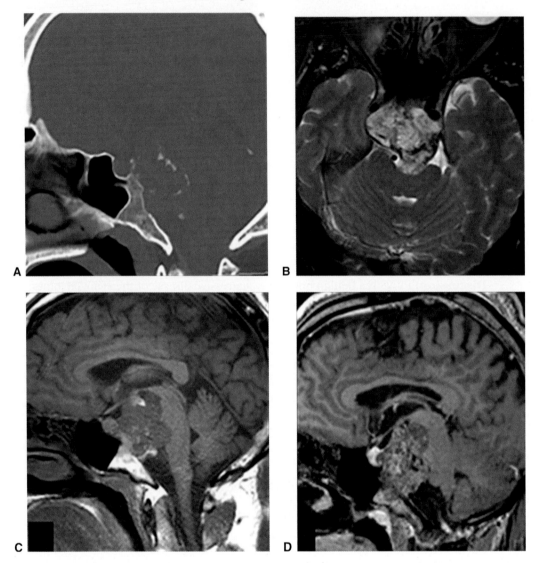

Imaging Findings: CT demonstrates a peripherally calcified mass in the prepontine cistern with scalloping of the superior dorsal clivus. On MRI, the mass arises from the dorsal clivus with an exophytic large soft tissue prepontine component, which enhances heterogeneously.

Discussion: Chordomas are slow growing, locally aggressive primary bone tumor arising from notochordal remnant. They rarely metastasize. They are midline tumors with nearly equal incidence in clivus region, sacrum, and rest of the spine.

Histologically, chordomas are classified into classic (most common), chondroid, and dedifferentiated types. In classic chordomas, the cells are in a mucopolysaccharide matrix. In chondroid type, the stroma resembles hyaline cartilage.

They can occur at any age but usually seen in adults with peak incidence in 4th decade of life and show male predilection by a factor of 2:1. In intracranial chordomas, given the proximity to several important structures, presenting compliant depends on the direction of tumor growth. Headache and 6th nerve paralysis are the most common presenting symptoms.

Intracranial chordomas commonly arise in the midline from spheno-occipital synchondrosis of the clivus. In about 15%, they can be paramedian arising from petrous apex. The rare sites of origin include sellar region, sphenoid sinus, nasopharynx, paranasal sinus region, and dura.

The classic appearance on imaging is destructive lobulated midline soft tissue mass centered in the clivus. It can spread anteriorly into sellar region and sphenoid sinus, laterally into petrous bone and middle cranial fossa, posteriorly into prepontine cistern, anteroinferiorly into nasopharynx, posteroinferiorly into foramen magnum, and superiorly into third ventricle and optic chiasm. Usually, more than one of these areas is involved. They rarely invade the brain parenchyma.

The internal imaging characteristics of the tumor depend to some extent on the histologic subtypes. Heterogeneity is common and results from hemorrhage, myxoid and gelatinous material, necrosis, and calcification. On CT, they are mildly hyperdense. On T1-weighted MR images, they are generally hypointense. The classic type is very hyperintense on T2-weighted images. In classic type, the apparent internal calcification is secondary to remaining portions of the destroyed bone rather than dystrophic calcification in the tumor. Low signal intensity septations and calcifications that separate high-intensity lobules are common. The chondroid and dedifferentiated types show somewhat low signal on T2 images. True calcification can be seen with chondroid subtype. Most of the tumors show moderate to marked heterogeneous contrast enhancement.

CTA/MRA is helpful in assessing vascular encasement. As these are soft tumors, vascular lumen tends to be preserved despite encasement.

Surgery and radiotherapy for the residual disease is the treatment of choice. Chordomas have high tendency for recurrence and warrant surveillance. They have overall worse prognosis than chondrosarcomas. Very high T2 signal of the tumor and enhancement are helpful features in assessing recurrence.

Differential diagnoses: Chondrosarcoma: generally off midline at petro-occipital fissure. Internal chondroid calcification. They tend to have much higher ADC than chordoma.

Invasive pituitary adenoma—sellar enlargement and inability to visualize pituitary gland separately from the mass are helpful features. Chordoma generally displaces the pituitary gland anteriorly.

Ecchordosis physaliphora—benign notochordal remnant. Generally small nonenhancing and prepontine in location. Show a stalk-like extension into the clivus.

References: Erdem E, Angtuaco EC, Van Hemert R, et al. Comprehensive review of intracranial chordoma. *Radiographics* 2003;23(4):995–1009. doi:10.1148/rg.234025176

Osborn AG. *Osborn's brain: Imaging, pathology, and anatomy*, 1st ed. Salt Lake City, UT: Amirsys Pub, 2013.

Yeom KW, Lober RM, Mobley BC, et al. Diffusion-weighted MRI: distinction of skull base chordoma from chondrosarcoma. *AJNR Am J Neuroradiol* 2013;34(5):1056–1061, S1. doi:10.3174/ajnr.A3333

18 Temporal Bone

SCOTT SORENSON • DANIEL THOMAS GINAT

QUESTIONS

1 Which letter corresponds to the lateral semicircular canal on the following image?

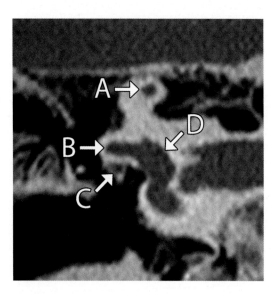

2 Which of the following corresponds to the facial nerve on the following oblique sagittal MRI?

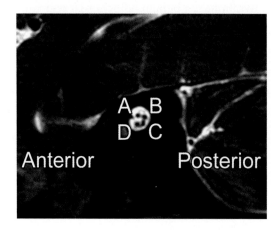

3 Which of the following is the most likely diagnosis based on the images below?

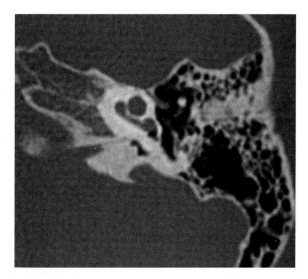

    A. Labyrinthine aplasia
    B. Common cavity
    C. Incomplete partition type 2
    D. Normal

4 Which of the following is the most likely diagnosis based on the image below?

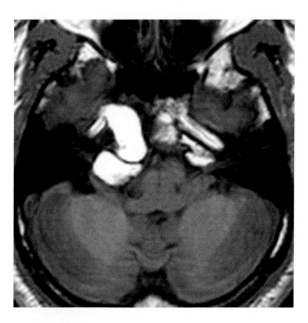

    A. Cholesterol granuloma
    B. Asymmetric petrous apex fat
    C. Vestibular schwannoma
    D. Meningioma

5   What is the most likely diagnosis based on the following image?

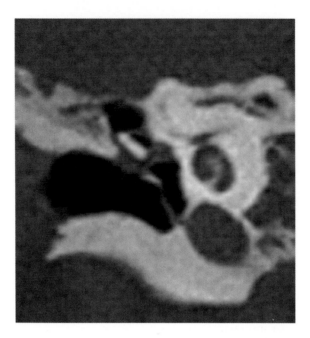

    A. External auditory canal cholesteatoma
    B. Pars flaccida cholesteatoma
    C. Pars tensa cholesteatoma
    D. Congenital cholesteatoma

6   Which of the following features of cholesteatoma are expected on MRI?

    A. Central enhancement and no restricted diffusion
    B. No central enhancement and no restricted diffusion
    C. Central enhancement and restricted diffusion
    D. No central enhancement and restricted diffusion

7   What is the most likely symptom experienced by the patient with the following imaging?

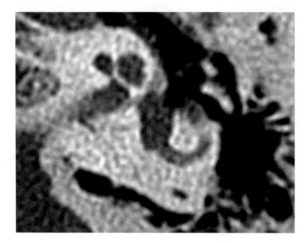

    A. Sensorineural hearing loss
    B. Conductive hearing loss
    C. Pulsatile tinnitus
    D. Otalgia

8 The most likely diagnosis based on the following images is?

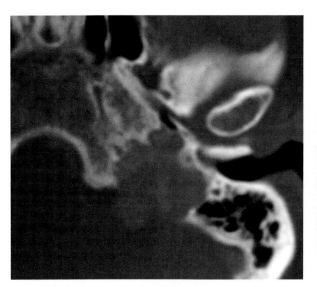 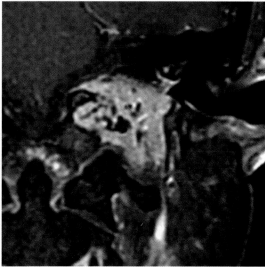

   A. Carotid body tumor
   B. Glomus vagale
   C. Glomus jugulare
   D. Glomus tympanicum

9 Glomus jugulare is supplied by which of the following arteries?

   A. Meningohypophyseal
   B. Lingual
   C. Facial
   D. Ascending pharyngeal

10 In this infant with fever, which of the following is the most likely diagnosis based on the image below?

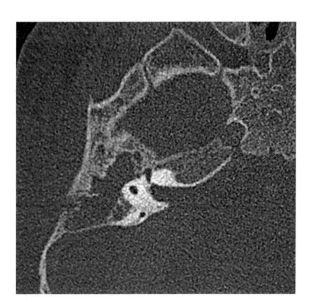

   A. Necrotizing otitis externa
   B. Petrous apicitis
   C. Coalescent mastoiditis
   D. Labyrinthitis

11 Which of the following best describes a potential complication of coalescent mastoiditis?

A. Ramsay Hunt syndrome
B. Bell palsy
C. Gradenigo syndrome
D. Bezold abscess

12 A 39-year-old male presents with tinnitus. Otoscopy reveals a right-sided red pulsatile retrotympanic mass. What is the most likely diagnosis?

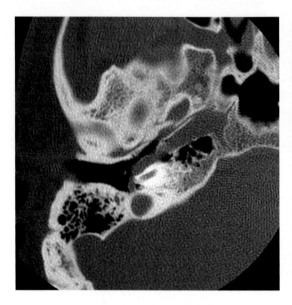 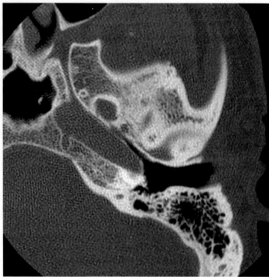

A. Cholesterol granuloma
B. High riding jugular bulb
C. Glomus tumor
D. Aberrant ICA

13 Which of the following entities may present with a red pulsatile retrotympanic mass on otoscopy?

A. Cholesterol granuloma
B. Congenital cholesteatoma
C. Dehiscent jugular bulb
D. Glomus tympanicum paraganglioma

14 What other vascular anomaly is most commonly associated with an aberrant ICA?

    A. Persistent hypoglossal artery

    B. Persistent otic artery

    C. Persistent stapedial artery

    D. Persistent trigeminal artery

15 Which corresponding bony foramen is absent in persistent stapedial artery?

    A. Foramen lacerum

    B. Foramen ovale

    C. Foramen rotundum

    D. Foramen spinosum

16 What complication from the temporal bone fracture is shown in the image below?

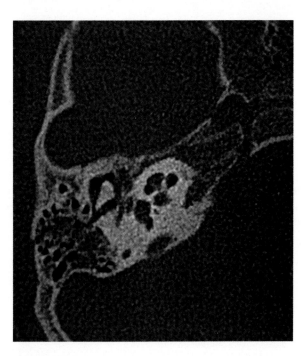

    A. Incudomalleal dislocation

    B. Sigmoid plate disruption

    C. Carotid canal disruption

    D. Pneumolabyrinth

ANSWERS AND EXPLANATIONS

1 **Answer B.**

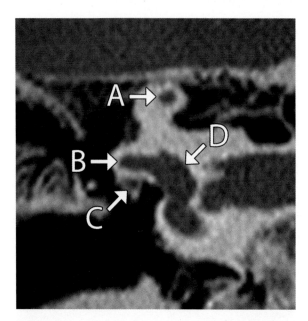

Imaging Findings: The coronal CT image shows the superior semicircular canal (A), the lateral semicircular canal (B), tympanic segment of the facial nerve canal (C), and vestibule (D).

2 **Answer A.**

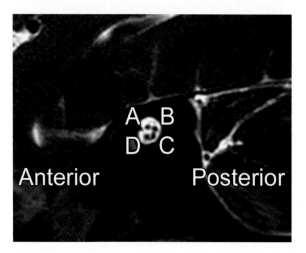

Imaging Findings: The oblique sagittal T2-weighted MRI through the internal auditory canal shows the facial nerve (A), superior vestibular nerve (B), inferior vestibular nerve (C), and cochlear nerve (D) in cross section.

Discussion: CT can provide detailed depiction of the temporal bone anatomy. The facial nerve courses from the internal auditory canal through the petrous bone via the labyrinthine segment, turns posteriorly at the geniculate ganglion, passes through the middle ear as the tympanic segment, and then turns inferiorly through the mastoid bone as the mastoid segment. The inner ear structures comprise the cochlear, which has approximately 2.5 turns; the vestibule, which is connected to the stapes footplate at the oval window; the horizontal, superior, and posterior semicircular canals, which are orthogonal to one another; and the vestibular aqueducts, which lead to the endolymphatic sac along the posterior aspect of the petrous temporal bone. The ossicular chain, which is located in the middle ear, comprises the malleus, incus, and stapes.

High-resolution T2-weighted MRI can resolve the four main cranial nerve branches in the internal auditory canal. The superior and inferior vestibular nerves are located in the posterior quadrants of the internal auditory canal, whereas the facial (seventh cranial nerve) is located in the anterosuperior quadrant and the cochlear nerve is located in the anteroinferior quadrant. A useful mnemonic for this is "seven up, coke down." The superior half of the internal auditory canal is separated from the inferior half by the falciform crest laterally.

Reference: Juliano AF, Ginat DT, Moonis G. Imaging review of the temporal bone: part I. Anatomy and inflammatory and neoplastic processes. *Radiology* 2013;269(1):17–33.

3 **Answer C.**   Incomplete partition type 2.

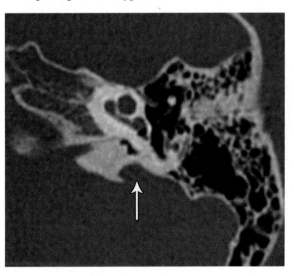

Imaging Findings: The axial CT image shows an enlarged vestibular aqueduct (arrow) and cystic cochlear apex.

Discussion: Incomplete partition type 2 is the most common congenital inner anomaly and results from developmental arrest in the 7th week of gestation. It is characterized by deficiency of the modiolus and the interscalar septum associated with the middle and apical turns, which consequently merge into a cystic cavity. In addition, vestibular aqueduct is often enlarged.

Labyrinthine aplasia is caused by developmental arrest of the otic placode during the 3rd gestational week and consists of complete absence of the inner ear structures and an atretic internal auditory canal.

A common cavity results from a developmental arrest in the 4th week of gestation and manifests as a combined cystic and featureless vestibule and cochlea.

Reference: Joshi VM, Navlekar SK, Kishore GR, et al. CT and MR imaging of the inner ear and brain in children with congenital sensorineural hearing loss. *Radiographics* 2012;32(3):683–698.

4 **Answer A.** Cholesterol granuloma.

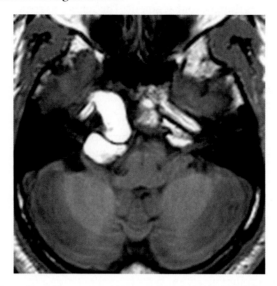

Imaging Findings: The T1-weighted MRI shows an expansile lesion centered in the right petrous apex with high signal internal components.

Discussion: Cholesterol granulomas are expansile, cystic lesions that contain blood products and chronic inflammatory material. The lesions are classically T1 hyperintense on MRI.

   Asymmetric petrous apex fat is also T1 hyperintense on MRI but can be differentiated from cholesterol granuloma by fat suppression techniques and the lack of bony expansion.

   Vestibular schwannomas enhance and are low signal on T1. These tumors can expand the internal auditory canal, but not the petrous bone.

   Meningiomas can cause hyperostosis rather than cystic changes and typically appears as enhancing tumors with dural tail.

Reference: Chapman PR, Shah R, Curé JK, et al. Petrous apex lesions: pictorial review. *AJR Am J Roentgenol* 2011;196(3 Suppl):WS26–WS37; Quiz S40–S43.

5 **Answer B.** Pars flaccida cholesteatoma.

6 **Answer D.** No central enhancement and restricted diffusion.

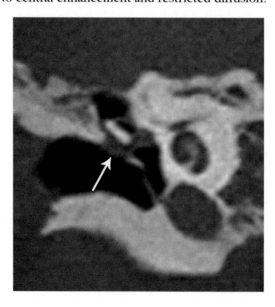

Imaging Findings: The coronal CT image shows an opacity (arrow) in the Prussak space and blunting of the scutum.

Discussion: Cholesteatomas are epidermal inclusion cysts that are most often acquired lesions resulting from eustachian tube dysfunction which cause negative pressure to build up in the middle ear cavity. This causes a retraction pocket to form in the loose upper part of the tympanic membrane also known as the pars flaccida. The retraction pocket begins in Prussak's space and can extend into the epitympanum. The present of a blunted scutum and ossicular erosion are helpful clues for making the diagnosis. If the cholesteatomas are sufficiently large, there can also be lateral semicircular canal and tegmen dehiscence. Congenital cholesteatomas are uncommon and typically located along the cochlear promontory.

MRI can be useful for differentiating cholesteatomas from other opacities. In particular, cholesteatomas typically display restricted diffusion and no internal enhancement and are T1 hypointense. An example is shown below with restricted diffusion and non-enhancing T1 hypointense signal compatible with a cholesteatoma.

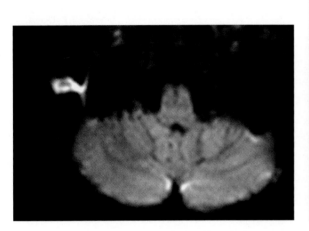
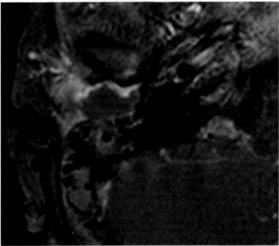

Reference: Baráth K, Huber AM, Stämpfli P, et al. Neuroradiology of cholesteatomas. *AJNR Am J Neuroradiol* 2011;32(2):221–229.

7 Answer B. Conductive hearing loss.

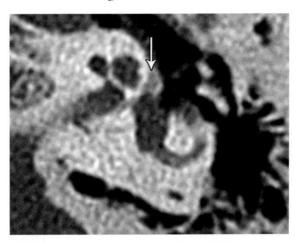

Imaging Findings: There is lucency in the otic capsule (arrow), in the region of the fissula ante fenestram, just inferior to the labyrinthine segment of the facial nerve.

Discussion: Otosclerosis is a process of bone remodeling that typically begins anterior to the oval window at the fissula ante fenestram. The fissula is a fold of connective tissue extending through the endochondral layer, between the oval window and the cochleariform process. Encroachment upon the stapes footplate can lead to conductive hearing loss. Lucent rather than sclerotic bony changes are the predominant feature throughout most of the disease process, which is why it is also known as otospongiosis. When the process surrounds the cochlea, it is called retrocochlear otosclerosis and can present with mixed or sensorineural hearing loss.

Reference: Juliano AF, Ginat DT, Moonis G. Imaging review of the temporal bone: part II. Traumatic, postoperative, and noninflammatory nonneoplastic conditions. *Radiology* 2015;276(3):655–672.

8   Answer C.   Glomus jugulare.

9   Answer D.   Ascending pharyngeal.

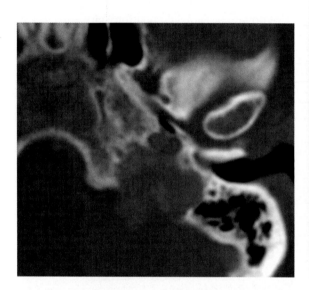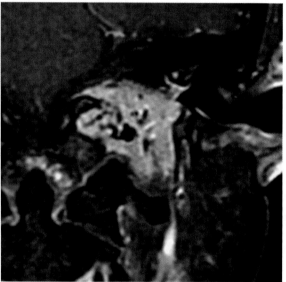

Imaging Findings: The axial CT image shows a lytic lesion centered in the left jugular foramen with irregular margins. The coronal postcontrast fat-suppressed MRI shows an avidly enhancing mass centered in the left jugular foramen with prominent flow voids.

Discussion: Glomus jugulare is a paraganglioma that arises from and can result in expansion and erosion of the jugular foramen and is supplied by the ascending pharyngeal artery. Paragangliomas are hypervascular tumors and classically display a salt-and-pepper appearance on MRI, in which the "pepper" component represents the multiple areas of signal void interspersed with the "salt" component that corresponds to hyperintense foci due to slow flow or hemorrhage.

Carotid body tumors splay the internal and external carotid arteries just above the bifurcation.

Glomus vagale arises from the nodose ganglion below the jugular foramen. The tumors displace the carotid artery anteromedially and the internal jugular vein posterolaterally, but do not splay the internal and external carotid arteries.

Glomus tympanicum refers to paragangliomas that are confined to the tympanic cavity along the cochlear promontory.

Reference: van den Berg R. Imaging and management of head and neck paragangliomas. *Eur Radiol* 2005;15(7):1310–1318.

10   Answer C.   Coalescent mastoiditis.

11 **Answer D.** Bezold abscess.

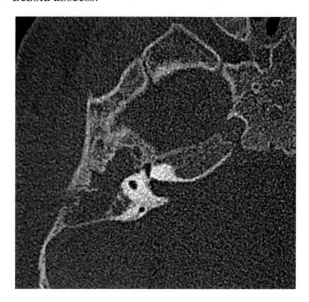

Imaging Findings: The axial CT image shows mastoid opacification, absence of the mastoid septations, and dehiscence of the lateral cortex.

Discussion: Coalescent mastoiditis is a complication of otitis media that results in erosion of the mastoid septa and potentially the cortex. Coalescent mastoiditis can be complicated by intracranial venous sinus thrombosis and subperiosteal abscesses as well as epidural abscess. In particular, Bezold abscess refers to extension of the infection deep to the sternocleidomastoid muscle and throughout the fascial planes of the neck.

Reference: Vazquez E, Castellote A, Piqueras J, et al. Imaging of complications of acute mastoiditis in children. *Radiographics* 2003;23(2):359–372.

12 **Answer D.** Aberrant ICA.

13 **Answer D.** Glomus tympanicum paraganglioma. Glomus tympanic paraganglioma and aberrant ICAs both present as red retrotympanic masses. Cholesterol granulomas and dehiscent jugular bulbs present as blue retrotympanic masses. Cholesteatomas present as white masses.

14 **Answer C.** Persistent stapedial artery. Up to 30% of aberrant ICAs may be associated with a persistent stapedial artery.

15 **Answer D.** Foramen spinosum. An absent ipsilateral foramen spinosum is associated with persistent stapedial artery. Did you notice the finding in the first figure?

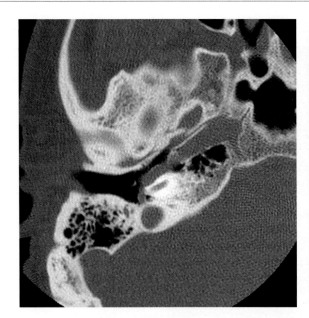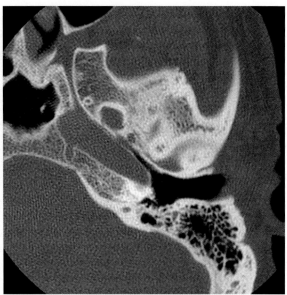

Imaging Findings: Bone window CT through the temporal bones reveals a tubular structure crossing the middle ear. There is an area of focal narrowing at the horizontal petrous internal carotid artery. Also seen is absence of the ipsilateral foramen spinosum. A persistent stapedial artery should be searched for in patients with aberrant ICA and absent foramen spinosum.

Discussion: When referrers see a red pulsatile retrotympanic mass, the two primary considerations are an aberrant ICA and glomus tympanic paraganglioma. As radiologists, it is important to distinguish between the two as misdiagnosis may lead to unnecessary biopsy, which may result in disastrous hemorrhage or even death. The two vessels that form the aberrant ICA are the inferior tympanic artery (a branch of the ECA) and the caroticotympanic artery. These two vessels enlarge and rejoin the horizontal segment of the ICA, which may be narrowed and results in tinnitus. Up to 30% of these patients may have a persistent stapedial artery. CT findings in persistent stapedial artery include absence of the ipsilateral foramen spinosum as well as an enlarged CNVII tympanic canal. Treatment is typically not necessary for both aberrant ICA and persistent stapedial artery.

References: Koch B, Hamilton BE, Hudgins P, et al. *Diagnostic imaging: head and neck*. Elsevier, 2016. ISBN: 9780323443012. https://www.elsevier.com/books/diagnostic-imaging-head-and-neck/koch/978-0-323-44301-2

Roll JD, Urban MA, Larson TC, et al. Bilateral aberrant internal carotid arteries with bilateral persistent stapedial arteries and bilateral duplicated internal carotid arteries. *AJNR Am J Neuroradiol* 2003;24(4):762–765.

16 **Answer D.** Pneumolabyrinth.

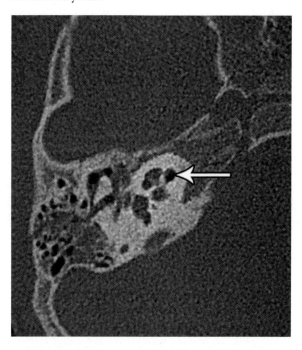

Imaging Findings: The axial CT image shows a right temporal bone fracture and air attenuation in the basal turn of the cochlea (arrow). There is also opacification of the mastoid air cells and middle ear.

Discussion: Temporal bone fractures have traditionally been classified as transverse, longitudinal, or oblique, and more recently as otic capsule sparing or violating. Regardless of the classification used, it is important to identify certain complications on imaging, such as pneumolabyrinth, ossicular chain disruption, facial canal involvement, and disruption of the carotid and jugular canals. In particular, compared with otic capsule sparing fractures, patients with otic capsule violating fractures are approximately two times more likely to develop facial paralysis, four times more likely to develop cerebrospinal fluid leak, and seven times more likely to experience profound hearing loss. They are also more likely to sustain intracranial complications including epidural hematoma and subarachnoid hemorrhage.

Reference: Collins JM, Krishnamoorthy AK, Kubal WS, et al. Multidetector CT of temporal bone fractures. *Semin Ultrasound CT MR* 2012;33(5):418-431.

CNS Angiography: Normal Anatomy and Vascular Diseases

DANIEL CHOW • ROBERT DARFLINGER

QUESTIONS

1 Regarding the images of a spinal angiogram shown below:

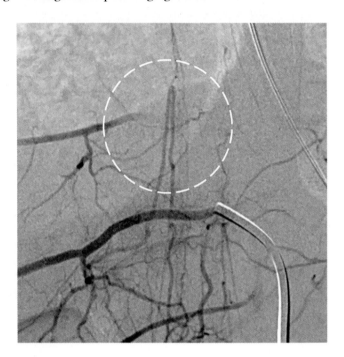

1a Which vessel is depicted?

A. Artery of Adamkiewicz
B. Artery of Lazorthes
C. Paravertebral artery
D. Segmental artery

1b Which of the following is true regarding this artery?

A. Most commonly arises above the 8th intercostal artery
B. Most commonly arises on the left
C. Can be sacrificed because of redundant blood supply of the cord
D. Contributes to the posterior spinal blood supply

2   Regarding the following angiographic image:

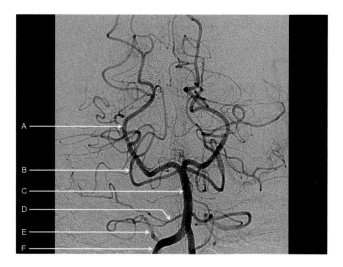

2a   Which structure corresponds to the superior cerebellar artery?

A.
B.
C.
D.
E.
F.

2b   Which structure corresponds to the anterior inferior cerebellar artery?

A.
B.
C.
D.
E.
F.

3   Regarding the following angiographic image:

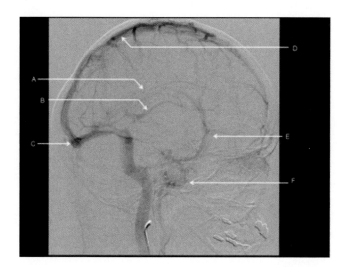

3a Which structure corresponds to the cavernous sinus?

    A.

    B.

    C.

    D.

    E.

    F.

3b Which structure corresponds to the internal cerebral vein?

    A.

    B.

    C.

    D.

    E.

    F.

4 Which of the following is part of the superficial venous system?

    A. Basal vein of Rosenthal

    B. Inferior petrosal sinus

    C. Vein of Galen

    D. Vein of Trolard

5 A 46-year-old female presenting 4 days after initial subarachnoid hemorrhage bleed.

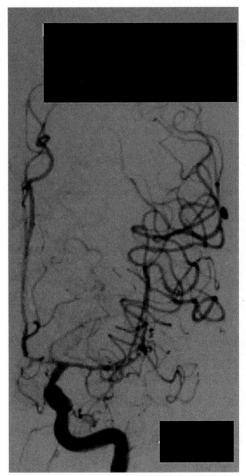

(Pretherapy)

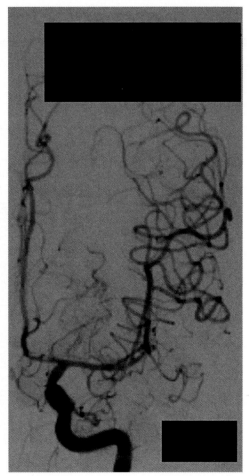

(Posttherapy)

5a What is true regarding the cause of pretherapy images?

A. More commonly encountered with a lower modified Fisher score
B. Peak probability seen within the first 24 hours
C. The risk steadily declines after the first 4 days.
D. May result in ischemia

5b What intra-arterial medication was most likely provided to this patient?

A. Alpha blocker
B. Beta-blocker
C. Calcium channel blocker
D. Tissue plasminogen activator (tPA)

6 A 17-year-old with recurrent nose bleeds demonstrates the following imaging findings. Family history of additional family members with recurrent epistaxis.

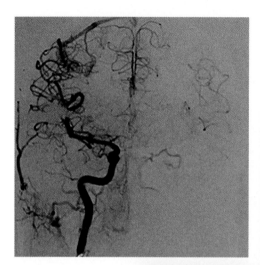
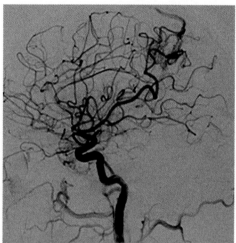
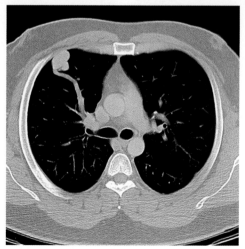

What is the diagnosis?

A. Encephalotrigeminal angiomatosis
B. CADASIL
C. Hereditary hemorrhagic telangiectasia
D. Subcortical arteriosclerotic encephalopathy

7   Which organ does hereditary hemorrhagic telangiectasia most commonly involve?

A. Cerebral parenchyma
B. Gastrointestinal
C. Nasal mucosa
D. Pulmonary

8   A 9-year-old female presents with recurrent transient ischemic attacks. What is the diagnosis?

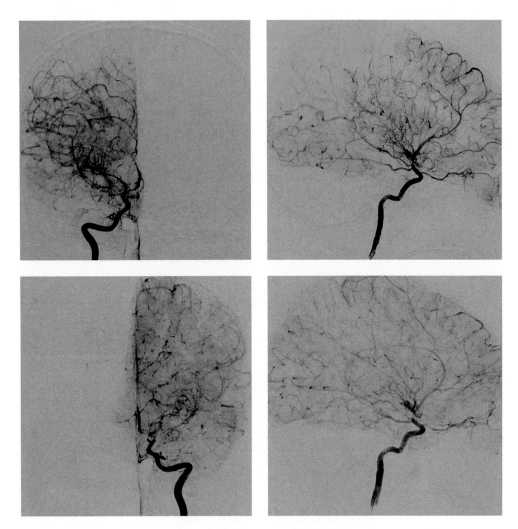

A. CADASIL
B. Fibromuscular dysplasia
C. Moyamoya disease
D. Reversible cerebral vasoconstriction syndrome

9   Which of the following is true regarding Moyamoya?

A. Bimodal age distribution
B. Children typically present with hemorrhage.
C. Posterior circulation more commonly involved relative to anterior circulation
D. Rarely presents with hemorrhage in adults

10 A male pediatric patient presents with recurrent nosebleeds; what is the diagnosis?

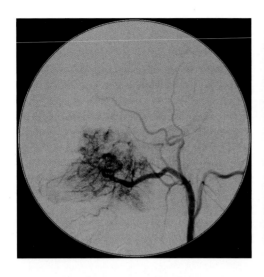
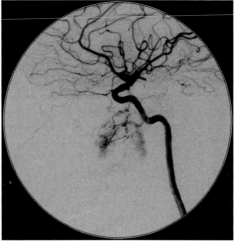

    A. Esthesioneuroblastoma
    B. Nasopharyngeal carcinoma
    C. Juvenile nasopharyngeal angiofibroma
    D. Rhabdomyosarcoma of the head and neck

11 Where do juvenile nasopharyngeal angiofibromas arise from?

    A. Pterygomaxillary fissure
    B. Pterygopalatine fossa
    C. Sphenopalatine foramen
    D. Vidian canal

12 A 58-year-old male presents with pulsatile tinnitus. What is the diagnosis?

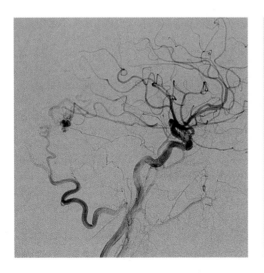
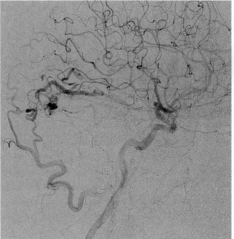

    A. Capillary telangiectasia
    B. Cerebral arteriovenous malformation
    C. Developmental venous anomaly
    D. Dural arteriovenous fistula

13 Regarding dural AVFs, which of the following is the most important risk factor for rupture?

   A. Antegrade venous drainage
   B. Cortical venous reflux
   C. Enlarged dural sinus
   D. Infratentorial location

14 A 40-year-old female presents with altered mental status.

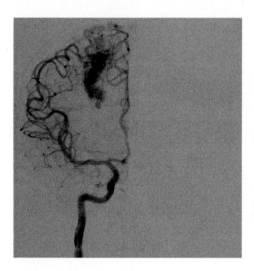
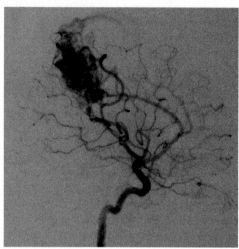

14a What is the diagnosis?

   A. Capillary telangiectasia
   B. Cerebral arteriovenous malformation
   C. Developmental venous anomaly
   D. Meningioma

14b Which of the following is a component of Spetzler-Martin classification?

   A. Presence or absence of aneurysms
   B. Presence or absence of intervening normal brain
   C. Superficial versus deep venous drainage
   D. Supratentorial versus infratentorial location

ANSWERS AND EXPLANATIONS

1a **Answer A.** Artery of Adamkiewicz.

1b **Answer B.** Most commonly arises on the left.

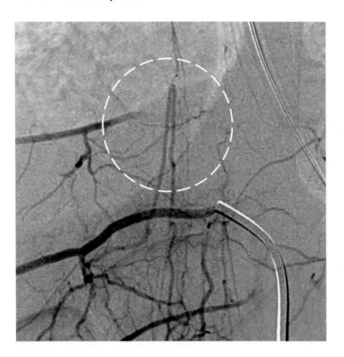

Imaging Findings: Diagnostic spinal angiogram in a 3-year-old child. The anterior spinal artery is visualized with injection of the right T9 intercostal artery following a classic hairpin turn, the artery of Adamkiewicz.

Discussion: The artery of Adamkiewicz, also known as the artery of the lumbar enlargement or great anterior radiculomedullary artery, is the largest anterior segmental medullary artery and supplies the anterior two-thirds of the spinal cord through the anterior spinal artery. Therefore, the distal cord is at risk to infarction if there is damage. It most commonly arises on the left at the level of the 9th through 12th intercostal artery. The vessel is named after Albert Adamkiewicz, a Polish pathologist.

Reference: Osborn AG, Jacobs JM, Osborn AG. *Diagnostic cerebral angiography*, 2nd ed. Philadelphia, PA: Lippincott-Raven, 1999:ix.

2a **Answer B.**

2b **Answer D.**

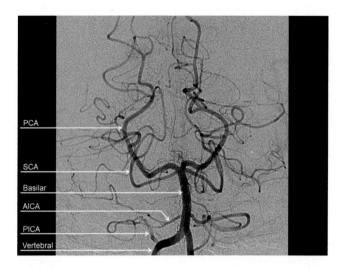

Imaging Findings: AP DSA images from a vertebral injection, which is fully annotated below.

Discussion: The two vertebral arteries combine to form the basilar artery. The posterior inferior cerebellar artery arises as the last branch of the vertebral artery (PICA). From the basilar artery two branches arise, the anterior inferior cerebellar artery (AICA) and the superior cerebellar artery (SCA). It also gives rise to pontine branches. The basilar artery bifurcates into the right and left posterior cerebral arteries (PCA).

Reference: Osborn AG, Jacobs JM, Osborn AG. *Diagnostic cerebral angiography*, 2nd ed. Philadelphia, PA: Lippincott-Raven, 1999:ix.

3a **Answer F.**

3b **Answer B.**

4 **Answer D.** Vein of Trolard

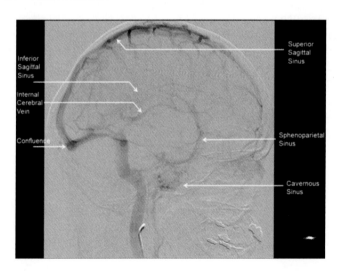

Imaging Findings: Lateral DSA images of venous anatomy, annotated below:

Discussion: It is important to recognize both superficial and deep venous structures. Briefly, the superficial (cortical) cerebral veins drain the cortex and subcortical white matter. In addition to the sagittal sinuses and cortical veins, named veins include the vein of Trolard (superior anastomotic vein), Labbe vein (inferior anastomotic vein), and sylvian (superficial middle cerebral vein). With regards to the deep venous system, this includes the internal cerebral vein, basal vein of Rosenthal, vein of Galen, and thalamostriate veins.

Reference: Osborn AG, Jacobs JM, Osborn AG. *Diagnostic cerebral angiography*, 2nd ed. Philadelphia, PA: Lippincott-Raven, 1999:ix.

5a   Answer D.   May result in ischemia.

5b   Answer C.   Calcium channel blocker (verapamil)

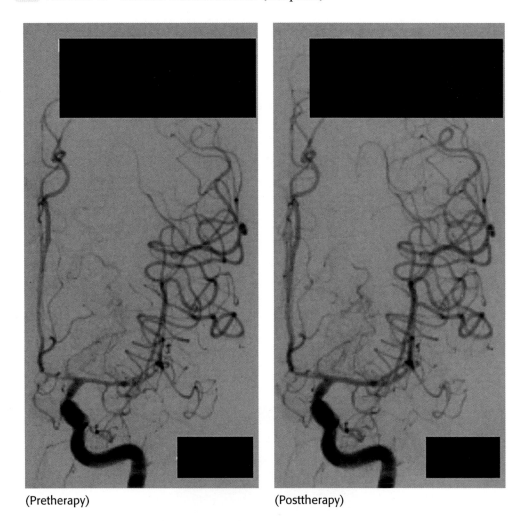

(Pretherapy)   (Posttherapy)

Imaging Findings: AP magnified image angiographic project of a left internal carotid artery injection demonstrates supraclinoid ICA narrowing, A1 segment narrowing, and M1 segment narrowing. Post–verapamil infusion images demonstrate improved luminal caliber.

Discussion: Complications of subarachnoid hemorrhage can be potentially life threatening. Classically, these are divided into the acute phase (days 0 to 4), subacute phase (days 4 to 30), and late phase (after day 30). With regard to the risk of vasospasm, the risk begins at days 3 and peaks at day 7 postbleed to approximately 4% to 5% and is seen most commonly between days 4 and 10. Therapy includes Triple

H (hemodilution, hypertension, and hypervolemia) to maintain cerebral perfusion pressure. Endovascularly, calcium channel blockers (e.g., verapamil) may be delivered.

Phase	Complications
Acute (days 0–4)	Rebleeding
	Acute hydrocephalus
Subacute (days 4–30)	Vasospasm
Chronic (beyond day 30)	Chronic hydrocephalus

Reference: Osborn AG, Jacobs JM, Osborn AG. *Diagnostic cerebral angiography*, 2nd ed. Philadelphia, PA: Lippincott-Raven, 1999:ix.

6 **Answer C.** Hereditary hemorrhagic telangiectasia (also known as Osler-Weber-Rendu).

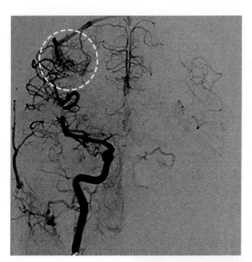
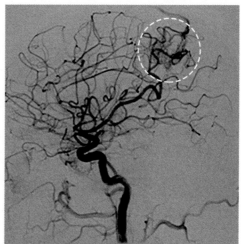
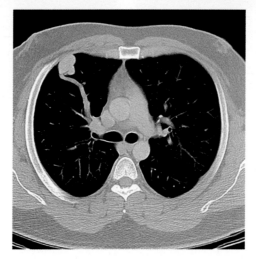

7 **Answer C.** Nasal mucosa

Imaging Findings: AP and lateral DSA images from a right internal carotid artery injection demonstrate cerebral arteriovenous malformation. Corresponding chest CT demonstrates a pulmonary AVM.

Discussion: Hereditary hemorrhagic telangiectasia (also known as Osler-Weber-Rendu) is an autosomal dominant disorder characterized by systemic angiodysplastic lesions. Although multiple organ systems may be involved, the most commonly involved are telangiectasia of nasal mucosa leading to recurrent epistaxis and telangiectasias of the oral cavity and skin, which also lead to recurrent bleeding. CNS manifestations typically include cerebral and spinal arteriovenous malformations.

Historically, Henri Rendu was a French physician who described a case of hereditary hemorrhagic telangiectasia in 1986. William Osler would describe additional cases 5 years later, and Frederick Weber would make additional contributions shortly after.

References: Henri Rendu (1844–1902). Rendu-Osler-Weber disease. *JAMA* 1966;197(7):583.

Osborn AG, Jacobs JM, Osborn AG. *Diagnostic cerebral angiography*, 2nd ed. Philadelphia, PA: Lippincott-Raven, 1999:ix.

8 **Answer C.** Moyamoya disease

9 **Answer A.** Bimodal age distribution

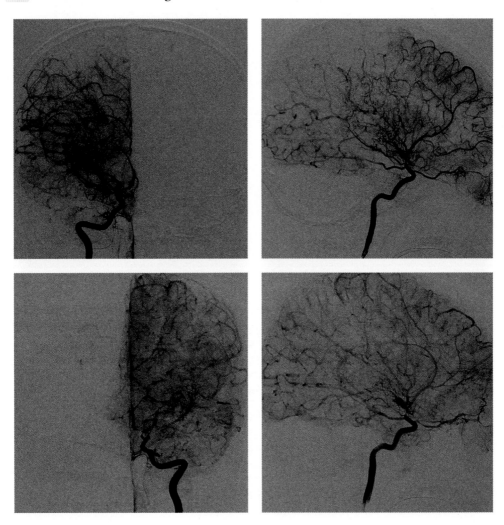

Imaging Findings: AP and lateral DSA images from a right and left internal carotid artery injection demonstrate narrowing of the proximal anterior and middle cerebral arteries bilaterally. There are innumerable tortuous collaterals that provide the classic "puff of smoke" appearance.

Discussion: True moyamoya disease presents with bilateral symmetric obliterative arteriopathy in the Southeast Asian population. The disease demonstrates a bimodal distribution, affecting those in early childhood and middle-aged adults. Radiographically, the presence of tortuous and tiny collaterals(lenticulostriate, thalamoperforator, leptomeningeal, and dural) gives rise to the classic "puff of smoke" appearance.

There are numerous conditions that may mimic this appearance, which is described as moyamoya syndrome. This may include phakomatoses such as NF1 and tuberous sclerosis as well numerous other disorders, including sickle cell, atherosclerosis, dissection, autoimmune diseases, Down syndrome, radiation, meningitis, protein C/S deficiency, and zoster.

References: Kuroda S, Houkin K. Moyamoya disease: current concepts and future perspectives. *Lancet Neurol* 2008;7(11):1056–1066.

Osborn AG, Jacobs JM, Osborn AG. *Diagnostic cerebral angiography*, 2nd ed. Philadelphia, PA: Lippincott-Raven, 1999:ix.

10 Answer C.   Juvenile nasopharyngeal angiofibroma

11 Answer C.   Sphenopalatine foramen

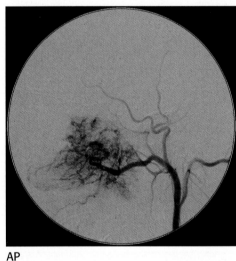
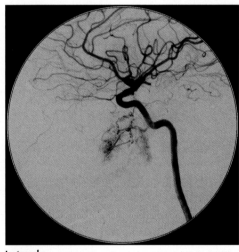

AP   Lateral

Imaging Findings: AP projection of left ECA injection demonstrates extensive vascular blush of the juvenile nasopharyngeal angiofibroma (JNA) from the sphenopalatine artery (distal internal maxillary artery). Lateral projection of the left internal carotid artery demonstrates additional supply to the JNA from the mandibulovidian artery (arising from petrous ICA) and artery of foramen ovale(arising from either internal maxillary or middle meningeal artery).

Discussion: Juvenile angiofibromas (JAFs) represent benign, vascular, nonencapsulated, and locally invasive nasal cavity mass. These tumors originate at the sphenopalatine foramen, where they may extend into the nasal cavity, nasopharynx, and pterygopalatine fossa. These tumors are almost exclusively seen in young adult males, and if found in a female should warrant genetic testing to evaluate for mosaicism. Clinically, these patients present with both nasal obstruction and recurrent epistaxis.

12 **Answer D.** Dural arteriovenous fistula

13 **Answer B.** Cortical venous reflux

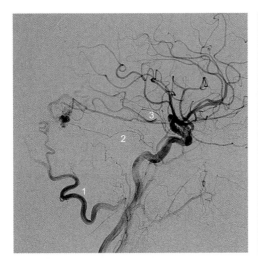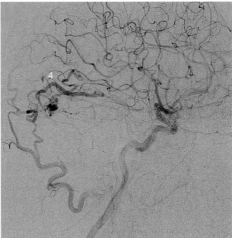

Imaging Findings: Lateral DSA projections in the early arterial phase from a left common carotid artery injection demonstrate a high risk left transverse sinus dural arteriovenous fistula with arterial supply from a left occipital artery (1), left middle meningeal artery (2), and left tentorial artery (3). There is cortical venous reflux into the left cortical vein (4) at the undersurface of the left temporal lobe.

Discussion: Dural arteriovenous fistulae are predominately acquired abnormal arterial connections to the dural venous sinuses, most frequently the transverse or sigmoid sinuses, although there are other less common entities. Most commonly, this represents a dural or pial artery or collection of arteries having formed an abnormal drainage into a series of channels within the wall of the dural sinus, although direct drainage into the sinus and the "parallel channel" type are also seen. Presence of "cortical venous reflux" increases the potential of hemorrhage.

Reference: Osborn AG, Jacobs JM, Osborn AG. *Diagnostic cerebral angiography*, 2nd ed. Philadelphia, PA: Lippincott-Raven, 1999:ix.

14a **Answer B.** Cerebral arteriovenous malformation

14b **Answer C.** Superficial versus deep venous drainage

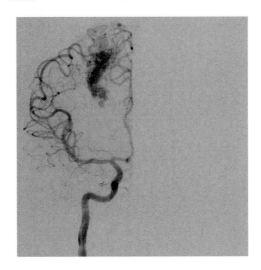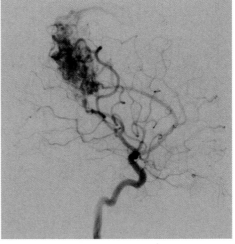

Imaging Findings: AP and lateral projections of an internal carotid injection demonstrate high-flow arteriovenous shunting with a large superior parietal arteriovenous malformation nidus with multiple superficial draining veins. The malformation is supplied by both anterior and middle cerebral artery branches.

Discussion: Arteriovenous malformations (AVMs) represent an abnormal vascular connection between arteries and veins through a vascular nidus that bypass the capillary system. As a point of distinction, these vascular lesions do not have intervening normal brain tissue. The most widely used classification scheme for these lesions is the Spetzler-Martin scale (see below). High-risk features to look for include flow-related aneurysms or venous outflow narrowing/restriction, which can increase the risk of hemorrhage.

Spetzler-Martin Scale

- Size
  - Small (<3 cm) = 1
  - Medium (>3 cm) = 2
  - Large (>6 cm) = 3
- Eloquence of Adjacent Brain
  - Noneloquent = 0
  - Eloquent = 1
- Venous Drainage
  - Superficial = 0
  - Deep = 1

Reference: Osborn AG, Jacobs JM, Osborn AG. *Diagnostic cerebral angiography*, 2nd ed. Philadelphia, PA: Lippincott-Raven, 1999:ix.

20 Noninterpretive Skills

DANIEL CHOW • PRACHI DUBEY

QUESTIONS

1   A radiologist misses a pulmonary embolus when evaluating a stroke CTA. Which type of error has occurred?

A. Cognitive
B. Perceptual
C. System error
D. Treatment

2   A radiology fellow mistakenly protocols an incorrect exam because of a complex drop-down menu. Considering the concept of "just culture," which of the following is the next best course of action?

A. Console the fellow, and work to improve the protocol interface.
B. Create incentives for better protocoling.
C. Remedial protocol training for the fellow
D. Punitive action with increased call

3   To save time, an MR technologist alters the axial DWI sequence from 2 skip 0 to 5 skip 1.5 knowing that this may reduce image quality. The final diagnosis was still able to be made, and no harm to the patient resulted from this action. Considering the concept of "just culture," which of the following is the next best course of action?

A. Reward the technologists for increasing efficiency.
B. Reprogram the technologists' console to prevent future adjustments.
C. Work with schedulers to allot more time for imaging.
D. Punitive action with suspension

4   While performing an epidural spinal injection, the fellow draws up lidocaine and contrast in separate syringes but fails to label them because he believes the risk is insignificant as he has placed them in separate areas of the procedure tray. The patient goes on to have the procedure without incident, but the nurse notices that the syringes were not appropriately labeled while cleaning up. Considering the concept of "just culture," which of the following is the next best course of action?

A. Console the fellow, as no harm occurred.
B. Coach the fellow to appropriately label syringes in the future.
C. Remedial training about the risks of unlabeled syringes
D. Punitive action with suspension

5 During a "time-out" prior to a lumbar puncture, which of the following is true regarding patient identifications?

A. Three identifiers are required.
B. The patient's room number may be used.
C. The accession number for the case may serve as an identifier.
D. A nurse who previously identified the patient may act as a source of patient identifier.

6 Which of the following is true regarding the various levels of sedation that may be required for some image-guided procedures?

A. ASA class I through IV may be safely sedated by radiologists or nurse practitioner without consultation with an anesthesiologist.
B. ASA class V patients should be sedated by anesthesiologists.
C. Patients with moderate sedation may have minimally impaired cognitive function, and coordination may be impaired, but ventilatory and cardiovascular functions are unaffected.
D. Patients with deep sedation retain a continuous and independent ability to maintain protective reflexes and a patent airway and are easily aroused by physical or verbal stimulation.

7 Which of the following is true regarding MRI safety zones?

A. Zone I—Where the MR scanner is located (the area of highest risk)
B. Zone II—Location where patients are screened
C. Zone III—Location of the scanner control room
D. Zone IV—Area of unrestricted access

8 A patient suffers cardiac arrest while undergoing an MRI of the brain. What is the next best step?

A. Quench the magnet to remove the electromagnetic field.
B. Perform ACLS at the scanner.
C. Perform CPR only at the scanner, and ACLS after the patient can be stabilized and moved out of the scanner.
D. Transfer the patient out of the scanner before beginning CPR.

9 A patient has a history of prior allergy to iodinated contrast administration for an elective outpatient scan. A referrer asks what a preferred appropriate premedication regimen is.

A. IV saline
B. Prednisone 50 mg by mouth at 13 hours, 7 hours, and 1 hour before contrast media injection, plus diphenhydramine 50 mg, IV, IM, or PO 1 hour before
C. Methylprednisolone sodium succinate 40 mg IV 1 hour before contrast administration
D. Dexamethasone sodium sulfate 30 mg IV 2 hours before contrast administration

10 A patient develops mild urticaria following contrast administration. Which of the following is recommended?

A. No treatment is necessary in most cases.
B. Prednisone 25 or 50 mg PO
C. Epinephrine IM
D. Epinephrine IV

11 A patient develops laryngeal edema following contrast administration. Which of the following is recommended?

    A. IM epinephrine (1:10,000) 1 to 3 mL
    B. IM epinephrine (1:1,000) 0.3 mL
    C. IV epinephrine (1:1,000) 1 to 3 mL
    D. IV epinephrine (1:10,000) 0.3 mL

12 While reading ER head CTs, you observe an acute intracerebral hemorrhage in a hypertensive patient. Which of the following is true regarding the appropriate communication of this finding?

    A. Must occur within 30 to 60 minutes of the time that the observation is made
    B. Finding may be communicated electronically.
    C. Must occur within 6 to 12 hours from when the imaging was performed
    D. Communication is not time sensitive but must be performed directly with the ordering primary physician.

13 Which is true regarding contrast administration *while breast-feeding*?

    A. Both gadolinium and iodinated contrast are not safe.
    B. Gadolinium is safe, but iodinated contrast is not.
    C. Iodinated contrast is safe, but gadolinium is not.
    D. Both gadolinium and iodinated contrast are safe.

14 What is the artifact shown in the following image?

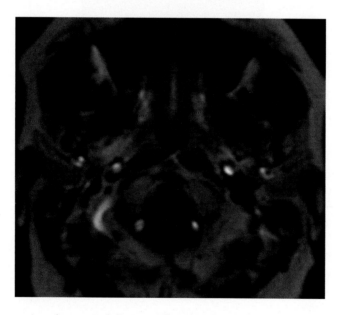

    A. T1 shortening due to gadolinium administration
    B. Flow-related signal due to time of flight technique
    C. Entry slice phenomenon
    D. Flow void

15 Below is an image from a noncontrast MR angiogram of the brain with time of flight technique. What is the artifact shown in the following image?

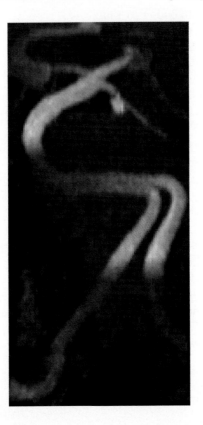

A. Inplane saturation
B. Motion artifact
C. Flow artifact
D. Flow void

16 B-value in diffusion weighted imaging relates to which of the following?

A. Magnetic field strength
B. Gradient
C. Echo time
D. Repetition time

17 Which of the following properties make a good screening tool?

A. High sensitivity
B. High specificity
C. High accuracy
D. High positive predictive value

18 A good confirmatory test for a disease should have which of the following properties?

A. High sensitivity
B. High specificity
C. High accuracy
D. High positive predictive value

19   What is the artifact shown in the following image?

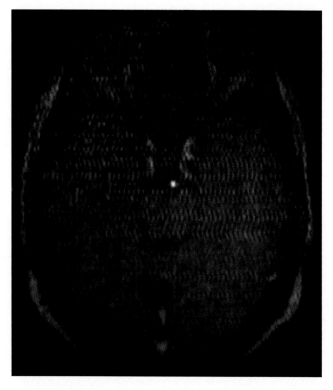

A. Eddy current artifact
B. Zipper artifact
C. Gibbs artifact
D. Motion artifact

20   Further imaging evaluation is inappropriate in which of the following scenarios?

A. Sudden onset of a severe headache without prodrome
B. Chronic headache with no new symptoms or neurologic deficit
C. Chronic headache with new left hand weakness
D. New headache in a pregnant woman

ANSWERS AND EXPLANATIONS

1   **Answer B.**   Perceptual. Errors in perception are by far the most common encountered by radiologists, accounting for 60% to 80% of errors. These errors occur within the initial detection phase of image interpretation. While not fully understood, several proposed risk factors are reader fatigue, distractions during image review, and "satisfaction of search." Cognitive errors (choice A) represent a faulty interpretation of information. System errors (choice C) are attributed to health system issues or issues within the context of care delivery (i.e., failure to communicate a finding). Lastly, treatment errors (choice D) represent an error in the performance of an operation or test.

2, 3, and 4   These questions relate to concept of "just culture," which seeks to improve patient safety by identifying system issues that lead individuals to engage in unsafe behaviors while balancing individual accountability with zero tolerance for reckless behavior. Introduced by David Marx, behavior is divided into three categories: human error, at-risk behavior, and reckless behavior.

2   **Answer A.**   Console the fellow, and work to improve the protocol interface. The behavior was a human error—an inadvertent mistake or slip.

3   **Answer D.**   Punitive action with suspension. The behavior is clearly reckless—a conscious disregard for an unjustifiable risk—and should be appropriately punished.

4   **Answer B.**   Coach the fellow to appropriately label syringes in the future. This presents an at-risk behavior, where the fellow takes a risk because he/she believes it to be insignificant and justified. These instances are best managed with coaching, to either remove incentives for poor behaviors or generate incentives for better choices.

5   **Answer D.**   A nurse who previously identified the patient may act as a source of patient identifier. Two patient identifiers are required for a formal "time-out" prior to a procedure. Acceptable identifiers may include the patient's name, medical record number, or telephone number. Sources of acceptable patient identifiers may also include a health care provider who has previously identified the patient. The patient's location, room number, or accession numbers cannot be used.

6   **Answer B.**   ASA class V patients should be sedated by anesthesiologists. Varying levels of sedation are required for diagnostic imaging procedures, including neurointerventional procedures. When considering sedation, the patient should be screened to determine his or her risk factors. Patients are classified per the American Society of Anesthesiologists (ASA) Physical Status Classification, which is as follows:

Class I	Normal healthy patient
Class II	Mild systemic disease
Class III	Severe systemic disease
Class IV	Severe systemic disease that is a threat to life
Class V	Moribund and not expected to survive without the operation
Class VI	Brain-dead patient whose organs are being removed for donor purposes

Classes I and II generally qualify for moderate sedation.

Classes III and IV may require additional consideration with anesthesiology consultation.

Class V should not be performed by nonanesthesiologists.

7　**Answer C.**　Zone III—Location of the scanner control room. The MRI suite is divided into four zones.

Zone I: Unrestricted access freely accessible to the public. This may include the image entrance area.

Zone II: The interface between zone I and strictly monitored zones III and IV. This may include the reception area and holding rooms. Patients in this area should be under the supervision of MR personnel.

Zone III: The first controlled area that is of potential danger between unscreened patients and the magnetic field. The technologist control and equipment rooms are typically in this area.

Zone IV: This zone is occupied by the scanner itself and is the highest risk.

8　**Answer D.**　Transfer the patient out of the scanner before beginning CPR. Should a medical emergency occur, the patient should first be moved to a magnetically safe environment while resuscitation or stabilization is begun (choice D). It is generally not advisable to perform CPR in proximity to the magnetic core (choices B and C). Quenching the magnet heats the magnetic coils and results in rapid liquid helium evaporation. This process floods the room with helium gas and displaces oxygen, which may result in asphyxiation of those left within the scanner.

9　**Answer B.**　Prednisone 50 mg by mouth at 13 hours, 7 hours, and 1 hour before contrast media injection, plus diphenhydramine 50 mg, IV, IM, or PO 1 hour before. Premedication may be used for patients at heightened risk for an allergic reaction to contrast. The two most frequently used protocols per the American College of Radiology Manual on Contrast Media are

1. Prednisone: 50 mg PO at 13 hours, 7 hours, and 1 hour before administration with diphenhydramine (Benadryl) 50 mg PO/IV/IM 1 hour before contrast media exposure
2. Methylprednisolone (Medrol) 32 mg by mouth 12 hours and 2 hours before

In instances where contrast is required within a shorter time, the following options exist, which are ordered in decreasing desirability:

1. Methylprednisolone (Medrol) 40 mg or hydrocortisone sodium succinate 200 mg IV q4h until administration with Benadryl 50 mg IV 1 hour prior
2. Dexamethasone sodium sulfate (Decadron) 7.5 mg or betamethasone 6.0 mg IV q4h until administration
3. Benadryl 50 mg IV alone

10 and 11   These questions are related to management of contrast reactions. Management of contrast reactions is a must-know. The reaction may be relatively benign such as urticaria (hives), which generally resolves without treatment. If treatment is necessary, consider Benadryl 25 or 50 mg orally. If this is administered, ensure the patient is not driving himself or herself home.

For severe laryngeal edema, the following treatment options should be administered after preserving IV access and providing oxygen via mask:

- IM epinephrine (1:1,000) 0.3 mL (0.3 mg)
- IV epinephrine (1:10,000) 3.0 mL (0.3 mg)

10   Answer A.   No treatment is necessary in most cases.

11   Answer B.   IM epinephrine (1:1,000) 0.3 mL (= 0.3 mg).

12   Answer A.   Must occur within 30 to 60 minutes of the time that the observation is made. For emergent results, there are three levels of communication based on the urgency of findings:

Level 1 (30 to 60 minutes): Findings that are life threatening or would require an immediate change in patient management. Examples in neuroimaging include herniation or an acute subarachnoid hemorrhage.

Level 2 (6 to 12 hours): New findings that may result in increased mortality or morbidity if not appropriately treated within 2 to 3 days. Examples in neuroimaging may include an impending pathologic vertebral fracture.

Level 3 (non–time-sensitive documentation): These findings may result in significant morbidity if not treated, but are not immediately life threatening. A new intracranial enhancing lesion may fall into this category.

13   Answer D.   Both gadolinium and iodinated contrast are safe. Both gadolinium and iodinated contrast are safe during breast-feeding. Only <0.05% of the maternal dose of gadolinium passes into breast milk. With regard to iodinated contrast, only 1% to 2% of oral contrast is absorbed into the bloodstream. Given these considerations, there is insufficient evidence to warrant stopping breast-feeding for either contrast agent.

14, 15, and 16   These questions are related to identification of common MRI artifacts.

14 **Answer C.**   Entry slice phenomenon.

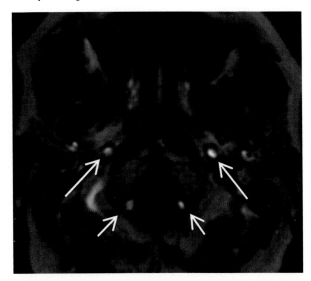

Imaging Findings: This is a T1-weighted axial image without contrast, (note the nasal mucosal surfaces showing absence of contrast enhancement) with hyperintense signal in the vessels. This signal is due to blood flowing into the slice with unsaturated spins also known as entry slice phenomenon. It is distinct from flow void, which refers to lack of signal due to flowing blood as seen in T2-weighted images. The phenomenon is utilized in generating time of flight MR angiogram; however, the image shown here is a routine spin echo T1-weighted axial image.

15 **Answer A.**   Inplane saturation.

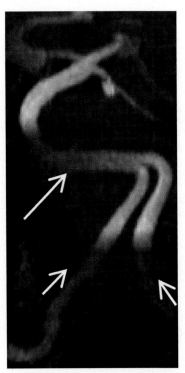

Imaging Findings: The above image shows loss of signal in the vertebral artery V3-V4 junction and basilar artery in a noncontrast MR angiogram with time of flight technique. This is due to horizontal course of the vessel in these segments with blood flowing in the imaging plane, which is prone to saturation like stationary spins, resulting in signal attenuation.

16 **Answer B.**   Gradient. The b-factor (b-value) summarizes the influences of the gradients (amplitude, duration of applied gradients, and spacing between pulsed gradients) on the diffusion-weighted images.

17 and 18   These questions relate to understanding sensitivity and specificity of diagnostic tools.

	Disease Present	Disease Absent	
Test Positive	True Positive (TP)	False Positive (FP)	Positive Predictive Value: TP/TP+FP
Test Negative	False Negative (FN)	True Negative (TN)	Negative Predictive Value: TN/TN+FN
	Sensitivity: TP/TP+FN	Specificity: TN/FP+TN	Accuracy: TP+TN/ TP+FP+FN+TN

17 **Answer: A.**   High sensitivity. A good screening test is one with high sensitivity, or ability to exclude disease. Sensitivity of a test is defined as the proportion with disease who are positive on the test: True Positive/(True Positive + False Negative).

18 **Answer B.**   High specificity. A good confirmatory test is one with high specificity, or high likelihood of having disease when test is positive. Specificity of a test is defined as the proportion without disease who are also negative on the test: True Negative/(False Positive + True Negative).

19 **Answer B.**   Zipper artifact.

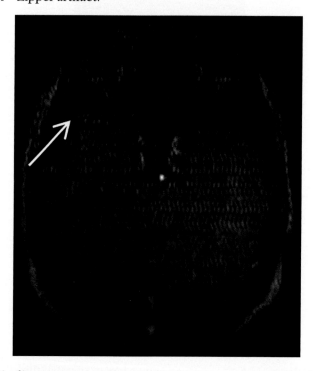

Imaging Findings: Zipper artifact as seen in the anterior aspect of this image is noise due to radiofrequency interference such as due to improper sealing of the scanning room allowing improper shielding from electronic devices. It can also be seen because of other hardware or software problems and typically affects all images acquired in the series.

20 **Answer B.** Chronic headache with no new symptoms or neurologic deficit. Based on the ACR appropriateness criteria, a patient with a headache without specific risk factors for underlying structural disease does NOT need further imaging. Specific risk factors that may warrant further evaluation with imaging include the other answer choices: sudden onset of severe ("thunderclap") headache, chronic headache with new neurologic deficits, and pregnant woman with a new headache.